Eating Disorders and Obesity

Guest Editors

BEATE HERPERTZ-DAHLMANN, MD
JOHANNES HEBEBRAND, MD

CHILD AND ADOLESCENT PSYCHIATRIC CLINICS OF NORTH AMERICA

www.childpsych.theclinics.com

Consulting Editor
HARSH K. TRIVEDI, MD

January 2009 • Volume 18 • Number 1

SAUNDERS an imprint of ELSEVIER, Inc.

W.B. SAUNDERS COMPANY
A Division of Elsevier Inc.

Elsevier Inc. • 1600 John F. Kennedy Boulevard • Suite 1800 • Philadelphia, Pennsylvania 19103-2899

http://www.childpsych.theclinics.com

CHILD AND ADOLESCENT PSYCHIATRIC CLINICS OF NORTH AMERICA Volume 18, Number 1
January 2009 ISSN 1056–4993, ISBN-13: 978-1-4377-0458-7, ISBN-10: 1-4377-0458-1

Editor: Sarah E. Barth

Child and Adolescent Psychiatric Clinics of North America (ISSN 1056-4993) is published quarterly by Elsevier Inc., 360 Park Avenue South, New York, NY 10010-1710. Months of issue are January, April, July, and October. Business and Editorial Offices: 1600 John F. Kennedy Boulevard, Suite 1800, Philadelphia, PA 19103-2899. Customer Service Offices: 6277 Sea Harbor Drive, Orlando, FL 32887-4800. Periodicals postage paid at New York, NY and additional mailing offices. Subscription prices are $238.00 per year (US individuals), $378.00 per year (US institutions), $122.00 per year (US students), $270.00 per year (Canadian individuals), $456.00 per year (Canadian institutions), $156.00 per year (Canadian students), $321.00 per year (international individuals), $456.00 per year (international institutions), and $156.00 per year (international students). International air speed delivery is included in all Clinics subscription prices. All prices are subject to change without notice. **POSTMASTER:** Send address changes to Child and Adolescent Psychiatric Clinics of North America, Elsevier Periodicals Customer Service, 11830 Westline Industrial Drive, St. Louis, MO 63146. **Customer Service: 1-800-654-2452 (US). From outside the United States, call 1-314-453-7041. Fax: 1-314-453-5170. E-mail: JournalsCustomerService-usa@elsevier.com (for print support) or journalsonlinesupport-usa@ elsevier.com (for online support).**

Reprints. For copies of 100 or more of articles in this publication, please contact the Commercial Reprints Department, Elsevier Inc., 360 Park Avenue South, New York, New York 10010-1710 Tel.: (212) 633-3812; Fax: (212) 462-1935, e-mail: reprints@elsevier.com.

Child and Adolescent Psychiatric Clinics of North America is covered in *MEDLINE/PubMed (Index Medicus), ISI, SSCI, Research Alert, Social Search, Current Contents,* and *EMBASE/Excerpta Medica.*

Printed in the United States of America.

Contributors

CONSULTING EDITOR

HARSH K. TRIVEDI, MD
Site Training Director and Director of Adolescent Services, E.P. Bradley Hospital;
Assistant Professor of Psychiatry and Human Behavior (Clinical), Brown Medical School;
President, Rhode Island Council for Child and Adolescent Psychiatry, East Providence,
Rhode Island

CONSULTING EDITOR EMERITUS

ANDRÉS MARTIN, MD, MPH

FOUNDING CONSULTING EDITOR

MELVIN LEWIS, MBBS, FRCPSYCH, DCH

GUEST EDITORS

BEATE HERPERTZ-DAHLMANN, MD
Professor, Director and Chair of Child and Adolescent Psychiatry and Psychotherapy,
University Clinics, RWTH Aachen, Aachen, Germany

JOHANNES HEBEBRAND, MD
Professor and Head, Department of Child and Adolescent Psychiatry, University
of Duisburg-Essen, Virchowstrasse, Germany

AUTHORS

CAROLYN BLACK BECKER, PhD
Associate Professor, Department of Psychology, Trinity University, San Antonio, Texas

HEIDI BRUTY, MD
Assistant Professor of Psychiatry and Behavioral Medicine, College of Medicine,
University of South Florida, Tampa, Florida

RACHEL BRYANT-WAUGH, BSc, MSc, DPhil
Consultant Clinical Psychologist, Honorary Senior Lecturer, Joint Head of the Feeding
and Eating Disorders Service, Department of Child and Adolescent Mental Health,
Great Ormond Street Hospital For Children NHS Trust, London, United Kingdom

CYNTHIA M. BULIK, PhD
Professor, Department of Psychiatry; Department of Nutrition, University of North Carolina
at Chapel Hill, Chapel Hill, North Carolina

IVAN EISLER, PhD
Reader in Family Psychology and Family Therapy, Section of Family Psychology and Family Therapy, Kings College, University of London, Institute of Psychiatry, London; and Head, Child and Adolescent Eating Disorders Service, South London and Maudsley NHS Foundation Trust, London, United Kingdom

MANUEL FÖCKER, MD
Department of Child and Adolescent Psychiatry and Psychotherapy, University of Duisburg-Essen, Essen, Germany

JOHANNES HEBEBRAND, MD
Professor and Head, Department of Child and Adolescent Psychiatry, University of Duisburg-Essen, Virchowstrasse, Germany

BEATE HERPERTZ-DAHLMANN, MD
Professor, Director and Chair of Child and Adolescent Psychiatry and Psychotherapy, University Clinics, RWTH Aachen, Aachen, Germany

ANKE HINNEY, PhD
Department of Child and Adolescent Psychiatry, Rheinische Kliniken Essen, University of Duisburg-Essen, Virchowstr, Essen, Germany

KRISTIAN HOLTKAMP, MD
Department of Child and Adolescent Psychiatry and Psychotherapy, University Clinics, RWTH Aachen, Aachen, Germany

ADRIENNE R. HUGHES, PhD
Lecturer, Department of Sports Studies, University of Stirling, Scotland, United Kingdom

DANIEL LE GRANGE, PhD
Associate Professor of Psychiatry, Section of Child and Adolescent Psychiatry, Department of Psychiatry, The University of Chicago; and Director, Eating Disorders Program, The University of Chicago Medical Center, Chicago, Illinois

SUZANNE E. MAZZEO, PhD
Assistant Professor, Department of Psychology; Department of Pediatrics, Virginia Commonwealth University, Richmond, Virginia

DASHA NICHOLLS, MBBS, MD
Consultant in Child and Adolescent Psychiatry, Honorary Senior Lecturer, Joint Head of the Feeding and Eating Disorders Service, Department of Child And Adolescent Mental Health, Great Ormond Street Hospital For Children NHS Trust, London, United Kingdom

TIMO D. MÜLLER
Department of Child and Adolescent Psychiatry and Psychotherapy, University of Duisburg-Essen, Essen, Germany

PAULINE S. POWERS, MD
Professor of Psychiatry and Behavioral Medicine, College of Medicine, University of South Florida, Tampa, Florida

JOHN J. REILLY, PhD
Professor of Paediatric Energy Metabolism, Division of Developmental Medicine, University of Glasgow, Yorkhill Hospitals, Glasgow, Scotland, United Kingdom

HARRIET SALBACH-ANDRAE, PhD
Department of Child and Adolescent Psychiatry, Psychosomatic and Psychotherapy, Charité- Universitätsmedizin Berlin, Campus Virchow Klinikum, Berlin, Germany

ULRIKE SCHMIDT, PhD, MRCPsych
Section of Eating Disorders, Institute of Psychiatry, London, United Kingdom

HEATHER SHAW, PhD
Senior Research Associate, Oregon Research Institute, Eugene, Oregon

HANS-CHRISTOPH STEINHAUSEN, MD, Dipl. Psych. PhD
Professor, Aalborg Psychiatric Hospital, Aarhus University Hospital, Denmark, Child and Adolescent Clinical Psychology, University of Basel; and Department of Child and Adolescent Psychiatry, University of Zurich, Postfach, Zurich, Switzerland

LAURA STEWART, PhD, RD
Dietitian, The Children's Weight Clinic, Edinburgh, Scotland, United Kingdom

ERIC STICE, PhD
Senior Research Scientist, Oregon Research Institute, Eugene, Oregon

BOYD SWINBURN, MB, ChB, FRACP, MD
Professor of Population Health, School of Exercise and Nutrition Sciences, Deakin University, Melbourne

JANET TREASURE
Professor, Department of Psychiatry, Guy's Hospital, London, United Kingdom

FREDERIQUE VAN DEN EYNDE, MD
Marie Curie Research Fellow, Institute of Psychiatry, Section of Eating Disorders, London, United Kingdom

Cover artwork Courtesy of Socorro Rivera G., Mexico City, Mexico

Contents

Foreword: Too little…too much …just right   **xv**

Harsh K. Trivedi

Preface   **xvii**

Beate Herpertz-Dahlmann and Johannes Hebebrand

Section I: Diagnostic Concerns

Diagnostic Issues in Eating Disorders and Obesity   **1**

Johannes Hebebrand

> A thorough understanding of weight related issues is required for the assessment of patients with obesity and eating disorders. Body weight adjusted for height is used for the diagnosis of both anorexia nervosa (AN) and obesity. For AN, the DSM IV A criterion refers to 85 % of expected weight as a guideline, for overweight and obesity BMI cut-offs are commonly used. Because the BMI distribution changes during childhood and adolescence, the 85th and 95th BMI centiles are used in the USA to classify children as at risk of overweight and obesity, respectively. 85 % of expected weight is approximately equivalent to the 10th BMI centile.

Eating Disorders of Infancy and Childhood: Definition, Symptomatology, Epidemiology, and Comorbidity   **17**

Dasha Nicholls and Rachel Bryant-Waugh

> This article describes a range of problem feeding and eating presentations seen in infants and children. In diagnostic terms some fall under the category of "feeding disorder," whereas others are childhood presentations of the eating disorders "anorexia nervosa," "bulimia nervosa," and atypical forms of these. Several other commonly occurring presentations that are difficult to fit into existing diagnostic categories are additionally described here, including "selective eating," "food avoidance emotional disorder," "food phobias," "functional dysphagia," and "food refusal."

Adolescent Eating Disorders: Definitions, Symptomatology, Epidemiology and Comorbidity   31

Beate Herpertz-Dahlmann

Eating disorders have morbidity and mortality rates that are among the highest of any mental disorders and are associated with significant functional impairment. This article provides an up-to-date review on recent developments and expanding knowledge in adolescent anorexia nervosa, bulimia nervosa, and related disorders. It covers diagnoses and assessment, recognition of typical symptoms, medical and psychiatric comorbidities, and current trends in epidemiology.

Psychological and Psychiatric Aspects of Pediatric Obesity   49

Johannes Hebebrand and Beate Herpertz-Dahlmann

A thorough dealing with psychological and psychiatric aspects of obesity requires careful consideration of causal implications. It is nowadays readily comprehensible that obesity can entail psychiatric symptoms, because stigmatization of obese children and adolescents, including teasing and bullying, is a common event. Sources include peers, teachers, parents, and health care providers. It would indeed seem peculiar if this ongoing and intense stigmatization did not affect mental well-being at a very early stage of life.

Section II: Etiologic and Neurobiologic Findings

Environmental and Genetic Risk Factors for Eating Disorders: What the Clinician Needs to Know   67

Suzanne E. Mazzeo and Cynthia M. Bulik

Patients and families often are aware of research on genetic factors influencing eating disorders. Accurate interpretations of research on environmental and genetic risk factors can be empowering to patients and families; however, misinterpretations could prove detrimental. Clinicians who are not versed in genetic research may believe they are ill prepared to discuss the nuances of genetic research with patients and families. In this article the authors discuss what is known about genetic and environmental risk factors with an emphasis on gene–environment interplay to improve clinicians' comfort level in discussing these complex issues with their patients.

Environmental and Genetic Risk Factors in Obesity   83

Johannes Hebebrand and Anke Hinney

Because of its high prevalence and the associated medical and psychosocial risks, research into the causes of childhood obesity has experienced a tremendous upswing. Formal genetic data based on twin, adoption, and family studies lead to the conclusion that at least 50% of the interindividual variance of the body mass index (BMI; defined as weight in kilograms divided by height in meters squared) is due to genetic factors. As a result of the recent advent of genome-wide association studies, the first polygenes involved in body weight regulation have been detected. Each of the predisposing alleles explain a few hundred grams of body weight. More polygenes will be detected in the near future, thus for the first time allowing in-depth analyses of gene–gene and gene–environment interactions. They also will enable developmental studies to assess the effect of such alleles throughout childhood and adulthood. The recent increase in obesity prevalence rates illustrates the extreme relevance of environmental factors for body weight. Similar to polygenes, the effect sizes of most such environmental factors are likely to be small, thus rendering their detection difficult. In addition, the validation of the true causality of such factors is not a straightforward task. Important factors are socioeconomic status and television consumption. The authors conclude by briefly assessing implications for treatment and prevention of childhood obesity.

Neuroimaging in Eating Disorders and Obesity: Implications for Research   **95**

Frederique Van den Eynde and Janet Treasure

Medicine and psychiatry have benefited from developments in investigational techniques. Neuroimaging is one such domain that has technically progressed enormously in recent years, resulting in, for example, higher temporal and spatial resolution. Neuroimaging techniques have been widely used in a range of psychiatric disorders, providing new insights into neural brain circuits and neuroreceptor functions in vivo. These imaging techniques allow researchers to study not only the configuration of brain structures but also aspects of normal and anomalous human behavior more accurately.

**Leptin-Mediated Neuroendocrine Alterations in Anorexia Nervosa:
Somatic and Behavioral Implications**   **117**

Timo D. Müller, Manuel Föcker, Kristian Holtkamp, Beate Herpertz-Dahlmann, and Johannes Hebebrand

Hypoleptinemia is a key endocrinological feature of anorexia nervosa (AN). Several symptoms in acute AN are related to the low circulating leptin levels including amenorrhea and semi-starvation–induced hyperactivity. The drop in leptin levels results from the loss of fat mass; once leptin levels fall below specific thresholds the hypothalamic-pituitary-gonadal and -thyroid axes are down-regulated; in contrast, the hypothalamic-pituitary-adrenal axis is up-regulated. Hypoleptinemia is the major signal underlying both somatic and behavioral adaptations to starvation. Because the mechanisms involved in this adaptation are similar in rodents and humans, rodent models can be used to investigate the relevant central pathways which underly the respective starvation-induced symptoms. During therapeutically induced weight gain, leptin levels can intermittently increase above normal concentrations. This hyperleptinemia could predispose to renewed weight loss.

Section III: Treatment Modalities

Overview of Treatment Modalities in Adolescent Anorexia Nervosa   **131**

Beate Herpertz-Dahlmann and Harriet Salbach-Andrae

> The aim of this article is to scrutinize and compare the benefits of distinct treatment settings for anorexia nervosa (AN) and to review the different treatment modalities that have proven helpful in the management of young patients with AN. Evidence-based findings on the effect of different treatment methods for AN are limited. Besides different treatment settings, a multimodal treatment approach comprising nutritional rehabilitation, nutritional counseling, individual psychotherapy and family-based interventions emphazising a group psychoeducation program for parents is presented.

Cognitive Behavioral Approaches in Adolescent Anorexia and Bulimia Nervosa   **147**

Ulrike Schmidt

> This article starts with what is known about cognitive behavior therapy (CBT) in adults with eating disorders and with some developmental considerations about CBT in children and adolescents. It then considers how CBT might be adapted for adolescents with eating disorders and reviews the current knowledge base on CBT in adolescents. The article finishes with some thoughts on future developments in this area.

Family Interventions in Adolescent Anorexia Nervosa   **159**

Daniel le Grange and Ivan Eisler

> Although our understanding of the mechanisms of change in eating disorder treatment remain limited, the empiric evidence for the effectiveness of family therapy for adolescent Anorexia Nervosa is gaining strength. A history of family involvement in psychiatric care, current approaches to family intervention in eating disorders and evidence for their efficacy are reviewed.

Pharmacotherapy for Eating Disorders and Obesity   **175**

Pauline S. Powers and Heidi Bruty

> Anorexia nervosa and bulimia nervosa are significant mental health problems in the adolescent population; however, there are no medications approved by the FDA for the treatment of adolescents with either of these disorders. Many medications are used off label for both the symptoms of eating disorders and their co-morbid conditions, particularly SSRIs and atypical anti-psychotics. The dosing, side effect profile, and long term effects of these medications in children and adolescents is unclear. Binge eating disorder, night eating syndrome, and sleep-related eating disorder often are associated with over-weight in adolescents. There are various pharmacological approaches to the treatment of obesity in the adolescent population some of which have FDA approval. In the article the authors discuss pharmacological approaches to guide

the treatment of eating disorders and obesity in the pediatric population, including risks of treatment, monitoring of potential side effects, and recent outcomes in the literature.

Evidence-Based Behavioral Treatment of Obesity in Children and Adolescents   189

Laura Stewart, John J. Reilly, and Adrienne R. Hughes

Obesity is the most common childhood disease and is widely acknowledged as having become a global epidemic. Well-recognized health consequences of childhood obesity exist, both during childhood and adulthood, affecting health and psychological and economic welfare. The importance of finding effective strategies for the management of childhood obesity has international significance with the publication of various expert reports and evidence-based guidelines in recent years.

Preventing Eating Disorders   199

Heather Shaw, Eric Stice, and Carolyn Black Becker

This article reviews eating disorder (ED) prevention programs, highlighting features that define successful programs and particularly promising interventions, and how they might be further refined. The field of ED prevention has advanced considerably both theoretically and methodologically compared with the earlier ED prevention programs, which were largely psychoeducational and met with limited success. Recent meta-analytic findings show that more than half (51%) of ED prevention interventions reduced ED risk factors and more than a quarter (29%) reduced current or future eating pathology (EP). A couple of brief programs have been shown to reduce the risk for future onset of EP and obesity. Selected interactive, multisession programs offered to participants older than 15 years, delivered by professional interventionists and including body acceptance or dissonance-induction content, produced larger effects. Understanding and applying these results can help inform the design of more effective prevention programs in the future.

Obesity Prevention in Children and Adolescents   209

Boyd Swinburn

Childhood and adolescent obesity has been increasing in most middle- and high-income countries, and, as with adult obesity, this has been driven by increasingly obesogenic environments, especially the food environment. This constitutes a "market failure," signaling the need for government interventions with policies, programs, and social marketing. Population prevention strategies are critical, and children and adolescents should be the priority populations. Food marketing to children is a central policy issue for governments to address, and comprehensive regulations are needed to provide substantive protection for children. Community-based intervention programs show some real promise in reducing childhood obesity, but the 2 big challenges ahead are to ensure that there is substantial ongoing funding so that the community capacity to promote healthy weights can be scaled up to a national level and to ensure that policies are in place to support these efforts. The social and cultural shifts that support healthy eating and physical activity occur differentially, and special efforts are needed to reduce the socioeconomic gradients associated with childhood obesity. A positive public health approach encompassing environmental, regulatory, sociocultural, and educational strategies offer the best chance of reducing obesity without increasing disordered eating patterns.

Outcome of Eating Disorders   225

Hans-Christoph Steinhausen

Both Anorexia Nervosa (AN) and Bulimia Nervosa (BN) are marked by a serious course and outcome in many of the afflicted individuals. In AN, there are an almost 18-fold increase in mortality including a high suicide rate, chronic courses in approximately 20 per cent of the cases, and more than half of the patients showing either a complete or a partial eating disorder in combination with another psychiatric disorder or another psychiatric disorder without an eating disorder. Mitigating factors of the outcome include onset of the disorder during adolescence and longer duration of follow-up. Vomiting, bulimia and purgative abuse, chronicity, and obsessive-compulsive features represent unfavourable prognostic factors in various studies. The longer-term outcome of BN is only slightly better result as compared to AN; however, the rate of mortality is low. Diagnostic crossover from bulimia nervosa to other eating disorders is a rather rare phenomenon, whereas the high rates of partial eating disorders may explain a large proportion of chronic courses. Social adjustment and the quality of personal relationship normalize in the majority of the affected patients. At present, the study of prognostic factors in bulimia nervosa does not allow any definite conclusions.

Index   243

FORTHCOMING ISSUES

April 2009
Childhood Bipolar Disorder
Jeffrey Hunt, MD, and
Daniel Dickstein, MD,
Guest Editors

July 2009
Early Childhood Mental Health
Mary Margaret Gleason, MD,
and Daniel S. Schechter, MD,
Guest Editors

October 2009
Sleep in Children and Adolescents
Jess P. Shatkin, MD, MPH,
and Anna Ivanenko, MD, PhD,
Guest Editors

RECENT ISSUES

October 2008
Treating Autism Spectrum Disorders
David J. Posey, MD, MS, and
Christopher J. McDougle, MD,
Guest Editors

July 2008
Refugee Mental Health
Schuyler W. Henderson, MD, MPH,
Guest Editor

April 2008
Attention Deficit Hyperactivity Disorder
Luis Augusto Rohde, MD,
and Stephen V. Faraone, MD,
Guest Editors

RELATED INTEREST

Psychiatric Clinics, March 2005 (Vol. 28, Number 1)
Obesity: A Guide for Mental Health Professionals
Thomas A. Walden, PhD, Albert J. Stunkard, MD, and Robert I. Berkowitz, MD,
Guest Editors

THE CLINICS ARE NOW AVAILABLE ONLINE!

Access your subscription at:
www.theclinics.com

Foreword
Too little…too much…just right

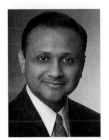

Harsh K. Trivedi, MD
Consulting Editor

Nearly 1 year into the consulting editor role, I find myself constantly trying to find "balance." Balance with regard to which topics we choose to cover. Balance in terms of how much of each topic we choose to bite off. Balance for the right mix of guest editors and contributors who provide both breadth and depth in a meaningful and cohesive package. Balance in finding the right proportion of evidence-based knowledge and mixing it with the right amount of practical application for clinical practice. This is a list that could go on for a few more pages.

In looking at the current issue, which marks the final transition between the editorship of Andrés Martin and myself, the importance of balance is driven home. The *Clinics* has covered the issue of eating disorders previously. In developing this issue, my predecessor intentionally chose to strike a new balance. The difference in our coverage this time around is the inclusion of obesity. As we face a national epidemic regarding obesity, and in particular childhood obesity, this is a topic that had to be discussed. The American Academy of Child and Adolescent Psychiatry estimates that up to one third of all children and adolescents in the United States are overweight[1]. Indeed, all of us can probably think of a number of patients in our practice who are dealing with issues regarding their weight.

At first glance, it may appear that having obesity and eating disorders covered within the same issue is but a *natural* extension. Therein lies the difficulty of finding balance. As our guest editors will show you throughout this issue, aside from certain common features, we are indeed talking about very different topics. To put it most bluntly- obesity is not an eating disorder nor is it a diagnosis in the DSM-IV-TR. And yet, the guest editors have managed to weave these topics together and to find the common thread. This is the beauty of the *Clinics* series: the ability to balance and rebalance, to take into account advances in the field, and to factor in the practicalities of clinical practice.

I extend my sincere gratitude to Beate Herpertz-Dahlmann and Johannes Hebebrand for rising to the occasion and creating such a wonderful issue. They not only have found balance in covering this topic but have also found clarity. I am also grateful

Child Adolesc Psychiatric Clin N Am 18 (2008) xv–xvi
doi:10.1016/j.chc.2008.10.001
1056-4993/08/$ – see front matter © 2008 Elsevier Inc. All rights reserved.

childpsych.theclinics.com

to the outstanding contributors for their insight and their expertise. As we look to help our patients, I hope that we learn much from this issue. Let this knowledge help them to find a new balance in their own lives: Neither too little, nor too much, but ultimately ...just right.

Harsh K. Trivedi, MD
Site Training Director and Director of Adolescent Services
E.P. Bradley Hospital
Assistant Professor of Psychiatry and Human Behavior (Clinical)
Brown Medical School
President, Rhode Island Council for Child and Adolescent Psychiatry
East Providence, RI 02915, USA

E-mail address:
harsh_trivedi@brown.edu.

REFERENCE

1. American Academy of Child and Adolescent Psychiatry. Obesity in children and teens. Available at: http://www.aacap.org/cs/root/facts_for_families/obesity_in_children_and_teens. Accessed September 3, 2008.

Preface

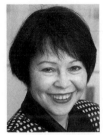 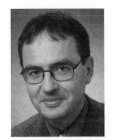

Beate Herpertz-Dahlmann, MD   Johannes Hebebrand, MD
Guest Editors

A little more than a year ago, Andrés Martin, the former Consulting Editor of *Child and Adolescent Psychiatry Clinics of North America*, asked us to act as Guest Editors for a special issue on eating disorders. We were both very delighted and surprised. Two researchers from Germany receiving the chance to co-edit an issue of this prestigious journal that publishes top expert reviews for application in clinical practice. We felt honored by this offer and at the same time were quite aware of the challenges that lay ahead of us. In our initial outline, we agreed to include obesity as one of the disorders covered in the issue.

Eating disorders and obesity are among the most prevalent clinical disorders of childhood and adolescence. They often take a chronic and disabling course with high morbidity and eventually mortality rates; the personal toll is high.

We were well aware of the fact that obesity cannot readily be viewed as an eating disorder; the clinical aspects and research issues differ. Nevertheless, several commonalities apply. Obesity in itself is a risk factor for the development of bulimia nervosa and is frequently associated with binge eating disorder. The elucidation of the pathways underlying appetite and weight regulation has resulted in a paradigm shift of our understanding of these disorders; we are now able to better grasp the neurobiologic complexity of these disorders, which in turn is beginning to influence our attitude toward patients. Environmental factors are of obvious importance in the development of both obesity and eating disorders. Today's environment reflecting the pursuit of thinness promotes dieting behavior, particularly among young females; current evidence suggests that this a major risk factor for eating disorders and that it may also contribute to the development of overweight and obesity.

Despite our vastly improved knowledge of epidemiology and neurobiology, including the discovery of major genes and polygenes involved in obesity, our treatment results for both eating disorders and obesity have not improved concomitantly. Children and adolescents with obesity, anorexia, or bulimia nervosa much too often become adults in whom these disorders persist.

It was our aim to provide readers with a comprehensive and up-to-date overview of three areas: (1) diagnostic and classification issues in eating disorders and obesity,

Child Adolesc Psychiatric Clin N Am 18 (2008) xvii–xix
doi:10.1016/j.chc.2008.09.001
1056-4993/08/$ – see front matter © 2008 Elsevier Inc. All rights reserved.

childpsych.theclinics.com

especially in light of the preparation of DSM-V; (2) important research findings in the neurobiology of both fields; and (3) the difficulty of finding effective treatment methods and prevention strategies.

Section I pertains to diagnostic issues and psychiatric and psychologic symptoms of eating disorders and obesity, with a focus on developmental aspects. In the first article, Hebebrand gives a general overview on definitions of both underweight and overweight, which serve as the basis for diagnosing both anorexia nervosa and obesity. He argues for use of body mass index (BMI) and BMI percentiles for defining both weight categories. The next article by Nicholls and Bryant-Waugh covers eating disorders of infancy and childhood, thereby elucidating the difficulty of applying DSM-IV criteria to eating disorders in younger subjects. In the third article, Herpertz-Dahlmann gives a brief overview on the different eating disorders in adolescence and points out the growing importance of "eating disorders not otherwise specified," the most common eating disorders encountered in clinical practice. In the last article of this section, Hebebrand and Herpertz-Dahlmann present data on the psychiatric comorbidity of obese children and adolescents in clinical and epidemiologic samples. They also address the emerging knowledge that depression in childhood may be associated with obesity in adulthood.

In Section II, we highlight the most recent etiologic and neurobiologic findings. Mazzeo and Bulik describe the interplay of "nature" and "nurture," providing their interpretation of formal genetic findings in eating disorders and discussing the implications for treatment. Hebebrand and Hinney summarize currently known genetic and environmental risk factors for the etiology of childhood obesity. In the third article, Van den Eynde and Treasure give a very thorough overview of recent findings obtained with modern neuroimaging techniques and their implications for further research. In the last article of the second section, Müeller and colleagues address important aspects of the neurobiology of anorexia nervosa by describing the role of the hormone leptin in the somatic and behavioral adaptation to the starvation process.

Section III comprises a selection of articles that summarize different treatment modalities and new findings pertaining to prevention strategies.

Although much progress has been made in improving treatment, there is still a rather high proportion of patients with anorexia nervosa who fail to respond to any kind of therapy. This dilemma (and its implications for treatment research) is addressed in the article by Herpertz-Dahlmann and Salbach. The article by Schmidt covers recent data and emerging new ideas in cognitive behavioral therapy for adolescents who have eating disorders, while Le Grange and Eisler summarize their extensive knowledge on family therapy and interventions. Powers and Bruty outline state-of-the-art pharmacotherapy for eating disorders and obesity—an area requiring much more research to improve the evidence basis for the use of currently employed medications, and potentially more important in the effort to come up with novel and more effective medications. Stewart and colleagues focus on the behavioral treatment of childhood and adolescent obesity; they provide a very practical overview of the different behavioral strategies. Further research is required to address the effectiveness of such interventions. The important and promising domain of prevention is presented by Shaw, Stice, and Black Becker for eating disorders and by Swinburn for obesity. Steinhausen concludes this issue with a review on recent data about outcome in eating disorders.

After our work has been finished, we would like to express our considerable gratitude to all contributors of this issue. This book is not a solo effort, but the work of many leading experts in the field of eating disorders and obesity who were willing to share their time, wisdom, and expertise. We have learned much by obtaining deep insight into the topics discussed.

We wish to thank Andrés Martin for his confidence in both of us to compile this issue, Harsh Trivedi for his editorial advice, and Sarah Barth at Elsevier for her constant and extraordinary support. Last but not least, we want to thank our patients and their families for teaching us about their disorders and their struggles.

We both hope that this issue will be valuable for all professionals in clinical practice who want to help their patients to find a way out of their disorder.

Beate Herpertz-Dahlmann, MD
Director and Chair of Child and Adolescent Psychiatry and Psychotherapy
University Clinics
RWTH Aachen University
Neuenhofer Weg 21
D-52074 Aachen, Germany

Johannes Hebebrand, MD
Director of the Department of Child and Adolescent Psychiatry and Psychotherapy
University of Duisburg-Essen
Virchowstr. 174
D-45147 Essen, Germany

E-mail addresses:
bherpertz-dahlmann@ukaachen.de (B. Herpertz-Dahlmann)
johannes.hebebrand@uni-duisburg-essen.de (J. Hebebrand)

Diagnostic Issues in Eating Disorders and Obesity

Johannes Hebebrand, MD

KEYWORDS

- Eating disorder • Obesity • Definition
- Body mass index • Review

OBESITY AND THE DEFINITION OF AN EATING DISORDER

The reasons for addressing diagnostic issues of eating disorders and obesity jointly in an introduction to this special issue are manifold: In clinical terms, eating disorders and obesity have merged in the sense that treatment centers during the past 20 years have increasingly focused on all the respective disorders, which apart from obesity include the Diagnostic and Statistical Manual of Mental Disorders (4th edition, text revision) (DSM-IV TR)[1] psychiatric disorders anorexia nervosa (AN) and bulimia nervosa (BN) and eating disorder not otherwise specified (EDNOS), including binge eating disorder (BED) for which, however, separate research criteria have been delineated. Recent discussions pertain to the definition of obesity or a subgroup(s) thereof as a psychiatric disorder.[2–4] It has become common practice to cover both eating disorders and obesity in textbooks, handbooks, journals, and articles. Finally, the biomedical explosion brought on by the discovery of leptin and the pathways involved in body weight regulation has proven fruitful for the understanding of obesity and eating disorders. However, despite this impressive merging in clinical and research terms, many differences addressed further in the diverse articles of this issue require attention. Additionally, dealing jointly with obesity and eating disorders requires a thorough understanding of the definition and concept of an eating disorder and the overlap with, but also distinction from, obesity.

In an adult a constant body weight is maintained if both energy intake and energy expenditure are in equilibrium.[5,6] Accordingly, in theory, an increment in body weight and, in the longer, term overweight and obesity, ensue from an increased energy intake while keeping energy expenditure constant or, alternatively, from a reduced energy expenditure with maintenance of previous energy intake. The same principles—albeit in opposite directions—apply for loss of body weight, which if continuous over time results in underweight. In biological and physiologic terms, however,

Department of Child and Adolescent Psychiatry, University of Duisburg-Essen, Virchowstrasse 174, 45147 Essen, Germany
E-mail address: johannes.hebebrand@uni-due.de

Child Adolesc Psychiatric Clin N Am 18 (2008) 1–16
doi:10.1016/j.chc.2008.07.007
1056-4993/08/$ – see front matter © 2008 Elsevier Inc. All rights reserved.

a change in energy intake almost automatically entails a compensatory change in energy expenditure (and vice versa), indicating that the 2 sides of the energy equation cannot be viewed separately from one another; they are jointly regulated through complex pathways. For example, caloric restriction leads to a disproportionately reduced resting energy expenditure in an attempt by the organism to curtail further weight loss and to enable rapid weight regain once the caloric restriction is lifted.[5]

The pathways underlying weight regulation have been the subject of intensive research over the past 15 years; the authors have come to realize that this regulatory system encompasses many tissues/organs, including the adipose tissue, the gastrointestinal tract, muscles, and, prominently, the brain.[7] The authors have witnessed the discovery of many anorexigens and orexigens, which act in concert to tightly control energy intake and expenditure. Specific brain regions, including the hypothalamus, and complex neuronal systems, such as the reward system, form the central weight regulatory system.[8] The respective circuits and pathways do not represent a distinct system but rather overlap with other systems underlying regulation of, for instance, lipid and glucose metabolism, blood pressure, body temperature, fertility, stress, mood, anxiety, libido, cognition, and memory.

The term "eating disorder" implies an aberrant eating behavior. Whether or not this behavior leads to or is associated with a body weight at the tails of weight distribution or a fluctuating weight is obviously of clinical importance but not a diagnostic requirement per se. Weight disorders overlap, but can clearly be distinct from eating disorders. If the definition of an eating disorder rests on an aberrant eating behavior, all weight alterations and the subsequently ensuing conditions/disorders, which solely or mainly result from alterations of energy expenditure, would not fit this definition.

For example, many obesity researchers believe that physical inactivity figures prominently in the development of obesity; it is also obvious that a genetically determined low resting energy expenditure can entail excessive weight gain over time. In both examples, eating behavior is not necessarily in any way grossly perturbed in the sense that the respective individual or an outside observer would be able to diagnose an aberrant eating behavior. Finally, it is well known that obesity can ensue over a period of many years or even decades with only small annual increments of body weight.[5] A daily energy intake 30 kcal in excess of energy expenditure will entail weight gain and eventually, overweight; however, such a small amount of overeating is not detectable to the outside observer and thus seemingly precludes classification as an eating disorder. This type of obesity results from a minimal deviation from the complex system responsible for the maintenance of a constant body weight over time.

Is the premise correct that eating disorders are by definition associated with aberrant eating behavior? Interestingly, this is not the case. Clearly, in both BN and BED aberrant eating behavior figures prominently with respect to the diagnostic criteria; both disorders are characterized by binge eating attacks. However, an aberrant eating behavior is not necessarily required for the diagnosis of AN. The DSM-IV TR diagnostic criterion A merely refers to the refusal to maintain body weight at or above a minimally normal weight for age and height;[1] criteria B-D make no reference to eating behavior. At least in theory, AN as based on this definition could result from excessively increasing physical activity while maintaining caloric intake. Indeed, the condition termed anorexia athletica[9] is compatible with the notion that some underweight athletes potentially lose weight or maintain their leanness through excessive energy expenditure and not or only to a slight degree through a curtailment of energy intake. It however seems reasonable to assume that those individuals who increase energy expenditure without concomitantly initiating a higher caloric intake experience hunger, which they do not respond to adequately.

Nevertheless, this brief discussion should suffice to illustrate the need to precisely define eating disorders. As the term in its narrow sense suggests, a quantitatively extreme or qualitatively altered eating behavior should be the cardinal feature of such disorders; the perturbed eating behavior should be described and figure prominently in the respective diagnostic criteria. As such, a recent proposal for revised criteria for AN was based on observable behavior and includes reference to symptoms of disordered eating.[10]

In contrast and in a broad sense, the term eating disorder could additionally encompass behavior resulting in a too low or too high energy intake for a given energy expenditure with ensuing effects over time on body weight. According to this broad definition, the authors could define any form of obesity as an eating disorder. The problem with this definition, however, is that in many cases, neither the individual nor an outside observer will be able to observe this behaviorally driven increase or decrease in energy intake due to its small magnitude.

WEIGHT CLASSES, BODY COMPOSITION, AND BODY FAT DISTRIBUTION

Overweight is present if body weight adjusted for height, age, and gender exceeds a specified cutoff, underweight in turn relates to an adjusted body weight less than a specified threshold value; the respective threshold values are based on convention. Both weight categories are defined independently of body composition. Nevertheless, it is evident that extreme underweight can only result if both fat mass and lean body mass are reduced. Similarly, extreme overweight implies elevated fat mass and lean body mass. In modern societies overweight usually implies that fat mass constitutes an above average percentage of total body mass. It is crucial to bear in mind that this is not necessarily so: an increased relative fat-free mass can result in overweight as for instance in an athletic individual.[11]

By definition, obesity implies an excessive fraction of total body weight composed of fat mass or, in other terms, adiposity is elevated above a threshold value. Accordingly, obesity can in theory only be diagnosed if fat and fat-free mass are determined; studies of children and adolescents have suggested the use of thresholds of 30% body fat in girls and 25% in boys based on medical indicators, such as blood pressure and blood lipids.[12–14] Matters are further complicated by the fact that the medical implications of fat are dependent on the body fat distribution pattern with mainly only central (also termed intra-abdominal, visceral, or android; "apple-shaped") fat entailing elevated risks for obesity-related medical sequelae (other than orthopedic disorders) as compared with gluteofemoral (gynoid; "pear-shaped") fat.[15]

Various models and indirect methods for estimation of body composition have been developed, all of which are imperfect and require several assumptions and age- and gender-specific considerations. For research purposes, body composition has been determined using techniques, such as total body water, dual-energy x-ray absorptiometry (DXA), total body imaging techniques, underwater weighing, total body electrical conductivity, and total body potassium.[16] In clinical studies, bioelectrical resistance and skinfold measurements are employed most frequently. Body fat distribution patterns are frequently and easily assessed by measuring waist and hip circumferences and additionally skinfolds (for US reference data and percentiles see http://www.cdc.gov). Primarily for research purposes, imaging techniques can precisely localize body fat in the whole body and at the level of single organs and tissues. Sex-specific body fat distribution patterns differ by ethnicity in obese adolescents,[17] potentially accounting for some of the ethnic differences in risks for the development of type 2 diabetes mellitus and other metabolic disorders associated with obesity.

In clinical practice, the body mass index (BMI; Quetelet's index) defined as weight in kilograms divided by height in meters squared (kg/m^2) has become widely accepted as the weight–height index throughout childhood and adulthood;[11,18] in adults the correlations between BMI and height and weight are in the range of −0.2 and 0.6 to 0.8.[19] In children these correlations vary somewhat according to sex and age, but in general terms they also provide relatively high correlations to weight and low correlations to height. BMI is commonly used as a surrogate measure of adiposity.[20] Indeed, the correlations between BMI and percent body fat as determined by DXA are typically high.[21,22] For example, for 196 healthy girls aged 4 to 16 years DXA-derived fat mass was highly ($r = 0.93$) correlated with BMI;[22] however, and not unexpectedly, correlations are lower if individuals of only one weight class are assessed. Particularly among underweight individuals, the correlation between BMI and percent body fat is substantially lower; for example, the correlation between BMI and fat mass as determined with DXA was $r = 0.46$ in a study of 23 AN patients with a mean age of 15.5 years and a mean BMI of 15.3.[23]

During childhood, adolescence, and adulthood the left flank of the BMI distribution is steep, whereas the right side is slanted, particularly in countries with high obesity prevalence rates. In other words, the BMI is not normally distributed. The BMI range between the median of a representative segment of the same-aged population and the extreme left tail is considerably smaller than that between the median and the extreme right tail, reflecting the fact that on an individual level, extreme overweight is biologically tolerated for extended periods of time, whereas individuals with BMI values at the extreme end of the left side of the distribution are at risk for death of starvation.

Table 1 delineates the cutoff values for defining different weight categories among adults according to the World Health Organization (WHO);[24] this categorization is widely accepted in Europe and the United States and reflects increased health risks at higher BMI. Note that the cutoff values for underweight and overweight are less than 18.5 kg/m^2 and 25 kg/m^2 or more, respectively. Overweight in turn is subcategorized into 4 different weight classes with obesity defined with a BMI of 30 kg/m^2 or more. Many investigators have used the term overweight synonymously with the WHO classification of pre-obesity, defined as a BMI between 25 and 29.9 kg/m^2.

An appropriate understanding of BMI and body composition requires knowledge of gender, ethnic/racial, social, and age-related aspects.[25] For any given BMI, percent body fat is on average higher for women than men and for Asians than whites.[26]

Table 1
Classification of relative body weight in adults according to BMI and risks of comorbidities[24]

Classification	BMI (kg/m^2)	Risk for Comorbidities
Underweight	<18.5	Low (but risks of other clinical problems increased)
Normal range	18.5–24.9	Average
Overweight	≥25	—
Pre-obese	25–29.9	Increased
Obese class I	30–34.9	Moderate
Obese class II	35–39.9	Severe
Obese class III	≥40	Severe

Because a low socioeconomic background is associated with overweight and obesity in many industrial societies,[27,28] caution is required on attributing an elevated BMI of a minority to ethnicity or race. To prove that an effect is indeed because of race/ethnicity, BMI or percent body fat must be adjusted for socioeconomic status (SES). In low-development countries, overweight and obesity are frequently encountered among the wealthy;[28] thus, the relationship between obesity and SES in many of these countries is opposite to that of industrialized countries.

A specific BMI at 2 different ages can, in epidemiologic terms, imply large differences in the percentage of individuals with a BMI more or less than the respective value. This holds true particularly for children, and also for adults. According to the 2005 through 2006 data from the National Health and Nutrition Examination Survey,[29] 33.3% and 35.3% of US adult men and women, respectively, had a BMI of 30 kg/m^2 or more. However, among those adults aged 40 to 59 years, approximately 40% of men were obese, compared with only 28% of men aged 20 to 39 years, and 32% of men aged 60 years and older. Among women, 41% of those aged 40 to 59 years were obese compared with 30.5% of women aged 20 to 39 years. According to the Centers for Disease Control and Prevention (CDC) growth charts for children and adolescents (**Fig. 1**)[30] a BMI of 30 at age 20 years is within the 90th to 95th BMI centile range for both genders. Accordingly, prevalence rates of obesity defined as a BMI of 30 kg/m^2 or more increase substantially with age during adulthood; rates in the United States are well below 10% at age 20 years and more than 40% during the age period 40 to 59 years.

The strong age dependency of, particularly, childhood and adolescent BMI implies that an adequate interpretation of the index of a young individual child requires knowledge of the BMI distribution of children of the same age and gender. Frequently, BMI centile curves as based on anthropometric data of a large and ideally representative sample are used for this purpose; older children and parents are readily able to grasp this epidemiologic concept as having good face value for educational purposes. BMI standard deviation scores (BMI-SDs) or Z-scores are commonly employed in clinical studies to further differentiate extreme overweight or underweight (>99th and <1st centile).

For children and adolescents, however, there is no clear-cut international consensus as to what cutoff should be used to define overweight and obesity; existing definitions are statistical rather than risk-based. In the United States, Himes and Dietz (1994)[31] have suggested use of the 85th and 95th centiles; in other countries the 90th and 97th centiles serve as the respective cutoffs (eg, Kromeyer-Hauschild et al,[32] **Fig. 2**). The 95th and 85th centiles based on the 2000 growth curves of the CDC have been recommended for classification of young individuals as being overweight or at risk for overweight in the United States (see **Fig. 1**, CDC[30,33]); the term obesity is avoided. However, these cutoffs are not consistent with those used in adulthood; for example, the centile of an 18-year-old girl with a BMI of 30.1 kg/m^2—thus fulfilling the adult criterion for obesity—is less than the 95th centile and would thus be at risk for "overweight" according to the CDC (see **Fig. 1B**).

Ideally, the cutoffs for defining overweight and obesity should reflect increased medical risks; however, there is no BMI or BMI centile cutoff at which medical risks differ substantially from slightly lower values or centiles. In addition, it seems likely that the medical risks of overweight and obesity are not fixed; potentially the normal course of an obesity-associated disorder, the effect of obesity on this disorder, and its treatment change over time.

Ethnic differences in obesity rates need to be taken into consideration; in US adolescents rates of overweight (defined by way of sex- and age-specific BMI ≥95th percentile based on the CDC growth charts) differ between non-Hispanic whites,

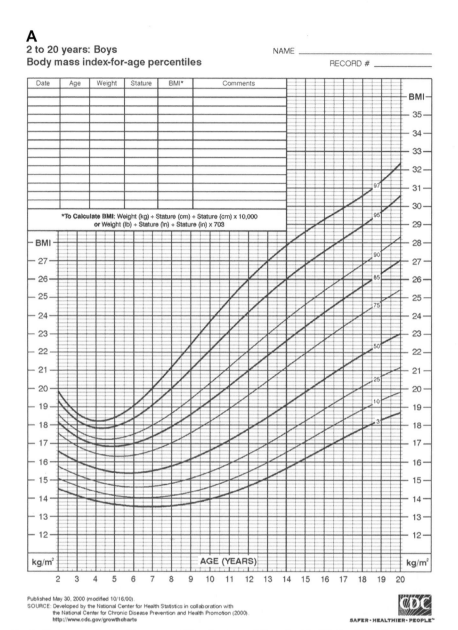

A

2 to 20 years: Boys
Body mass index-for-age percentiles

NAME _____

RECORD # _____

*To Calculate BMI: Weight (kg) ÷ Stature (cm) ÷ Stature (cm) x 10,000
or Weight (lb) ÷ Stature (in) ÷ Stature (in) x 703

Published May 30, 2000 (modified 10/16/00).
SOURCE: Developed by the National Center for Health Statistics in collaboration with
the National Center for Chronic Disease Prevention and Health Promotion (2000).
http://www.cdc.gov/growthcharts

Fig. 1. Body mass index-for-age centiles for boys (*A*) and girls (*B*) for the US population. (*Courtesy of* the National Center for Health Statistics, Hyattsville, MD.)

non-Hispanic blacks, and Mexican Americans particularly among females. The respective rates for boys and girls were 19.1%, 18.5%, and 18.3% and 15.4%, 25.4%, and 14.1%, respectively, according to the National Health and Nutrition Examination Survey (NHANES) 2003–2004.[34] Accordingly, non-Hispanic black adolescent girls have the highest prevalence rate of overweight.

In developed countries the definition of threshold BMI centiles for underweight has received comparatively much less attention. It makes intuitive sense to label the same

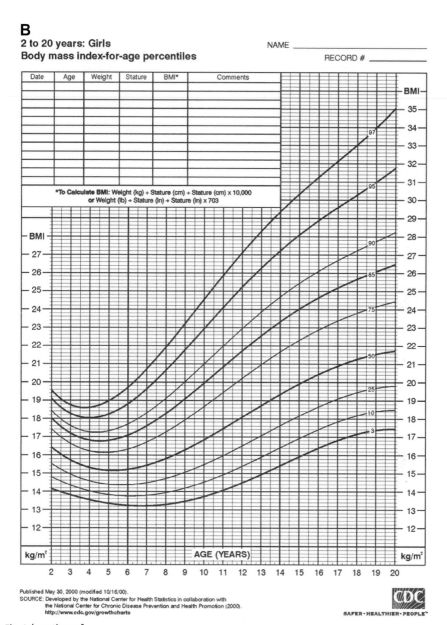

B

2 to 20 years: Girls
Body mass index-for-age percentiles

NAME _____

RECORD # _____

*To Calculate BMI: Weight (kg) ÷ Stature (cm) ÷ Stature (cm) x 10,000
or Weight (lb) ÷ Stature (in) ÷ Stature (in) x 703

Published May 30, 2000 (modified 10/16/00).
SOURCE: Developed by the National Center for Health Statistics in collaboration with
the National Center for Chronic Disease Prevention and Health Promotion (2000).
http://www.cdc.gov/growthcharts

SAFER·HEALTHIER·PEOPLE™

Fig. 1 (*continued*)

proportions of the population as underweight and overweight. Accordingly, underweight can be defined with a BMI less than 15th or less than 10th centile. A more severe degree of underweight would thus entail a BMI less than 5th or 3rd centile.

Use of specific centiles as cutoffs for the definition of weight classes obviously requires a consensus as to the reference population. International comparisons of the absolute BMI values constituting centiles in the lower to middle range typically reveal only a slight degree of divergence among reference populations ascertained in different industrialized countries.[35] However, large differences exist in the upper

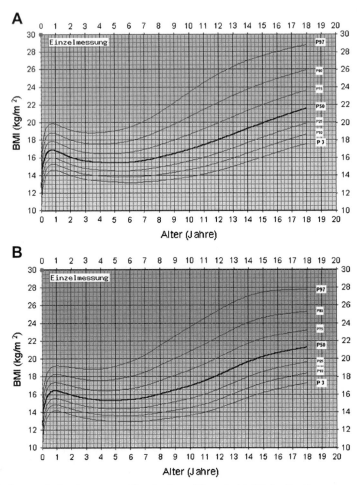

Fig. 2. Body mass index-for-age centiles for boys (*A*) and girls (*B*) for the German population. (*From* Kromeyer-Hauschild K, Wabitsch M, Kunze D, et al. Perzentile für den Bodymass-Index für das Kindes- und Jugendalter unter Heranziehung verschiedener deutscher Stichproben. Monatsschr Kinderheilkd 2001;149:807–18; with permission.)

centile range; BMI values corresponding to the 90th or 97th centile are, for example (substantially) higher in the United States than in European countries (compare US with German BMI centiles; see **Figs 1** and **2**).

Because of secular trends for height and moreso for weight, centile curves based on a formerly representative population-based survey do not reflect the true BMI distribution of the current population. For instance, the measurement data used to construct the nationally representative CDC 2000 growth charts were obtained from a series of national health examination surveys conducted by the National Center for Health Statistics from 1963 to 1994 and from supplemental data sources; more recent data were excluded to avoid an upward shift in the BMI-for-age curves.[36]

In an attempt to define internationally acceptable centile cutoffs for overweight and obesity, the International Obesity Task Force (IOTF) averaged the national curves from 6 different countries passing through BMI of 25 and 30 kg/m² at age 18 years.[37] Application of the cutoff points to the national datasets on which they were based gave a wide range of prevalence estimates at age 18 years of 5% to 18% for overweight and 0.1% to 4% for obesity. It remains to be seen if these cut-offs are adopted sufficiently for international comparisons of rates of childhood over-weight and obesity.

SYNOPSIS OF DEVELOPMENTAL ASPECTS RELATED TO BODY WEIGHT AND BODY COMPOSITION

Viewed across the lifespan, the developmental pattern of BMI is similar to that of per-cent body fat. Typically BMI increases steeply during the first 6 months of life primarily because of an increase in fat mass, to then decline until age 6 to 8 years as a result of a strong increase in height (see **Fig. 1**) and a decrease in fat mass. The time point dur-ing childhood at which BMI again increases has been termed adiposity rebound; the earlier it occurs, the higher the risk for subsequent development of obesity and vice versa.[38] BMI increases throughout the rest of childhood and adolescence; this increase continues—albeit more slowly—during adulthood. In males, the BMI increase during adolescence is, on average, the result of proportional increases in both fat-free mass and fat mass; percent body fat between ages 5 to 15 years remains fairly stable at 16% to 29% depending on the respective study. In contrast, the BMI increase in girls aged 6 to 11 years is disproportionately based on an increase in fat mass; percent body fat increases from 17% to 24% in 3- to 5-year-olds to 24% to 40% in girls of the age range 6 to 11 years; during the age range 12 to 19 years, percent body fat increases substantially less than between the other 2 age periods and averages 28% to 39%.[21] In adults, percent body fat averages 25% to 45%;[25] higher percent-ages apply to older adults.

BMI in infancy is minimally correlated with BMI at age 35 years ($r \approx 0.15$;[39]). Accord-ingly, an overweight infant is only at a minimally elevated risk for obesity in adulthood provided that parental obesity is not present (**Fig. 3**). The greatest variation in rates of weight gain is seen in the first 1 to 2 years of life, when infants may show significant

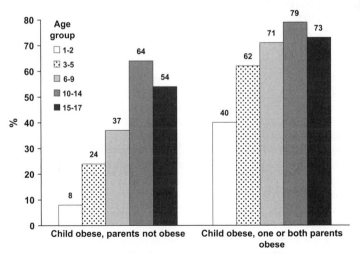

Fig. 3. Risk for persistence of childhood obesity into adulthood. Obesity in childhood and young adulthood (21–29 years of age) was defined with a BMI more than or equal to 85th centile for age and sex and a BMI at or more than 27.8 kg/m² for men and 27.3 kg/m² for women, respectively. (*Data* from Whitaker RC, Wright JA, Pepe MS, et al. Predicting obesity in young adulthood from childhood and parental obesity. N Engl J Med 1997;337(13):869–73.)

"catch-up" or "catch-down" growth as a consequence of intrauterine restraint or enhancement of fetal growth. By age 2 years, growth usually follows the genetic trajectory.[40] Small-for-date babies who rapidly gain weight after birth (catch-up growth) are at an elevated risk for adult obesity and cardiovascular disorders.[41] At age 10 years BMI is correlated with BMI at age 35 years in the magnitude of 0.35; during late adolescence BMI tracks well into adulthood (correlation with BMI at age 35 years: $r = 0.7$).[39] If a child is obese, the risk for persistence into adulthood increases with the degree of adiposity, age of the child, and parental obesity (see **Fig. 2**).[42,43]

EATING DISORDERS AND BODY WEIGHT

As pointed out above, eating disorders are not synonymous with weight disorders; diagnostic criteria related to body weight are not relevant to BED and BN. Clinically relevant aspects pertaining to body weight in these 2 disorders can be summarized as follows.

Bulimia Nervosa

The National Comorbidity Replication,[44] a nationally representative face-to-face household survey (n = 9282) conducted in 2001 to 2003 in the United States, revealed that individuals who received a lifetime diagnosis of BN had a BMI distribution similar to that of non-affected participants. In some clinical samples, rates of both current and lifetime overweight and obesity have been reported in excess of population-based rates.[45] In BN, weight fluctuations in excess of those observed in healthy individuals can occur.[46] Both on a short- and long-term basis, substantial weight fluctuations can occur in these patients because of changes in eating behavior (such as the weekly number of binge eating attacks) and attempts to counter-regulate (such as fasting, physical activity, purging frequency, use of laxatives). Whereas some of the weight fluctuations reflect strong shifts in hydration status, larger weight gains and losses are necessarily related to quantitative alterations of body fat and fat-free mass. Dieting or the ensuing weight loss can seemingly trigger the development of binge eating attacks[47] and subsequently BN. It is estimated that roughly 10% of women with AN subsequently develop BN;[48,49] accordingly, strong weight fluctuations and in particular weight loss can set in before development of BN. In addition, women with BN can (repeatedly) dip into the underweight range during the course of BN; if in such cases the weight criterion for AN is met and amenorrhea lasts for at least 3 months, the diagnosis would change from BN to AN of the binge eating/purging type. In an individual patient percent body fat can be reduced to subnormal values despite a body weight still higher than the AN weight criterion, thus contributing to the elevated rates of amenorrhea in BN patients. Both childhood and parental obesity have been detected more frequently in patients with BN than in healthy controls,[50] indicating that obesity in itself or a genetic predisposition to overweight is a risk factor for the development of BN.

Binge Eating Disorder

Investigators have recently argued that BED should become a formal eating disorder in DSM-V.[51,52] In clinically ascertained BED patients obesity is common. However, in a community sample only half of the BED subjects were obese; because in this study obesity was defined with a BMI more than 27.5 kg/m^2 the association would be even weaker if the WHO cutoff of 30 kg/m^2 had been employed.

A more recent epidemiologic study performed in St. Louis[53] reported a mean BMI of 33.6 kg/m^2 for subjects who scored positive for BED; 30% of these had a BMI less than 30 kg/m^2; almost 20% had a BMI 40 kg/m^2 or more, roughly 4 times the rate in individuals who screened negatively for BED. An odds ratio of 2.6 was observed for a BMI of 40 kg/m^2 or more in the National Comorbidity Replication.[44] There is general consensus that BED is present in up to one third of patients seeking weight loss treatment.[54] Only about 5% of obese subjects meet criteria for BED.[55]

Little is known about why weight is in the normal range in a substantial subgroup of individuals with BED. Caloric intake during a binge might not be that high. In theory, the increased caloric intake during the attacks could result in prolonged satiation, so that, for instance, net weekly caloric intake is not increased. Additionally or alternatively, energy expenditure is increased through engagement in physical activity or an increased resting energy expenditure. Finally, it seems possible that the body weight of such individuals increases as a result of binge eating attacks, albeit to a level still within the normal range. In an experimental study, the more-obese subjects with BED ate significantly more than the less-obese BED subjects when they were asked to binge; this relationship was not observed when subjects were asked to eat normally. Intake of the binge meal was significantly and positively correlated with BMI among subjects with BED.[56]

Anorexia Nervosa

The only eating disorder for which body weight is relevant in diagnostic terms is AN;[1] underweight is the first of the 4 DSM-IV TR criteria. Both ICD-10[57] and DSM-IV TR refer to a weight below a minimally normal weight for age and height; 85% of expected weight is provided as an "arbitrary but useful guide." The average body weights for age, height, and gender reported in the Blood and Build Pressure Study[58] have frequently been referred to in AN-related research.[59] Unfortunately however, the criterion of 85% of expected weight was never rigorously defined; different investigators have assessed body weights of their patients by referring to, for example, average body weight, ideal body weight, or expected body weight. In many cases, the reference basis for these definitions was not provided, leading to noncomparability of weight-related results in clinical studies of AN.

Another disadvantage of the weight criterion is that it is not based on the BMI, which as shown here is widely used for classification of weight classes.[24] As a consequence, weight-related research in AN remains apart from weight-related research in general, thus entailing unwarranted research barriers. Both DSM-IV and ICD-10, however, refer to an alternative weight criterion based on a BMI less than 17.5 kg/m^2, which is 1 BMI unit less than the cutoff value for underweight according to the WHO classification. Because the manifestation age of AN ranges from childhood to adulthood, the weight criterion should be applicable to all age groups or, alternatively, provide separate thresholds based on age. The BMI criterion based on a BMI less than 17.5 kg/m^2 is only applicable to adults; in, for example, 10-year-old girls, this BMI is above the 50th centile (see **Fig. 1**), thus clearly documenting its inapplicability in children and young adolescents.[60]

Unfortunately, the DSM-IV TR threshold definition does not indicate the extent of overlap with underweight in non-anorectic individuals of the respective sex, age, and population. The authors have shown that 85% expected body weight corresponds to absolute BMI values between the 5th and 10th age centiles as based on former population-based studies in the United States (NHANES-I) and Germany.[35] Because the secular trend toward increasing rates of overweight and obesity observed in many populations is largely based on weight increments in the upper half of the BMI distribution, the absolute BMI values constituting the 5th or 10th centiles have remained fairly stable over time. Thus, the BMI values depicted in **Table 1** skew between the 3rd and 10th centile of the CDC BMI centiles (see **Fig. 1**).

Accordingly, the authors suggest the use of the 10th BMI centile in developed countries as the threshold value for a revised version of the AN weight criterion.[10]

BMI values at admission of AN patients for inpatient treatment typically range from 12 to 17 kg/m^2; in single cases BMI is less than 10 kg/m^2. In a study encompassing 272 adolescent and adult patients, 5 and 100 patients had a BMI less than 10 kg/m^2 and 13 kg/m^2, respectively.[61] In marasmic women ascertained at a treatment center during the 1992 to 1993 famine in Somalia, the risk for mortality increased sharply at the time BMI values dropped below 11 kg/m^2.[62] In males, death set in at somewhat higher BMI values. Single individuals were alive at BMI values less than 10 kg/m^2. It must be borne in mind that the dieting habits of even extremely ill patients with AN usually differ substantially from those of individuals subjected to severe famine, thus accounting for the ability of AN patients to survive at BMI values less than 12 kg/m^2. Nevertheless, based on the aforementioned study[61] (**Table 2**) 7 of the 14 patients with a referral BMI below 11 kg/m^2 died during the follow-up period. Because 11 of the 100 patients with a BMI less than 13 kg/m^2 died in contrast to 1 of the 172 patients with a BMI of 13 kg/m^2 or more, the authors conclude that a referral BMI of less than 13 entails a strongly elevated mortality risk. In any case such a low BMI indicates that the underweight is potentially of a life-threatening degree.

Single groups have shown that the premorbid body weight or BMI distribution of AN patients does not differ substantially from that of healthy controls.[63,64] On admission for inpatient treatment, patients' BMIs are correlated ($r = 0.63$) with premorbid BMI centiles:[64] the higher the premorbid body weight the higher the BMI at admission. Not unexpectedly, the magnitude of weight loss is higher in patients with premorbid overweight. The correlation between the premorbid BMI centile and weight loss is $r = 0.66$.[64] The BMI at referral also predicts future body weight (see **Table 2**).[61] Among the aforementioned 272 patients with AN, the correlation between referral BMI and BMI at follow-up was 0.33; particularly those 100 patients presenting with a BMI less than 13 kg/m^2 frequently remained underweight. Only 4.4% of the 272 patients had a BMI 25 kg/m^2 or more at follow-up, indicating that overweight and obesity are infrequent outcomes of AN. In addition, the obvious preponderance of follow-up BMI in the lower range indicates that the low body weight in AN tracks into adulthood independent of whether or not patients recover.

The fourth DSM-IV TR criterion for a diagnosis of AN relates to secondary amenorrhea in postmenarcheal women. Amenorrhea is in most cases induced by a drop of

Table 2
Relationship between BMI less than 13 kg/m^2 and 13 kg/m^2 or more at referral for inpatient treatment and BMI at follow-up in 272 patients with anorexia nervosa

	BMI at Referral	
BMI at Follow-up	<13 kg/m^2 $n = 100$	≥13 kg/m^2 $n = 172$
≤17.5 kg/m^{2a}	35%	12.8%
≤5th centile[a]	44%	19.8%
≤10th centile[a]	56%	29.0%
≥25 kg/m^2	1%	3.4%
Deceased	11%	0.6%

The mean follow-up duration was 9.5 years (for details see Ref. 61).
[a] Including deceased patients.

serum leptin levels to less than a critical range.[65] This hypoleptinemia results in a downshift of the hypothalamic–pituitary–gonadal axis with amenorrhea ensuing in clinical terms; weight regain initially leads to increments of leptin followed by follicle stimulating hormone and luteinizing hormone.[66] Application of recombinant leptin to low normal weight women with hypothalamic amenorrhea over a 3-month period resulted in ovulations in single women and a general improvement in the reproductive axis.[67] Due to the critical role of hypoleptinemia in the induction of amenorrhea further studies are necessary to provide us with a reference range for women with AN, thus potentially enabling us to use hypoleptinemia as a diagnostic criterion in AN.[10]

REFERENCES

1. American Psychiatric Association. Diagnostic and statistical manual of mental disorders—DSM-IV-TR. [text revision]. 4th edition. Washington, DC: American Psychiatric Association; 2000.
2. Bornstein SR, Schuppenies A, Wong ML, et al. Approaching the shared biology of obesity and depression: the stress axis as the locus of gene-environment interactions. Mol Psychiatry 2006;11(10):892–902.
3. Kishi T, Elmquist JK. Body weight is regulated by the brain: a link between feeding and emotion. Mol Psychiatry 2005;10(2):132–46.
4. Volkow ND, O'Brien CP. Issues for DSM-V: should obesity be included as a brain disorder? Am J Psychiatry 2007;164(5):708–10.
5. Weigle DS. Appetite and the regulation of body composition. FASEB J 1994;8(3):302–10.
6. Friedman JM, Halaas JL. Leptin and the regulation of body weight in mammals. Nature 1998;395(6704):763–70.
7. Friedman JM. Modern science versus the stigma of obesity. Nat Med 2004;10(6):563–9.
8. Zheng H, Berthoud HR. Eating for pleasure or calories. Curr Opin Pharmacol 2007;7(6):607–12.
9. Sudi K, Ottl K, Payerl D, et al. Anorexia athletica. Nutrition 2004;20(7–8):657–61.
10. Hebebrand J, Casper R, Treasure J, et al. The need to revise the diagnostic criteria for anorexia nervosa. J Neural Transm 2004;111(7):827–40.
11. Gray DS. Diagnosis and prevalence of obesity. Med Clin North Am 1989;73(1):1–13.
12. Sweeting HN. Measurement and definitions of obesity in childhood and adolescence: a field guide for the uninitiated. Nutr J 2007;6:32.
13. Williams DP, Going SB, Lohman TG, et al. Body fatness and risk for elevated blood pressure, total cholesterol, and serum lipoprotein ratios in children and adolescents. Am J Public Health 1992;82(3):358–63.
14. Dwyer T, Blizzard CL. Defining obesity in children by biological endpoint rather than population distribution. Int J Obes Relat Metab Disord 1996;20(5):472–80.
15. Bouchard C, Després JP, Mauriège P. Genetic and nongenetic determinants of regional fat distribution. Endocr Rev 1993;14(1):72–93.
16. Goran MI. Measurement issues related to studies of childhood obesity: assessment of body composition, body fat distribution, physical activity and food intake. Pediatrics 1998;101:505–18.
17. Liska D, Dufour S, Zern TL, et al. Interethnic differences in muscle, liver and abdominal fat partitioning in obese adolescents. PLoS ONE 2007;2(6):e569.

18. Dietz WH, Robinson TN. Use of the body mass index (BMI) as a measure of overweight in children and adolescents: periods of risk in childhood for the development of adult obesity—what do we need to learn? J Pediatr 1998;132(2):191–3.
19. Watson PE, Watson ID, Batt RD. Obesity indices. Am J Clin Nutr 1979;32(4): 736–7.
20. Barlow SE, Dietz WH. Obesity evaluation and treatment: expert committee recommendations. The maternal and child health bureau, health resources and services administration and the department of health and human services. Pediatrics 1998;102(3):E29.
21. Mei Z, Grummer-Strawn LM, Pietrobelli A, et al. Validity of body mass index compared with other body-composition screening indexes for the assessment of body fatness in children and adolescents. Am J Clin Nutr 2002;75(6):978–85.
22. Goulding A, Gold E, Cannan R, et al. DEXA supports the use of BMI as a measure of fatness in young girls. Int J Obes Relat Metab Disord 1996;20(11):1014–21.
23. Kerruish KP, O'Connor J, Humphries IR, et al. Body composition in adolescents with anorexia nervosa. Am J Clin Nutr 2002;75(1):31–7.
24. World Health Organization. Obesity. Preventing and managing the global epidemic. Geneva (Switzerland); 1998.
25. Chumlea WC, Guo SS, Kuczmarski RJ, et al. Body composition estimates from NHANES III bioelectrical impedance data. Int J Obes Relat Metab Disord 2002; 26(12):1596–609.
26. Wang J, Thornton JC, Russell M, et al. Asians have lower body mass index (BMI) but higher percent body fat than do whites: comparisons of anthropometric measurements. Am J Clin Nutr 1994;60:23–8.
27. Shrewsbury V, Wardle J. Socioeconomic status and adiposity in childhood: a systematic review of cross-sectional studies 1990–2005. Obesity (Silver Spring) 2008;16(2):275–84.
28. McLaren L. Socioeconomic status and obesity. Epidemiol Rev 2007;29:29–48.
29. Available at: http://www.cdc.gov/nchs/data/databriefs/db01.pdf. Accessed August 25, 2008.
30. 2000 CDC growth charts: United States. Available at: http://www.cdc.gov/ growthcharts. Accessed August 25, 2008.
31. Himes JH, Dietz WH. Guidelines for overweight in adolescent preventive services: recommendations from an expert committee. The expert committee on clinical guidelines for overweight in adolescent preventive services. Am J Clin Nutr 1994;59(2):307–16.
32. Kromeyer-Hauschild K, Wabitsch M, Kunze D, et al. Perzentile für den Body-mass-Index für das Kindes- und Jugendalter unter Heranziehung verschiedener deutscher Stichproben. Monatsschr Kinderheilkd 2001;149:807–18.
33. Kuczmarski RJ, Ogden CL, Guo SS, et al. 2000 CDC growth charts for the United States: methods and development. Vital Health Stat 11 2002;246:1–190.
34. Available at: http://www.cdc.gov/nccdphp/dnpa/obesity/childhood/prevalence. htm. Accessed August 25, 2008.
35. Hebebrand J, Himmelmann GW, Heseker H, et al. Use of percentiles for the body mass index in anorexia nervosa: diagnostic, epidemiological and therapeutic considerations. Int J Eat Disord 1996;19(4):359–69.
36. Available at: http://www.cdc.gov.growthcharts; see link *interactive training modules*. Accessed August 25, 2008.
37. Cole TJ, Bellizzi MC, Flegal KM, et al. Establishing a standard definition for child overweight and obesity worldwide: international survey. BMJ 2000;320(7244): 1240–3.

38. Rolland-Cachera MF. Rate of growth in early life: a predictor of later health? Adv Exp Med Biol 2005;569:35–9.

39. Guo SS, Roche AF, Chumlea WC, et al. The predictive value of childhood body mass index values for overweight at age 35 y. Am J Clin Nutr 1994;59(4):810–9.

40. Ong KK, Ahmed ML, Emmett PM, et al. The Avon Longitudinal Study of Pregnancy and Childhood Study Team. Association between postnatal catch-up growth and obesity in childhood: prospective cohort study. BMJ 2000;320(7240): 967–71.

41. Eriksson JG, Forsén T, Tuomilehto J, et al. Catch-up growth in childhood and death from coronary heart disease: longitudinal study. BMJ 1999;318(7181): 427–31.

42. Serdula MK, Ivery D, Coates RJ, et al. Do obese children become obese adults? A review of the literature. Prev Med 1993;22(2):167–77.

43. Whitaker RC, Wright JA, Pepe MS, et al. Predicting obesity in young adulthood from childhood and parental obesity. N Engl J Med 1997;337(13):869–73.

44. Hudson JI, Hiripi E, Pope HG Jr, et al. The prevalence and correlates of eating disorders in the national comorbidity survey replication. Biol Psychiatry 2007; 61(3):348–58.

45. Hebebrand J, Fichter M, Gerber G, et al. Genetic predisposition to obesity in bulimia nervosa: a mutation screen of the melanocortin-4 receptor gene. Mol Psychiatry 2002;7(6):647–51.

46. Kendler KS, MacLean C, Neale M, et al. The genetic epidemiology of bulimia nervosa. Am J Psychiatry 1991;148(12):1627–37.

47. Polivy J, Herman CP. Dieting and binging. A causal analysis. Am Psychol 1985; 40(2):193–201.

48. Fichter MM, Quadflieg N, Hedlund S. Twelve-year course and outcome predictors of anorexia nervosa. Int J Eat Disord 2006;39(2):87–100.

49. Herpertz-Dahlmann BM, Wewetzer C, Schulz E, et al. Course and outcome in adolescent anorexia nervosa. Int J Eat Disord 1996;19(4):335–45.

50. Fairburn CG, Welch SL, Doll HA, et al. Risk factors for bulimia nervosa. A community-based case-control study. Arch Gen Psychiatry 1997;54(6):509–17.

51. Striegel-Moore RH, Franko DL. Should binge eating disorder be included in the DSM-V? A critical review of the state of the evidence. Annu Rev Clin Psychol 2008;4:305–24.

52. Latner JD, Clyne C. The diagnostic validity of the criteria for binge eating disorder. Int J Eat Disord 2008;41(1):1–14.

53. Grucza RA, Przybeck TR, Cloninger CR. Prevalence and correlates of binge eating disorder in a community sample. Compr Psychiatry 2007;48(2):124–31.

54. Dingemans AE, Bruna MJ, van Furth EF. Binge eating disorder: a review. Int J Obes Relat Metab Disord 2002;26(3):299–307.

55. Spitzer RL, Yanovski S, Wadden T, et al. Binge eating disorder: its further validation in a multisite study. Int J Eat Disord 1993;13(2):137–53.

56. Guss JL, Kissileff HR, Devlin MJ, et al. Binge size increases with body mass index in women with binge-eating disorder. Obes Res 2002;10(10):1021–9.

57. Available at: http://www.who.int/classifications/icd/en/. Accessed August 25, 2008.

58. Documenta Geigy. Scientific tables. (reprinted from Society of Actuaries 1959; Build and Blood Pressure Study). 7th edition. Basle (Switzerland): Geigy; 1973.

59. Russell G. The prognosis of eating disorders: a clinician's approach. In: Herzog W, Deter HC, Vandereycken W, editors. The course of eating disorders. Berlin: Springer Verlag; 1992. p. 198–213.

60. Hebebrand J, Wehmeier P, Remschmidt H. Weight criteria for diagnosis of anorexia nervosa. Am J Psychiatry 2000;157:1024.
61. Hebebrand J, Himmelmann GW, Herzog W, et al. Prediction of low body weight at long-term follow-up in acute anorexia nervosa by low body weight at referral. Am J Psychiatry 1997;154(4):566–9.
62. Collins S. The limit of human adaptation to starvation. Nat Med 1995;1(8):810–4.
63. Nielsen S. Evaluation of growth in anorexia nervosa from serial measurements. J Psychiatr Res 1985;19(2–3):227–30.
64. Coners H, Remschmidt H, Hebebrand J. The relationship between premorbid body weight, weight loss, and weight at referral in adolescent patients with anorexia nervosa. Int J Eat Disord 1999;26(2):171–8.
65. Köpp W, Blum WF, von Prittwitz S, et al. Low leptin levels predict amenorrhea in underweight and eating disordered females. Mol Psychiatry 1997;2(4):335–40.
66. Ballauff A, Ziegler A, Emons G, et al. Serum leptin and gonadotropin levels in patients with anorexia nervosa during weight gain. Mol Psychiatry 1999;4(1):71–5.
67. Welt CK, Chan JL, Bullen J, et al. Recombinant human leptin in women with hypothalamic amenorrhea. N Engl J Med 2004;351(10):987–97.

Eating Disorders of Infancy and Childhood: Definition, Symptomatology, Epidemiology, and Comorbidity

Dasha Nicholls, MBBS, MD *, Rachel Bryant-Waugh, BSc, MSc, DPhil

KEYWORDS
- Feeding disorder • Eating disorder • Child • Diagnosis
- Epidemiology

Feeding and eating disorders occur in normally developing children, in those with chronic or serious medical conditions, and in those with developmental disabilities or disorders. They are usually multifactorial in nature, involving different bodily systems and specific aspects of individual and interpersonal functioning, and can therefore be conceptualized as biopsychosocial disorders. They require a multidisciplinary approach for assessment and treatment, with components of intervention individually tailored according to the formulation and presenting features. Treatment approaches include those focused on the child; those focused on caregivers; those focused on relationships between the child and caregivers and other family members; and those focused on the child's wider context, for example, school.

This article is restricted to those feeding and eating difficulties that are not fully accounted for at the time of presentation by an underlying medical problem, although such a problem may have contributed to the development of the disorder; and to feeding or eating problems that are clinically significant in terms of their impact on physical, social, or emotional development. The authors use the term "eating disorder" to mean eating difficulties associated with morbid preoccupation with weight and shape. At this time there is no satisfactory widely accepted terminology to describe the other

Department of Child And Adolescent Mental Health, Great Ormond Street Hospital For Children NHS Trust, London WC1N 3JH, UK
* Corresponding author.
E-mail address: nichod@gosh.nhs.uk (D. Nicholls).

Child Adolesc Psychiatric Clin N Am 18 (2008) 17–30
doi:10.1016/j.chc.2008.07.008
1056-4993/08/$ – see front matter © 2008 Elsevier Inc. All rights reserved.

childpsych.theclinics.com

clinically significant eating difficulties seen in childhood, described below, and therefore little in the way of empiric research on many of these clinical presentations.

FEEDING DISORDERS OF INFANCY AND EARLY CHILDHOOD

The fourth edition of the Diagnostic and Statistical Manual of Mental Disorders (DSM-IV)[1] distinguishes 3 feeding disorders: a broad diagnostic category named "feeding disorder of infancy or early childhood" (**Box 1**) and two distinct subtypes; "pica" and "rumination disorder," discussed separately below. The ICD-10 Classification of Behavioural and Mental Disorders classification system[2] also has a broad category called "feeding disorder of infancy and childhood" (**Box 2**), which includes rumination. These diagnostic systems exclude presentations where the feeding disorder is directly attributable to a medical condition or another psychiatric disorder. The systems require the child to have lost weight or failed to gain weight. However, two of the commonest clinical presentations in younger children are selective eating (also known as faddy eating, and perseverative feeding disorder) and food aversion secondary to prolonged enteral feeding, neither of which is usually associated with low weight.

Subclassification and Measurement of Feeding Disorders and Feeding Problems

Two major areas of difficulty related to feeding problems are classification and measurement. In many cases the problem is initially identified and described by caregivers and although assessment often includes some observation of the child's feeding, usually in a clinical setting, few investigators report objective measurement. This is perhaps unsurprising because feeding is generally considered to occur in a relational context, with variables relating to caregiver and child having an impact on the nature and severity of the feeding problem.[3] The emphasis in the literature has been on describing different types of presenting problems based on clinical observation and parental report, rather than on deriving clear diagnostic subgroups by way of robust empiric means. Until approaches for identification, measurement, and classification of feeding disorders can be agreed on, studies of epidemiology, treatment, course, and prognosis remain difficult.

The traditional distinction between organic and nonorganic feeding problems is problematic because it assumes that either feeding disorders are related to physical, structural, or functional abnormalities or they are triggered by social and environmental factors. Such a stark dichotomy does not reflect the complexity of the factors that combine to result in complex feeding problems. In addition, the term "nonorganic" may be taken to imply that rigorous assessment has excluded organic contributions, which is not always the case. Reilly and colleagues[4] found that of 47 children

---

Box 1
DSM-IV criteria for feeding disorder of infancy and early childhood

A. Feeding disturbance as manifested by persistent failure to eat adequately with significant failure to gain weight or significant loss of weight over at least 1 mo.

B. The disturbance is not because of an associated gastrointestinal or other general medical condition (eg, esophageal reflux).

C. The disturbance is not better accounted for by another mental disorder (eg, rumination disorder) or by lack of available food.

D. The onset is before age 6 yr.

Box 2
ICD-10 criteria for feeding disorder of infancy and childhood (research criteria)
A. Persistent failure to eat adequately, or persistent rumination or regurgitation of food.
B. Failure to gain weight or loss of weight or other significant health problem over a period of at least 1 mo (in view of the frequency of transient eating difficulties, researchers may prefer a minimum duration of 3 mo for some purposes).
C. Onset of the disorder before age 6 yr.
D. Absence of other mental and behavioral disorders in ICD-10 (other than mental retardation).
E. No organic disease sufficient to account for the failure to eat.
From World Health Organization. The ICD-10 classification of mental and behavioural disorders: diagnostic criteria for research. Geneva: World Health Organization, 1992; with permission.

diagnosed with nonorganic failure to thrive, 36% had oral motor dysfunction, concluding that the term "nonorganic" in such children was questionable.

Attempts have been made to classify feeding difficulties that arise primarily from psychological and relationship difficulties, rather than as a result of organic or developmental problems. Chatoor[5] and colleagues have proposed criteria for subgroups of feeding disorders, including "feeding disorder of state regulation," "feeding disorder of reciprocity" (previously "feeding disorder of attachment"), "infantile anorexia," "sensory food aversions," "feeding disorder associated with concurrent medical condition," and "posttraumatic feeding disorder." It is unclear what proportion of children presenting to multidisciplinary pediatric feeding clinics could be accounted for by these clinical presentations. Crist and Napier-Phillips[6] used a behavioral feeding questionnaire to attempt to empirically derive feeding problem subtypes. In 96 control and 249 clinically referred children, 5 presentations accounted for 55% of the cases: "picky eaters," "toddler refusal – general," "toddler refusal – textures," "older children refusal – general," and "stallers." Nearly half the group did not fall into one of these subgroups. Burklow and colleagues[7] also identified 5 categories of clinical feeding disorder presentations but did not attempt to separate organic from nonorganic. They were "structural abnormalities," "neurologic conditions," "behavioral and psychosocial problems," "cardiorespiratory problems," and "metabolic dysfunction." Of 103 referred children, 85% were coded as having a significant behavioral component to their presentation, underlining the fact that even feeding problems with significant medical or developmental contributions may be amenable to psychological interventions.

Feeding Problems in the Context of Neurodevelopmental Disorders or Learning Disability

Feeding difficulties in children with autistic spectrum disorders (ASD) most commonly focus on selectivity by texture, taste, brand, presentation, or appearance, which may or may not result in failure to gain weight or weight loss. Such children may also present with food refusal, failure to eat the usual family diet, inappropriate rate of eating, obsessive eating patterns, failure to accept novel foods and inappropriate mealtime routines, which may be a result of common ASD features (eg, attention to detail, perseveration, fear of novelty, sensory impairments, and biological food intolerances). Schreck and Williams[8] have challenged the view that these behaviors are entirely related to ASD, suggesting that the family's reported eating preferences may be more relevant. Furthermore, selective eating, such as that found in children with ASD, is also seen in children without diagnosed developmental disorder (see Selective Eating). Organic contributions may also be a factor in this group of children. Schwarz and colleagues[9] found that in 79 children with moderate to severe developmental disability, 56% (44) demonstrated gastroesophageal reflux and 27% (21) had oropharyngeal dysphagia.

Facial and oral hypersensitivity can be found along with neurological difficulties, such as epilepsy, and are also associated with situations where oral desensitization has failed to occur, such as prolonged tube feeding.

Enteral Feeding

Increasingly, children presenting to clinical services are started on enteral feeding for any of several reasons and have difficulty making the transition from tube feeding to oral feeding. Although not a diagnosis in itself, "tube feeding" can lead to specific difficulties requiring psychological intervention. Problems created by enteral feeding include reduction of appetite and thirst, leading to lack of recognition of hunger and thirst drive; absence of normal response to sight/smell of food, for instance, salivation and lack of pleasure; reduced opportunities to practice the routine and skills required for oral feeding, such as chewing or using cutlery; and fear of and revulsion at certain textures, tastes, and smells. Careful assessment will identify the extent to which each of these has become a factor.

Epidemiology and Comorbidity

Estimates of the incidence and prevalence of feeding disorder and feeding difficulties in children are difficult to ascertain with any reliability. More than 50% of parents report one problem feeding behavior and more than 20% report multiple problems in children aged 9 months to 7 years,[6] in line with the widely quoted figure that 1 in 4 children in pediatric populations have a feeding disorder.[10] Using more stringent criteria, Dahl and Sundelin,[11] found a prevalence rate of 1.4% in infants aged between 3 and 12 months. Most of them (82%) were underweight for their age.

The prevalence of parent-reported feeding problems in children with disabilities is higher, estimated at around 40%–70% in association with developmental disabilities and chronic medical conditions,[12] and as high as 89% in children with neurologic impairment.[13] Ledford and Gast[14] report that up to 89% of children with ASD have problem feeding behaviors. Other high-risk groups include infants of premature birth, children with craniofacial anomalies, and those with certain genetic syndromes (such as Russell-Silver syndrome). Levels of comorbidity differ across the varying presentations of feeding problems. Axis II developmental disorders and axis III physical conditions are commonly associated with feeding disorders.

PICA

Pica is a term used to denote the persistent eating of nonnutritive substances over an extended period of time. Pica tends to be diagnosed at the time the behavior reaches clinical significance, for example, intervention might be required in relation to the ingestion of toxic substances. It is not usually diagnosed before the age of 18 months (24 months if using ICD-10 criteria). Some clinicians also use the term to include the eating of foodstuffs in a raw or unprepared form, such as flour or raw potatoes, although technically such substances may be nutritive. In the clinical setting the main questions to be addressed relate to possible physical, psychological, and developmental underlying causes, complications resulting from the ingestion of nonnutritive substances, and an assessment of the child's psychosocial environment. The most common harmful outcomes of pica in children include lead poisoning, other accidental poisoning, parasitic infestation, infections, gastrointestinal obstruction, and gastrointestinal lacerations. It can also be associated with sleep walking, nightmares, night terrors, and head banging or rocking in sleep.[15]

Epidemiology and Comorbidity

There are prevalence figures for pica in institutionalized adults (eg, 9.2% of 607 such adults[16]), but rates for infants and young children are less clear, and the literature is largely comprised of case reports. Pica can be associated with developmental disorders, including learning disability and pervasive developmental disorders. In cases where pica occurs during the course of another mental disorder, such as pervasive developmental disorder or Kleine–Levin syndrome, a diagnosis of pica should only be made if severe enough to require additional and independent treatment.

The risk for pica is also increased in vulnerable individuals subject to poverty, neglect, deprivation, and lack of supervision. Pica is also well known to occur in individuals with nutritional deficiencies; cases have been reported of iron deficiency due to celiac disease presenting as pica.[17] Finally, pica also occurs in older individuals of normal intelligence, for example, in pregnancy and as part of culturally sanctioned practice (eg, eating soil is not uncommon in some African countries and in India and would not be considered a disorder).

RUMINATION DISORDER

Rumination disorder is characterized by the regurgitation of recently ingested food, which is re-chewed before being swallowed again, or in some cases spat out, in a process repeated several times. The experience seems to be pleasurable or soothing, with rumination in infants often being understood as a form of self-stimulation. Some investigators have described a typical posture characterized by an arched back, backward tilt to the head, and contraction of abdominal muscles, representing attempts to regurgitate part of the digested food. Rumination can be associated with weight loss and vomiting,[18] and complications include malnutrition as a result of inadequate nutrient or calorie retention, halitosis, dental damage, electrolyte abnormalities, and abdominal pain. The diagnosis requires that there should have been a period of normal feeding of at least 1 month's duration before the regurgitation. It has been linked to severe medical and psychosocial conditions, including malnutrition, aspiration pneumonia, and complete social withdrawal. Assessment aimed at identifying situations and emotions that trigger the symptoms can be helpful.

Epidemiology and Comorbidity

Rumination is seen in three distinct populations: infants (the most common); individuals with psychiatric and neurologic disorders, particularly developmental disabilities; and adults who do not have overt psychiatric or neurologic disorders.[19] Variability in the use of terms in relation to rumination disorder makes clear statements about incidence and prevalence difficult. Sensory and emotional deprivation are associated with rumination in children, which may explain the increased incidence of rumination in institutionalized children,[19] infants in intensive care units, and in normal infants with attachment disorders. Alternative causes of regurgitation or vomiting need to be ruled out, the most obvious being gastrointestinal conditions, such as gastroesophageal reflux pyloric stenosis or gastrointestinal infections. Many infants experience periods of vomiting or posseting, which can be distinguished from rumination disorder by the absence of the characteristic preparatory movements and apparent pleasure derived from the behavior. Regurgitating and spitting out food have also been well described as symptoms of an eating disorder in older individuals;[20] eating disorders therefore need to be ruled out.

SELECTIVE EATING

Selective eating is a term that has been used to describe extreme faddy eating, which may persist into middle childhood and beyond. Other terms sometimes used include picky or choosy eating,[21] or perseverative feeding disorder.[22] Variations in terminology make comparisons across the literature difficult, but all these descriptions include two essential features: eating a highly limited range of foods and extreme reluctance to try new foods. Because the preferred foods are often soft carbohydrate-based finger foods, the child may not have developed chewing skills or learnt to use a knife and fork. Difficulties in sensory integration may be a factor to a greater or lesser degree. In addition, this type of eating pattern has often led to exclusion from social norms around eating. Feeding as a point of parent–child communication has often become distorted by conflict and resistance.

Many investigators use the term food neophobia (fear of trying new foods) and picky eating interchangeably.[23] Others, such as Galloway and colleagues,[24] make a clear distinction between picky eating and neophobia, asserting that whereas pickiness is predicted primarily by environmental or experiential factors, neophobia is predicted by more enduring and dispositional factors. As noted above, picky eating is a common feature in toddlers and generally this is a phase that children "grow out of," but for a minority of children, food neophobic behaviors do not improve with maturity.[23] Food neophobia is a dimensional trait that Pliner and Loewen[25] conceptualize as a personality trait, embedded in other aspects of the child's temperament. Overall rates of food neophobia in the population are low,[26] with boys having higher rates than girls, and reducing with age. Studies in adults have shown high neophobia to be positively correlated with trait anxiety and negatively correlated with novelty seeking. In children, Pliner and colleagues[25] found correlations between shyness and emotionality and reluctance to try unfamiliar foods.

Consistent with this, anxiety symptoms are sometimes, but not always, a feature of children and young adolescents with selective eating presenting to clinical services.[27] In selective eating, food neophobia is of such a marked degree that concern about the impact on the child's social activities or conflict as a result of the child's highly rigid eating patterns has arisen. Timimi and colleagues[28] noted that although mealtimes are a battleground in families of younger selective eaters, many parents of older children with selective eating seemed to have given up trying to change their children's eating habits. Concern about the impact of restricted diet on physical health or social development is usually the presenting concern. In general, measures of well-being, such as growth and pubertal development, are unaffected by a highly limited nutritional range, because these children are not usually underweight.[27]

Over a period of years children with selective eating develop an avoidance-reinforced anxiety associated with new foods. There may be anticipatory nausea (with sight or smell triggers), fear of vomiting (textures), or a fear of choking.

Epidemiology and Comorbidity

There have been no long-term outcome studies focusing specifically on selective eating and little is known about its prevalence in older children and adults. Picky eating is the only type of early feeding problem that has been linked to later eating disorders, specifically anorexia nervosa.[29] Clinical cases are more commonly seen in boys than girls,[27] although picky eating in normal populations has a more even gender distribution.[30] In a cohort of 20 children (age, 4–7 years) with extremely selective eating, 30% had obsessions and compulsions and 40% had social and school attendance difficulties.[28] As noted, the population in which selective eating is a common feature is children with autistic spectrum disorder (ASD).[31] Many children with ASD have, in common with many children with selective eating, increased sensitivity to texture and smell, a well-developed sense of disgust, and difficulties with messy play. A proportion will also have subtle neurodevelopmental difficulties, such as mild dyspraxia, or delayed language development, not sufficient to meet the criteria for developmental disorder.[27]

FOOD AVOIDANCE EMOTIONAL DISORDER

The term food avoidance emotional disorder (FAED) has been used to describe avoidance of food to a marked degree in the absence of the characteristic psychopathology of eating disorders in terms of weight and shape cognitions.[32] It excludes children who are chronically low in weight and is of uncertain nosologic status, other than being clearly distinguishable from anorexia nervosa.[33]

Unlike patients with anorexia nervosa, children with FAED know that they are underweight, would like to be heavier, and may not know why they find this difficult to achieve. A child with FAED may give any number of reasons for not being able to eat: fear of being sick, "not hungry," "can't eat," "hurts my tummy," etc. A question of whether some of the cultural variants of anorexia nervosa that have been described would be best conceptualized as FAED,[34,35] or whether they are indeed variants of anorexia nervosa remains unanswered at this point, and little is known about the course and outcome. It is likely that a few cases are a precursor to "true" eating disorders, but for others the presentation may be distinct.

Epidemiology and Comorbidity

No published epidemiologic data on FAED exist at present. Food avoidance often exists as an isolated symptom, but comorbid obsessional anxiety or depression may be present. This term excludes loss of appetite due to low mood – the food avoidance and anxiety related to eating can be as marked in FAED as in anorexia nervosa. We have come to use the term FAED when food avoidance is marked and merits treatment intervention in its own right, regardless of comorbidities.

These children often have other medically unexplained symptoms, and occasionally weight loss is attributed to undiagnosed physical disorder. Addressing these concerns with a comprehensive physical assessment and an open mind is essential if a therapeutic alliance is to be successfully achieved. Inevitably some cases will actually have previously unidentified organic pathology, the commonest being inflammatory bowel diseases, food allergies, and intracranial pathology.[36]

FOOD PHOBIAS

Phobias involving food can occur in isolation or as part of a more generalized anxiety disorder. The nature of the specific fear varies with, among other things, the child's developmental stage. Fears that are common are fear of vomiting (emetophobia), fear of contamination or poisoning, fear of choking or swallowing (sometimes known as functional dysphagia – discussed further below), and fear of the consequences of hypercholesterolemia.[37] Food phobias are usually secondary events and follow a period of normal eating for the developmental stage. Clear trigger events may be identified in some but not all cases, for example, choking events, or may be directly linked to the fear, such as a fear of cholesterol developing in a child who saw his/her father die of a myocardial infarction. Presenting features include rigid eating patterns, which may have led to parent–child conflict; a restricted range of foods; and in more extreme cases, a restricted quantity of food leading to weight loss. The extent to which obsessional rituals have taken hold will depend on contextual factors, such as parental responses to the child's anxiety and the temperament of the child. Reports suggest that phobias of this kind can be chronic and lead to significant functional impairment.[38]

In some children, food phobias may be a feature of more pervasive anxiety disorder or obsessive compulsive disorder (OCD). OCD can present as food-related obsessions in the absence of weight and shape concerns. For example, a child may develop obsessional fear about the content of food or about the freshness of food, such that food intake is limited to those sources that are of "known" safety in terms of cleanliness, and only certain family members are entrusted to prepare food. The association between anorexia nervosa and OCD is well recognized[39] and is thought to be particularly common in childhood anorexia nervosa presenting in boys.

Epidemiology and Comorbidity

No studies to our knowledge have studied food phobia separately from other childhood anxiety disorders. Common problems associated with food phobias include depression, panic attacks, social anxiety, compulsions, and difficulties with separation. In addition, phobic eating patterns can be associated with food allergies, through an understandable generalization of "food can be dangerous" associated cognitions.

FUNCTIONAL DYSPHAGIA

Functional dysphagia (also known as globus hystericus or phagophobia [see, for example, Okada and colleagues[40]]) is a term used to describe swallowing difficulties associated with a fear of choking. It can be found as an isolated symptom of acute onset, often following trauma or as a feature of other disorders. Functional dysphagia is probably more valid as a symptom descriptor than a separate nosologic entity. As a symptom, it needs to be recognized and managed appropriately, through a combination of psycho-education, graded desensitization and exposure, behavioral rewards, family therapy, and in some cases anxiolytic medication.

Epidemiology and Comorbidity

Functional dysphagia is found clinically in patients with FAED, selective eating, food refusal, and sometimes anorexia nervosa and isolation. It is also associated with other anxiety symptoms and with somatization or conversion disorder. Data on the population epidemiology of dysphagia are scarce. One study found lifetime self-reported dysphagia in 16% of a sample of more than 600 adults (peak age, 40–50 years). Intermittent dysphagia was associated with anxiety, whereas progressive dysphagia was associated with depression.[41] The methodology of this study did not enable organic disease as a contributor to be excluded, which makes the findings all the more interesting.

FOOD REFUSAL

Food refusal as an isolated behavior is an experience most parents encounter at some point during their child's development. The behaviors identified with food refusal in toddlers include whining or crying, tantrums, and spitting out food.[6] This refusal pattern is often general in nature as opposed to food specific and linked to other types of oppositional behavior. Food refusal in older children is often associated with other defiant behaviors, such as delaying eating by talking, trying to negotiate what food will be eaten, getting up from the table during meals, and refusing to eat much at a meal, but requesting food immediately afterward. Much of the nutritional intake of these children is gained through snacking between meals. These behaviors mostly seem to reflect general disruptive behavior, rather than possible oral motor difficulties.[6]

In addition to food refusal as a form of oppositional behavior, it can occur in children of otherwise biddable and compliant temperament. This might typically be in situations where an initial trigger event results in food avoidance (such as illness or trauma) and subsequent events serve to perpetuate the symptom, serving some psychological function (such as the expression of anger, frustration, or rejection). If not addressed it can progress to become severe and extreme. Pervasive refusal syndrome[42] is a term sometimes used to describe "profound and pervasive refusal to eat, walk, talk, or engage in self care." This rare condition has been conceptualized as an extreme posttraumatic stress reaction in cases of evident or suspected abuse[42] and as a form of learned helplessness.[43] The term pervasive refusal, though evocative to anyone who has met these children, may be problematic in the development of a therapeutic alliance with young persons or their families.

Epidemiology and Comorbidity

Food refusal is common, especially at certain developmental stages. The literature includes case reports and series where food refusal occurs in various conditions, including cerebral palsy, and in children with learning disabilities and other developmental disorders. One might hypothesize that food refusal is one of the few ways in which some children are able to communicate that something is either physically or emotionally wrong. Profound disturbances, such as pervasive refusal syndrome, are extremely rare.

CHILDHOOD EATING DISORDERS
Anorexia Nervosa

Anorexia nervosa is seen clinically from about age 7 upward. By definition, its presentation is similar to that of older sufferers, with some important developmental differences. Several articles have described these differences in presentation between children and adolescents,[33,44–49] which lie in psychological, behavioral, and physical domains.

Key psychological and behavioral differences include the fact that children have limited capacity for self-appraisal or reflection and may have difficulty putting the thoughts and feelings driving behavior into words. Thus, a child with behaviors characteristic of anorexia nervosa, such as specific avoidance of fatty foods, excessive exercising after meals, and even vomiting, may not voice dissatisfaction with weight and shape. Developmentally sensitive, reliable instruments, such as the child adaptation of the Eating Disorders Examination,[50,51] have improved our ability to assess core psychopathology, but as with adolescents and adults, they cannot always be relied on to make a clinical diagnosis of anorexia nervosa. It has been proposed that diagnosis in children might more usefully take into account parental report, the child's subjective experience, and direct clinical observation, yet standardized approaches to how these components might best be integrated to inform diagnostic evaluation in children are still lacking.[52]

The second main area of developmental difference is in terms of physical impact. Much has been written about the way that childhood anorexia nervosa can have a detrimental and even irreversible effect by interrupting physical development.[53] This complex area is one in which individualized assessment of a young person's previous growth and maturational trajectory, multisystem evaluation, and genetic potential all need to be taken into consideration, not simply direct comparison to population-based norms.

Epidemiology and comorbidity

Epidemiologic studies have tended to group children and adolescents or focus on the peak age ef at onset (around 15 years), making few incidence estimates available for the younger age group. Data from a general practitioner register study reported an incidence of anorexia nervosa of 17.5/100,000 in 10- to 19-year olds and 0.3/100,000 in 0- to 9-year olds.[54] Currin and colleagues[55] found no cases of anorexia nervosa in children younger than age 10 years in a UK primary care study undertaken in the early 1990s, whereas Van Son and colleagues[56] reported 1 case in 10 years in a Netherlands primary care study. Retrospective studies from the United States and Denmark have suggested higher figures, for instance, 9–27/100,000 for 10 to14-year old girls and 3.7/100,000 for boys.[57,58] The proportion of boys with childhood onset anorexia nervosa is higher than in older adolescent samples, before the gender-specific effects of puberty have come into play. Comorbidities mirror those in older patients, the commonest being OCD and depression. Increasingly, autistic spectrum traits are being recognized in conjunction with anorexia nervosa.

Bulimia Nervosa and Binge Eating

Although some adults retrospectively report premenarcheal onset of bulimia nervosa,[59] there are no other reports in the literature of childhood bulimia nervosa. In our experience, on the rare occasions when bulimia nervosa presents before adolescence, it is usually in young people who have reached developmental maturity at a young age. Binge eating in children on the other hand would appear to be common, particularly in children whose parents seek treatment for their overweight.[60] Traits of childhood overeating are more common in women with bulimia nervosa, although the same is not true for anorexia nervosa.[61] Prevention strategies for childhood obesity and overweight may therefore be useful in preventing bulimia nervosa. Increasingly there has been a focus on the factors that may contribute to "loss of control eating" in children,[62] in the hope that prevention of future eating disorders may be tackled through this avenue. For example, there is some suggestion that when parents control their child's intake too much, this can potentiate preferences for high-fat, energy-dense foods, limit children's acceptance of a variety of foods, and disrupt children's regulation of energy intake by altering responsiveness to internal cues of hunger and satiety.[63]

Epidemiology and comorbidity

Binge eating is reported as occurring in about 6.2% of 6- to 13-year-old normal and overweight children.[64] The experience of loss of control over eating, independent from the amount of food consumed, seems to affect between 15% and 18% of children and adolescents seeking treatment for overweight.[65,66] Currin and colleagues[55] found no cases of bulimia nervosa in children younger than age 10 years in a UK primary care study, whereas Van Son and colleagues[56] reported 1 case in 10 years in a Netherlands primary care study.

SUMMARY

The authors have described the range of feeding and eating problems presenting clinically in preadolescent children, with the exception of childhood obesity, which is addressed elsewhere. This is a complex area, but also one of overlaps and similarities. Many of the problems described are of uncertain nosologic status and linked to this is a lack of systematic research in the area. Priority areas for future research include epidemiologic studies of childhood problem eating behaviors to enable a better understanding of the range of normal eating in childhood and early adolescence. This might form the basis of a dimensional approach to defining problem feeding and eating behavior. There is also a need for prospective longitudinal clinical studies to clarify the course of feeding and eating problems in this age group and explore continuities and discontinuities between the various presentations described.

Services for feeding and eating problems of childhood are generally lacking and highly variable in nature.[67] This may reflect a perception that these conditions are rare or not serious and there may be different views as to whether they are best managed by generic or specialist services. Although the authors have tried in this article to focus on those areas whereby psychological skills are essential, not all mental health professionals believe they are skilled in this area.

REFERENCES

1. American Psychiatric Association. Diagnostic and statistical manual of mental disorders—DSM-IV. 4th edition. Washington, DC: American Psychiatric Association; 1994.
2. WHO. ICD-10 classification of mental and behavioural disorders. London: Churchill Livingstone; 1991.
3. Davies WH, Satter E, Berlin KS, et al. Reconceptualizing feeding and feeding disorders in interpersonal context: the case for a relational disorder. J Fam Psychol 2006;20:409–17.
4. Reilly SM, Skuse DH, Wolke D, et al. Oral-motor dysfunction in children who fail to thrive: organic or non-organic? Dev Med Child Neurol 1999;41:115–22.
5. Chatoor I. Feeding disorders in infants and toddlers: diagnosis and treatment. Child Adolesc Psychiatr Clin N Am 2002;11:163–83.
6. Crist W, Napier-Phillips A. Mealtime behaviors of young children: a comparison of normative and clinical data. J Dev Behav Pediatr 2001;22:279–86.
7. Burklow KA, Phelps AN, Schultz JR, et al. Classifying complex pediatric feeding disorders. J Pediatr Gastroenterol Nutr 1998;27:143–7.
8. Schreck KA, Williams K. Food preferences and factors influencing food selectivity for children with autism spectrum disorders. Res Dev Disabil 2006;27:353–63.
9. Schwarz SM, Corredor J, Fisher-Medina J, et al. Diagnosis and treatment of feeding disorders in children with developmental disabilities. Pediatrics 2001;108: 671–6.
10. Babbitt RL, Hoch TA, Coe DA, et al. Behavioral assessment and treatment of pediatric feeding disorders. J Dev Behav Pediatr 1994;15:278–91.
11. Dahl M, Sundelin C. Early feeding problems in an affluent society. I. Categories and clinical signs. Acta Paediatr Scand 1986;75:370–9.
12. Byars KC, Burklow KA, Ferguson K, et al. A multicomponent behavioral program for oral aversion in children dependent on gastrostomy feedings. J Pediatr Gastroenterol Nutr 2003;37:473–80.
13. Sullivan PB, Lambert B, Rose M, et al. Prevalence and severity of feeding and nutritional problems in children with neurological impairment: Oxford feeding study. Dev Med Child Neurol 2000;42:674–80.

14. Ledford JR, Gast DL, Luscre D, et al. Observational and incidental learning by children with autism during small group instruction. J Autism Dev Disord 2008; 38:86–103.

15. Stein MA, Mendelsohn J, Obermeyer WH, et al. Sleep and behavior problems in school-aged children. Pediatrics 2001;107:E60.

16. McAlpine C, Singh NN. Pica in institutionalized mentally retarded persons. J Ment Defic Res 1986;30(Pt 2):171–8.

17. Korman SH. Pica as a presenting symptom in childhood celiac disease. Am J Clin Nutr 1990;51:139–41.

18. Khan S, Hyman PE, Cocjin J, et al. Rumination syndrome in adolescents. J Pediatr 2000;136:528–31.

19. Olden KW. Rumination. Curr Treat Options Gastroenterol 2001;4:351–8.

20. Birmingham CL, Firoz T. Rumination in eating disorders: literature review. Eat Weight Disord 2006;11:e85–9.

21. Jacobi C, Agras WS, Bryson S, et al. Behavioral validation, precursors, and concomitants of picky eating in childhood. J Am Acad Child Adolesc Psychiatry 2003;42:76–84.

22. Harris G, Booth IW. The nature and management of eating problems in pre-school children. In: Cooper PJ, Stein A, editors. Feeding problems and eating disorders in children and adolescents. Monographs in Clin Pediatr No 5. Chur (Switzerland): Harwood Academic Publishers; 1992. p. 61–85.

23. Carruth BR, Skinner JD. Revisiting the picky eater phenomenon: neophobic behaviors of young children. J Am Coll Nutr 2000;19:771–80.

24. Galloway AT, Lee Y, Birch LL. Predictors and consequences of food neophobia and pickiness in young girls. J Am Diet Assoc 2003;103:692–8.

25. Pliner P, Loewen ER. Temperament and food neophobia in children and their mothers. Appetite 1997;28:239–54.

26. Koivisto UK, Sjoden PO. Food and general neophobia in Swedish families: parent-child comparisons and relationships with serving specific foods. Appetite 1996;26:107–18.

27. Nicholls D, Christie D, Randall L, et al. Selective eating: symptom, disorder or normal variant? Clin Child Psychol Psychiatry 2001;6:257–70.

28. Timimi S, Douglas J, Tsiftsopoulou K. Selective eaters: a retrospective case note study. Child Care Health Dev 1997;23:265–78.

29. Marchi M, Cohen P. Early childhood eating behaviors and adolescent eating disorders. J Am Acad Child Adolesc Psychiatry 1990;29:112–7.

30. Jacobi C, Schmitz G, Agras WS. Is picky eating an eating disorder? Int J Eat Disord 2008, in press.

31. Schreck KA, Williams K, Smith AF. A comparison of eating behaviors between children with and without autism. J Autism Dev Disord 2004;34:433–8.

32. Higgs JF, Goodyer IM, Birch J. Anorexia nervosa and food avoidance emotional disorder. Arch Dis Child 1989;64:346–51.

33. Cooper PJ, Watkins B, Bryant-Waugh R, et al. The nosological status of early onset anorexia nervosa. Psychol Med 2002;32:873–80.

34. Tareen A, Hodes M, Rangel L. Non-fat-phobic anorexia nervosa in British South Asian adolescents. Int J Eat Disord 2005;37:161–5.

35. Lee HY, Lock J. Anorexia nervosa in Asian-American adolescents: do they differ from their non-Asian peers. Int J Eat Disord 2007;40:227–31.

36. De Vile CJ, Sufraz R, Lask B, et al. Occult intracranial tumours masquerading as early onset anorexia nervosa. Br Med J 1995;311:1359–60.

37. Lifshitz F. Nutritional dwarfing in adolescents. Growth, Genetics and Hormones 1987;3:1–5.
38. Lipsitz JD, Fyer AJ, Paterniti A, et al. Emetophobia: preliminary results of an internet survey. Depress Anxiety 2001;14:149–52.
39. Shafran R, Bryant-Waugh R, Lask B, et al. Obsessive-compulsive symptoms in children with eating disorders: a preliminary investigation. Eating Disorders: Journal of Treatment and Prevention 1995;3:304–10.
40. Okada A, Tsukamoto C, Hosogi M, et al. A study of psycho-pathology and treatment of children with phagophobia. Acta Med Okayama 2007;61:261–9.
41. Eslick GD, Talley NJ. Dysphagia: epidemiology, risk factors and impact on quality of life–a population-based study. Aliment Pharmacol Ther 2008;27:971–9.
42. Lask B, Britten C, Kroll L, et al. Pervasive refusal in children. Arch Dis Child 1991; 66:866–9.
43. Nunn KP, Thompson S. The pervasive refusal syndrome: learned helplessness and hopelessness. Clin Child Psychol Psychiatry 1996;1:121–32.
44. Gowers SG, Crisp AH, Joughin N, et al. Premenarcheal anorexia nervosa. J Child Psychol Psychiatry 1991;32:515–24.
45. Bryant-Waugh R, Lask B. Eating disorders in children. J Child Psychol Psychiatry 1995;36:191–202.
46. Jacobs BW, Isaacs S. Pre-pubertal anorexia nervosa: a retrospective controlled study. J Child Psychol Psychiatry 1986;27:237–50.
47. Arnow B, Sanders MJ, Steiner H. Premenarcheal versus postmenarcheal anorexia nervosa: a comparative study. Clin Child Psychol Psychiatry 1999;4:403–14.
48. Peebles R, Wilson JL, Lock JD. How do children with eating disorders differ from adolescents with eating disorders at initial evaluation? J Adolesc Health 2006;39: 800–5.
49. Bravender T, Bryant-Waugh R, Herzog D, et al. Classification of child and adolescent eating disturbances. Workgroup for Classification of Eating Disorders in Children and Adolescents (WCEDCA). Int J Eat Disord 2007;40(Suppl): S117–22.
50. Bryant-Waugh R, Cooper P, Taylor C, et al. The use of the eating disorder examination with children: a pilot study. Int J Eat Disord 1996;19:391–7.
51. Watkins B, Frampton I, Lask B, et al. Reliability and validity of the child version of the eating disorder examination: a preliminary investigation. Int J Eat Disord 2005;38:183–7.
52. Couturier J, Lock J, Forsberg S, et al. The addition of a parent and clinician component to the eating disorder examination for children and adolescents. Int J Eat Disord 2007;40:472–5.
53. Katzman DK. Medical complications in adolescents with anorexia nervosa: a review of the literature. Int J Eat Disord 2005;37(Suppl):S52–9.
54. Turnbull S, Ward A, Treasure J, et al. The demand for eating disorder care. An epidemiological study using the general practice research database. Br J Psychiatry 1996;169:705–12.
55. Currin L, Schmidt U, Treasure J, et al. Time trends in eating disorder incidence. Br J Psychiatry 2005;186:132–5.
56. van Son GE, van Hoeken D, Bartelds AI, et al. Time trends in the incidence of eating disorders: a primary care study in the Netherlands. Int J Eat Disord 2006;39: 565–9.
57. Pfeiffer RJ, Lucas AR, Ilstrup DM. Effect of anorexia nervosa on linear growth. Clin Pediatr 1986;25:7–12.

58. Joergensen J. The epidemiology of eating disorders in Fyn County, Denmark, 1977–1986. Acta Psychiatr Scand 1992;85:30–4.

59. Kent A, Lacey JH, McCluskey SE. Pre-menarcheal bulimia nervosa. J Psychosom Res 1992;36:205–10.

60. Decaluwe V, Braet C, Fairburn CG. Binge eating in obese children and adolescents. Int J Eat Disord 2003;33:78–84.

61. Micali N, Holliday J, Karwautz A, et al. Childhood eating and weight in eating disorders: a multi-centre European study of affected women and their unaffected sisters. Psychother Psychosom 2007;76:234–41.

62. Tanofsky-Kraff M, Goossens L, Eddy KT, et al. A multisite investigation of binge eating behaviors in children and adolescents. J Consult Clin Psychol 2007;75: 901–13.

63. Birch LL, Davison KK. Family environmental factors influencing the developing behavioral controls of food intake and childhood overweight. Pediatr Clin North Am 2001;48:893–907.

64. Tanofsky-Kraff M, Yanovski SZ, Wilfley DE, et al. Eating-disordered behaviors, body fat, and psychopathology in overweight and normal-weight children. J Consult Clin Psychol 2004;72:53–61.

65. Goossens L, Braet C, Decaluwe V. Loss of control over eating in obese youngsters. Behav Res Ther 2007;45:1–9.

66. Levine MD, Ringham RM, Kalarchian MA, et al. Overeating among seriously overweight children seeking treatment: results of the children's eating disorder examination. Int J Eat Disord 2006;39:135–40.

67. Puntis JW. Specialist feeding clinics. Arch Dis Child 2008;93:164–7.

Adolescent Eating Disorders: Definitions, Symptomatology, Epidemiology and Comorbidity

Beate Herpertz-Dahlmann, MD

KEYWORDS

- Eating disorders • Adolescence • Anorexia nervosa
- Bulimia nervosa • Epidemiology • Comorbidity • Review

Eating is a biological need, the importance of which is taken for granted by most human beings. However, eating disorders have morbidity and mortality rates that are among the highest of any mental disorders and are associated with significant functional impairment. Anorexia nervosa (AN) is the third most common chronic illness of adolescence, and bulimia nervosa (BN) affects more than 1% of adolescent girls.[1] In addition, many adolescents do not fulfill criteria for these distinct diagnoses, but are affected by subthreshold disorders of eating (eating disorder not otherwise specified, EDNOS), which are often as severe and long lasting as the classical conditions. With increasing incidence rates of obesity across all age groups, binge eating disorder (BED) has been a growing concern. Although subsumed under the diagnosis of EDNOS in the Diagnostic and Statistical Manual of Mental Disorders, Fourth Edition (DSM-IV), binge eating disorder is described in more detail in the article by Hebebrand.

This article provides an up-to-date review on recent developments and increasing knowledge in adolescent AN, BN, and related disorders. It covers diagnoses and assessment, recognition of typical symptoms, medical and psychiatric comorbidities, and current trends in epidemiology (see also, the article by Hebebrand and Herpertz-Dahlmann, elsewhere in this issue).

DEFINITION AND CLASSIFICATION

AN, BN, and EDNOS all are characterized by the same distinct core of psychopathology—a morbid preoccupation with weight and shape. Fear of fatness dominates the

This research was supported by the German Ministry for Education and Research (01GV0602 360372).

Department of Child and Adolescent Psychiatry and Psychotherapy, RWTH Aachen University, Neuenhofer Weg 21, 52074 Aachen, Germany.

E-mail address: bherpertz-dahlmann@ukaachen.de

life of the adolescent, and self-esteem is predominantly contingent on the ability to control one's weight and figure.

Anorexia Nervosa

In AN, the exaggerated wish for thinness leads to significant weight loss; individuals fall below a minimally normal weight for their age and height. Younger AN patients probably have not lost weight, but may weigh less than is expected with the corresponding growth in height. Low body weight is the result of severe and selective food restriction and/or excessive exercise. This exercise is not only voluntary in character, but is seemingly also in part triggered by starvation-induced biological changes.[2] Most of the patients experience their symptoms as ego-syntonic, and accordingly most, but not all, do not regard their state as an illness and deny serious associated medical complications. Weight loss is pursued beyond the bounds of reason and to the exclusion of other age-appropriate activities. It is often followed by social isolation and withdrawal, and emaciation is mostly interpreted as an achievement without feelings of remorse or suffering.

According to the DSM-IV, AN sufferers can be classified into two subgroups: restricting and binge eating/purging type. Patients with binge eating/purging type may engage in bingeing *and* purging, *only* bingeing (with intermittent periods of fasting or of excessive exercising), or *only* purging (ie, practicing self-induced vomiting, laxative abuse, or other extreme forms of weight control). It is still under debate whether the binge eating/purging type is associated with a worse outcome than the restricting type.[3,4]

In contrast to AN in adults, the diagnosis of adolescent AN should take into account normal pubertal growth and growth-related increases in weight. For this reason, a fixed body mass index (BMI, calculated as weight in kilograms divided by height in meters^2) criterion in children and adolescents is misleading; instead BMI centiles should be used to define "underweight." In Germany, a BMI lower than the 10th percentile is considered the threshold for a diagnosis of AN. If the patient has a BMI lower than the third percentile, many clinicians believe that she should be admitted to inpatient treatment (for a more detailed survey on weight and its definitions see Hebebrand).

Amenorrhea may be primary, because menarche will be postponed by starvation. Moreover, an adolescent will be considered to have amenorrhea when her menstruation occurs only after administration of sexual hormones (**Box 1**).

In anticipation of the revision of the DSM, there has been a lot of discussion about the usefulness of DSM-IV (and Tenth Revision of the International Classification of Diseases [ICD-10]) criteria for AN.

First, the hallmark criterion of AN—that is, maintenance of low body weight—is also found in some healthy individuals.[5,6] In addition "refusal to maintain body weight at or

---

Box 1
Diagnostic criteria for AN according to DSM-IV (abbreviated form)

- Refusal to maintain a minimal body weight for age and height (less than 85% of that expected)
- Intense fear of gaining weight or becoming fat
- Disturbance in the way in which one's body weight or shape is experienced
- Amenorrhea

Subtypes: Restricting and Binge Eating/Purging Type.

above a minimally normal weight," implies an active and purposeful process. However, at least at some point in the course of starvation, many patients admit that they are no longer in control of their body weight, and in several cases, an unintentional weight loss (eg, by a somatic disease) marks the beginning of the disorder. Criterion B according to the DSM-IV (fear of gaining weight) relies only on thoughts or feelings and cannot be easily objectified. Moreover, patients with a low premorbid body weight obviously demonstrate little drive for thinness,[7] and although some of the patients do not deny the seriousness of their current condition (criterion C), they do not want to change it. Amenorrhea (criterion D) is not unique to AN, but is found in many conditions linked to a reduced energy intake. Furthermore, patients who still menstruate psychopathologically closely resemble those in their course of illness who do not.[8]

In sum, several investigators have recently expressed the need for alternative diagnostic criteria for AN that are more empirically based and endorse observation, than relying on interpretations of the patient's behavior (eg, see Bulik et al,[5] and Hebebrand et al[6]).

Bulimia Nervosa

Bulimic patients are mostly within the normal weight range, although many have a body weight in the low normal range and some are slightly overweight. In BN, periods of dieting and fasting are interrupted by binge eating episodes accompanied by a feeling of loss of control. During binges, a large amount of food ("more than most people would eat in similar circumstances and similar periods of time") is consumed. Bingeing is compensated by self-induced vomiting, laxative, diuretic, or other medication abuse or – more rarely – by non-purging strategies like exercising and dieting. Binges and purging behaviors are practiced mostly in secret. Patients are reluctant to seek help and feel ashamed of their behavior. Similar to AN, a morbid fear of becoming fat and overvaluation of shape and weight are core symptoms of BN. BN (**Box 2**) is also divided into two subgroups, the purging and non-purging type (see earlier discussion).

The frequency of binge attacks needed to make the diagnosis is based on convention. In the current DSM, a minimum frequency of 2 binges per week is required. However, there is no evidence that this is a valid criterion, because individuals with fewer binge attacks (eg, once a week) may have similar psychopathology or outcomes.[9] In addition, there is a lack of specification for the "amount of food that is larger than most people would eat." According to observations by Keel and colleagues,[10] several self-identified binge-eaters did not eat more during a so-called "attack" than did "normal" college women, and those with binge attacks that were not objectively large did not differ from those with large binge attacks in terms of general and specific

---

Box 2
Diagnostic criteria for BN according to DSM-IV (abbreviated form)

- Recurrent episodes of binge eating
- Recurrent inappropriate compensatory behavior, for example, self-induced vomiting, laxative abuse, or fasting
- Frequency of binge eating at least twice a week for 3 months
- Self-worth is contingent on shape and weight
- Bulimic symptoms do not exclusively occur during the context of AN

Subtypes: Purging and non-purging type.

psychopathology. Moreover, the binge-eating criterion is questionable because of the lack of empiric evidence for its sub-criterion "loss of control."

In sum, several of the diagnostic criteria for BN involving the frequency and duration of bingeing and the amount of food consumed are questionable because of little empiric support. In addition, some investigators support the subtyping of BN into two categories (with and without a history of AN) because patients with a history of AN seem to be more likely to have a protracted illness with repeated relapses into AN.[11]

Eating Disorder Not Otherwise Specified

NOS diagnoses are residual categories by definition. Consequently, EDNOS is a heterogeneous diagnosis merging all those patients who narrowly miss full criteria for AN or BN, in addition to those with broader eating disorder spectrum symptoms ("partial ED"). According to Fairburn and colleagues Cooper[12] and other investigators, EDNOS—although a "residual" category—is "the most common eating disorder diagnosis encountered in clinical practice." This fact is not only true for adults, but also for adolescents. In their comparison of different classification systems for eating disorders in childhood and adolescence, Nicholls and colleagues[13] reclassified 226 children referred to a specialist clinic between the age of 7 and 16 years according to DSM-IV criteria. More than 50% of their sample fell into the DSM-IV category of EDNOS. In a very recent US study,[14] 280 adolescents (mean age: 16 years, range: 12–19 years) seeking outpatient treatment through a specialized service were assessed for the diagnosis of an eating disorder. Again, more than 50% presented with EDNOS, most of whom could be best described as subthreshold AN or BN. Moreover, the investigators reported that individuals with EDNOS had higher levels of specific eating pathology and general psychopathology than those with DSM-IV AN. Moreover, the natural course did not differ between young women with partial or full syndrome of AN or BN.[15] In our own investigation with a large representative sample in Germany comprising 1,800 11- to 17-year-olds, about one-third of the girls and 15% of the boys reported a partial eating disorder syndrome, which was most prevalent in overweight youth.[16] There was also a significant association between partial eating disorder syndromes and psychopathology, including internalizing and externalizing behavioral problems.

Classification of Childhood and Adolescent Anorectic and Bulimic EDs

It has already been emphasized that many children and adolescents have to be classified in the residual category of EDNOS, but for different reasons from adults. Younger subjects are often not able to describe or even understand the nature of their disturbed eating behavior. Because several of the diagnostic criteria for DSM-IV AN or BN rely on feelings or thoughts, many of these youngsters will not fulfill them. Moreover, young individuals often fail to recognize the harmful nature of weight loss and purging behaviors and feel overwhelmed by their fear of gaining weight. The importance of weight- and shape-related self-esteem to core symptoms of AN or BN often cannot be validated in younger age groups. Additionally, the insubstantial usefulness of a fixed BMI criterion in developing weight-losing subjects has already been discussed.

Potential strategies have been proposed for changing classification criteria in childhood and adolescence. They include an amendment to classic eating disorder criteria for this age group, a specific classification category for eating disorders with onset in childhood or adolescence, or a broad classification, whereby a subcategory of eating disorders in young age could be subsumed. Finally, diagnostic criteria could be primarily based on objective parameters like certain behaviors antagonistic to the maintenance of a normal body weight (eg, reduced intake, such as fasting or purging), elevated energy expenditure (eg, exercise) or physiologic measurements indicating semi-starvation (subnormal leptin levels, bradycardia, low T3[6]) (for a review see reference 17).

SYMPTOMS

As mentioned above, *anorectic* patients are intensely preoccupied by thoughts of food and their fear of fatness. The disorder almost always begins with dieting: girls often become vegetarians, skip meals, and confine themselves to "healthy stuff" like fruit, vegetables, and whole grain bread. A minority of anorectic patients are overweight before the onset of their illness. Many individuals celebrate their small meals, take a long time to finish them, and practice rituals while eating. Others have strange eating habits and cut their food into small pieces, rearrange food items several times on their plates, or take very small bites. Some develop an extensive interest in recipes and cooking. Younger adolescents or children may even refuse to drink because of an overwhelming fear of becoming fat.[18]

Several times a day these girls step on the scales, look in mirrors to assess their shape, and express concern about weight gain. Paradoxically the pursuit of thinness escalates despite the increasing weight loss. Continuous weight loss is considered a triumph. Many of the patients are physically hyperactive and practice sports or commit themselves to fitness training or gymnastics. Exercising and stepping on the scales can become highly ritualized and obsessive. Although mostly content and cheerful in the beginning, anorectic individuals often develop depressive symptoms and social withdrawal with increasing starvation. Several of them have delayed psychosexual development and an age-inadequate bonding to their family.

Moreover, many of these symptoms are not voluntarily driven, but are induced by prolonged semi-starvation. There is an inverted u-shaped relationship between leptin and activity levels, suggesting that hyperactivity is largely triggered by hypoleptinemia.[19]

In the so-called "Minnesota-experiment" conducted in the 1940s, many of the "typical" symptoms of anorexia or BN could be provoked in healthy young men during a 24-week laboratory–semi-starvation program.[20]

Bulimic patients are usually older than anorectic patients. About one-fourth have a history of AN. They enter the bulimic cycle of fasting, bingeing, and purging by giving in to the intense urge to eat during a period of starvation. Only rarely does the binge–purge cycle begin de novo. Failure to adhere to a planned small amount of food is often followed by a binge attack to have enough food in the stomach to make vomiting easier. For the same purpose patients drink a lot of water during meals. A binge attack might comprise up to 11,000 kcal and mostly consists of food that is easy to swallow without much chewing. In contrast to anorectic individuals, many bulimic patients admit to having a strong appetite and a desire to eat. Overeating is nearly always a solitary and secretive habit. Although binge attacks are often provoked by emotional stress or feelings of emptiness at the beginning, they become more and more habitualized during the course of the disorder, which makes treatment more difficult.

Although most bulimic patients are of normal weight, mild, moderate, and severe forms of obesity have been noticed in bulimic patients. Amongst a community-based cohort of bulimic females, childhood and parental obesity were reported in more than one third of the cases, which significantly exceeds the respective rates in healthy and psychiatric controls.[21]

EPIDEMIOLOGY

It has often been proclaimed in the media that eating disorders are on the rise. However, changes in referral practices and diagnostic criteria often influence the results and lead to discrepant interpretations.

Anorexia Nervosa

Previous studies indicate that there was a global increase in the prevalence and incidence of AN until the 1970s, with more stable rates since then.[22] In adolescents and young women, most studies found a *point prevalence* rate for AN according to DSM-IV between 0.3 and 0.9.[23] These rates were assessed according to the current standard of a 2-stage selection model.[23] In the first step, a large population is investigated by means of a screening questionnaire to select the at-risk individuals. The persons at risk are then interviewed personally together with probands from a randomly selected sample of the general (not at risk) population (second step). In a recent study of 12- to 23-year-old girls and women attending public schools in Portugal, the exact point prevalence rate for adolescent AN was 0.39%.[24]

Lifetime prevalence rates for 20- 40-year-old women are estimated to be between 1.2% and 2.2%.[23,25] In community studies, it has been estimated that up to 50% of diagnosed cases are previously undetected by the health care system.[25]

Recent *incidence rates* show an overall stabilization, but report an increase in the adolescent and young adult group. In a recent study from England, the general incidence rate derived from general practitioners was 4.7/100,000 persons (CI, 3.6–5.8) in the year 2000;[22] in a Dutch study it was estimated to be 7.7/100,000 (CI, 5.9–10.0[23]) during the years 1995-1999. In all studies, incidence rates were highest for female adolescent girls between 15 and 19 years of age. According to Hoek,[23] they constitute about 40% of all identified new cases. In the Netherlands a significant increase from 56 to 110/100,000 was observed in this age group between the time periods of 1985 to 1989 and 1995 to 1999.[26]

Bulimia Nervosa

For BN, the *point prevalence* is calculated as being 1% to 2%. The rates differ substantially depending on the level of medical care (epidemiologic estimates vs. clinical estimates) with only a minority of individuals seeking mental health care.[23] In the above mentioned study based on data derived from general practices in the UK, [22] there was an increase in the *incidence* of bulimia up until 1996 followed by a decline to 6.6/100,000 persons in 2000. For 10- to 19-year-old girls and women, the incidence was rated 35.8/100,000 (CI, 22.3–48.6). The decrease in incidence of BN was confirmed by a recent US study that investigated prevalence rates from 1982 through 2002[27] and by a 2-stage survey (see above) reporting a prevalence rate of only 0.3% in Portuguese adolescents.[24] However, it has to be kept in mind that changes in patients' referrals or service use (eg, increase in self-help groups vs. medical advice) and a reduced recognition of symptoms according to a decreased media representation could bias these findings.

Very few studies report epidemiologic data for men. The men-to-women ratio for AN is estimated at about 1:10 to 1:15 and at 1:15 to 1:20 for BN.[22,27] According to recent studies, there has not been appreciable change in this ratio over time.

Eating Disorder Not Otherwise Specified

Although EDNOS represents the most common eating disorder in specialized eating disorder services, there are very few reports on its prevalence and incidence in the general population.

A recent 2-stage survey of a nationwide representative sample of 2,000 12- to 23-year-old Portuguese girls and women[24] (see earlier discussion) found a prevalence rate for EDNOS of 2.37%, using a reliable well-known screening instrument (EDE-Q) and an expert-rated interview (EDE).

COMORBIDITY
Medical Comorbidity

Eating disorders have a high rate of medical complications. In AN, mortality is significantly increased with 5% to 6% of patients suffering a premature death.[3] In BN, the mortality rate is lower and is estimated to be about 2%.[28]

The annual costs of treating eating disorders in the US[29] and in Germany[30] are very high and are even more expensive than the treatment of schizophrenia. For AN, the cost of illness in Germany based on data from the year 1998 was estimated to be about €195 million Euros (direct costs of €73 million for hospitalization and rehabilitation services, indirect costs of €124 million Euros for inability to work and premature death) and €124 million Euros for BN (€12 million direct and €112 million indirect costs).[30]

The severity of comorbid medical illness commonly depends on the rapidity and extent of weight loss, the current degree of underweight, the duration of the eating disorder (eg, habituation to starvation), and the intensity of purging. In addition to typical medical problems in adults, AN has a severe impact on growth and pubertal development in children and adolescents. The most important physiologic changes and complications (but not all) are given in **Table 1**.

AN, and to a lesser extent BN, lead to a variety of endocrine changes. In general, these abnormalities are a consequence of semi-starvation, of abnormal eating behavior, or of both with poorly balanced meals and thus are mostly assigned as adaptive mechanisms to conserve energy and protein. Amenorrhea is one of the core symptoms of AN and is indexed as a diagnostic guideline in both the ICD-10 and DSM-IV. Besides the alterations of the hypothalamic–pituitary-gonadal axis, disturbances of hypothalamic-pituitary-adrenal axis, hypothalamic–pituitary-thyroid axis, and hypothalamic-pituitary-growth-hormone-IGF-1 axis are typical sequelae of adolescent eating disorders. Many of these endocrinologic changes are associated with changes in neuropeptides, such as leptin or ghrelin, which is described in more detail by Hebebrand Müeller and colleagues, elsewhere in this issue.

Osteopenia and osteoporosis

Adolescents with eating disorders are at risk to develop osteopenia or osteoporosis associated with a 2- to 7-fold higher fracture risk in later life. Most of the bone mass is built up during adolescence. Any process interfering with normal bone mineral accrual in this critical period may lead to permanent deficits. Multiple factors contribute to a reduction of bone mass in AN (and to a lower extent in BN): hypogonadism, hypercortisolemia, low levels of insulin-like growth factor, malnutrition (eg, low protein or calcium intake), or excessive exercise, and bed rest (eg, as a "therapeutic strategy" during inpatient treatment). In addition, a critical role of neuropeptides like leptin, ghrelin, and peptide YY in bone metabolism has been discussed.[2] Normalization of body weight is believed to be the most important factor in counteracting bone loss in adolescent AN. However, there is still an ongoing debate about whether recovery from an

Table 1
Medical alterations in adolescent eating disorders

	AN	BN
Physical examination findings	Dry skin, lanugo hair formation (only with severe weight loss), acrocyanosis, alopecia, low body temperature, dehydration, retardation of growth and pubertal development	Erosion of dental enamel, parotid/salivary gland enlargement, scars on the skin of the back of the hand resulting from inducing the gag reflex, dehydration
Cardiovascular system	Bradycardia, ECG abnormalities (mostly prolonged QT-interval), pericardial effusion, edema (before or during refeeding)	ECG-abnormalities (cardiac arrhythmia, prolonged QT-interval)
Gastrointestinal system	Impaired gastric emptying, pancreatitis, constipation	Esophagitis, pancreatitis, delayed gastric emptying
Blood	Leukocytopenia, thrombocytopenia, anemia	
Biochemical abnormalities	Hypokalemia, hyponatremia, hypomagnesiemia, hypocalcemia, hypophosphatemia (during refeeding), low glucose levels, AST↑, ALT↑ (with severe fasting or beginning of refeeding), cholesterol ↑	Hypokalemia, hyponatremia, hypomagnesiemia (caused by diarrhea), hypocalcemia, metabolic alkalosis (in case of severe purging), metabolic acidosis (in case of severe laxative abuse)
Endocrine system	Cortisol ↑	n (↑)
	FSH, LH ↓	n (↓)
	Estradiol ↓	n (↓)
	FT3 ↓	n (↓)
	FT4 n (↓)	n (↓)
	TSH n (↓)	n
	GH ↑(n)	n (↑)
	IGF-1 ↓	n (↓)
	Leptin ↓	n (↓)

eating disorder is in fact associated with a complete restoration of bone mass[31] (for a review, see Misra and Klebanski[32]).

PSYCHIATRIC COMORBIDITY

It is well known that both AN and BN are often accompanied by other psychiatric conditions – either during the acute state or in the long-term course. The most frequent disorders are depression (major depressive disorder—MDD and dysthymia), anxiety disorders with a special emphasis on obsessive-compulsive disorder, substance abuse, and personality disorders. Several of these disorders are substantially affected by starvation and abnormal eating patterns.[33] Thus, one should always question whether depressive or anxious states are primarily the result of the physiologic consequences of malnutrition or had set in before the onset or after recovery from the eating disorder.

In addition, it should be kept in mind that rates of comorbidity are usually significantly higher in clinical settings than in field studies. This point is especially true for comorbid affective illnesses that enhance the probability of an individual seeking treatment. Thus, prevalences in most clinical samples are subject to a referral bias.

Affective Disorders

A wide range of depressive symptoms such as depressed mood, emotional emptiness, social withdrawal, loss of libido, and low self-esteem are prominent in malnourished anorectic patients. Studies that have used structured diagnostic interviews according to DSM-III-R or DSM-IV have reported a wide range of estimates, between 15% and 60%, for the percentage of treatment-seeking individuals with AN who meet lifetime criteria for a depressive disorder.[34] In adolescent AN, up to 80% of patients suffer from MDD during the acute stage of the illness[35–37] with no significant difference between epidemiologic and clinical samples.[38]

In bulimic patients, prevalence rates of MDD are similar to AN.[39] Keys and colleagues [20] were some of the first scientists to note mental changes during semi-starvation, such as emotional irritability, loss of libido, anhedonia, and difficulty making decisions. These changes may not only be evident in AN and BN patients with substantial weight loss, but also in bulimic girls with "only" erratic eating behavior. Thus, therapists should always wait for the effect of refeeding (because the mood of patients tends to lift with weight gain) or absence of purging before they start a specific "antidepressant" treatment.

There also seems to be a high prevalence of mood disorders in family members of eating disordered patients. However, a meta-analysis of several of these family studies revealed several methodological problems, so that the value of the results has to be questioned.[40] There is still an ongoing debate about whether shared genetic factors contribute to a common etiology of depression and eating disorders;[41] family study and twin data do not always support a shared genetic diathesis.[42]

Earlier investigations indicate that depression sometimes antedates the eating disorder[43,44] and may even begin in childhood.[45] Others suggest that the eating disorders precede depressive disorders.

In the latter case, the eating disorder may in fact produce depressive symptomatology by effecting neurobiological changes. In the author's work on the effects of steroid hormones on the anatomy of the developing brain during puberty, growth of limbic structures was significantly associated with increasing estrogen levels.[46] Consequently, one could imagine that anorectic patients with long-lasting deficient estrogen levels are more vulnerable to typical psychiatric disorders associated with dysfunctions in limbic brain areas, such as mood or anxiety disorders.

The incidence of *suicide* and *suicidal attempts* is also a serious problem in eating disorders. About 10% to 20% of individuals with AN and 25% to 35% of patients with bulimia report a history of attempted suicide. Those with purging or bingeing/purging behavior admit to significantly more suicide attempts than those with the restricting subtype. Suicidal behavior is also related to severity of the eating disorder and the presence of a cluster-B personality disorder.[47,48] The standardized mortality rate (representing the ratio of the observed number of deaths to the expected number of deaths in a matched population) for suicide in AN is estimated to be up to 5, whereas it does not appear to be elevated in BN. Unfortunately, data regarding rates for completed suicide and suicide attempts are lacking in adolescent AN and BN.

Anxiety Disorders (Other than OCD)

A wide range of anxiety disorders are common in patients with AN. Comparable to findings in depression estimates of comorbidity between 20% and 60% are suggested.[34,49,50] In adolescent AN, similar rates are found.[35]

During the acute phase of the illness, fears associated with eating, such as consuming certain foods, changing shape, and an avoidance of situations involving eating (eg, eating in a restaurant, at a party, at school), are prominent. In addition, typical anxiety disorders, such as agoraphobia, panic disorder, general anxiety disorder, PTSD, and especially social phobia are significantly more frequent in individuals with AN than in the general population.

In a study by Godart and colleagues[51] using a predominantly adolescent sample, the most frequent lifetime anxiety disorder was social phobia (55%) followed by simple phobia (45%). However, the sample size was rather small, and it was based only on retrospective diagnoses.

At the time a comorbid anxiety disorder is present, it commonly predates the eating disorder and has its onset in childhood.[49,51] In a very interesting study by Shoebridge and Gowers,[52] the investigators reported significant differences between anorectic patients and healthy controls concerning "high concern" of mothers and separation anxiety in the children: anorectic patients had more infant sleep difficulties, severe distress at first separation from their parents, and a later age for first sleeping away from home. Mothers of patients reported higher trait anxiety levels and higher personal engagement in child care without the participation of the father in contrast to the control mothers.

In BN, prevalence rates of anxiety disorders also vary between 25% and 75% (see Swinbourne and Touyz[53] for a review) with social phobia again being the most prevalent disorder, present in up to 70% of cases.[53] Because bulimic patients are usually older than anorectic individuals, prevalence rates in exclusively adolescent samples are difficult to find.

In sum, current literature suggests that there is an important association between eating disorders and anxiety disorders that probably carries significant implications for etiology and treatment. Because of the high prevalence of social phobia in adolescent AN, the authors have implemented social competence training in the treatment protocol, containing situations with and without eating in public.

Obsessive-Compulsive Disorder (OCD)

Numerous studies have revealed a high rate of obsessive-compulsive disorder among patients with eating disorders. Some have even argued that eating disorders, especially AN, are variants of the obsessive-compulsive spectrum of illness.

For the restrictive anorectic patient, food-related obsessive-compulsive features, such as cutting food into a certain number of pieces, eating vegetables separately from meat, or having meals exactly at the same time of the day, are very common. As has been demonstrated by Keys and colleagues,[20] food-restricted rituals arise in laboratory-induced starvation states and are alleviated with refeeding.

However, there are additional thoughts and behaviors in eating disordered patients that would qualify for a comorbid diagnosis of true OCD. The most frequent phenomena identified in eating disordered patients are ordering and washing rituals and obsessions with things going wrong. Anorectic individuals are also often characterized by certain traits such as rigidity, perfectionism, and scrupulosity.

There is still an ongoing debate as to whether prevalence rates of OCD are higher in restrictive AN than the binge–purge type or when compared with BN. However, recent studies have found similar rates of comorbid OCD in both AN and BN.[49] In the latter study, about 40% of the adult individuals received a lifetime diagnosis of OCD. In adolescent samples, about 20% of anorectic individuals suffer from OCD.[35,51] The onset is mostly in childhood. In the study by Kaye and colleagues,[49] 23% of the subjects with eating disorders had childhood-onset OCD in contrast to only 2% of the community sample.

Although OCD co-occurs in individuals and families with eating disorders, there are still no distinct data that would clearly support a shared genetic etiology.[42]

In sum, although the findings of prevalence rates of anxiety disorders are strikingly inconsistent, the comorbidity of both disorders brings up many important questions regarding the nature of the relationship. Childhood anxiety disorders (including OCD) may represent a risk factor for later eating disorders, suggesting that preventive strategies might be of value in this specific population. In addition, anxiety disorders are often still prominent in recovered eating disordered subjects,[54,55] so that specific treatment strategies that also address anxiety disorders are warranted.

Substance Abuse

Substance abuse and eating disorders co-occur at a rate that is greater than by chance; however, the risk for comorbidity is lower than that of anxiety or mood disorders. For AN, it is important to distinguish between the binge–purge and the restricting subtype, because there seems to be no elevated risk for substance abuse in the latter. This was confirmed by a recent study on personality traits and comorbid disorders, which demonstrated that the obsessional (perfectionistic) personality type was protective against the development of substance abuse.[56]

Unfortunately, few investigations have examined substance abuse in adolescent samples. In 1 study, among adolescent girls who were AN patients, about 8% suffered from substance abuse.[35] The disorder was 18 times as likely to co-occur with the AN binge-purging type than with the restricting type. In an adolescent sample suffering from bulimia, nearly two-thirds of individuals had tried alcohol at least once. A total of 40% of this sample reported using alcohol more than once per month, with 4% using it 2 to 4 days per week.[57] About one-third had tried illegal drugs at least once. The most commonly used drug was marijuana followed by cocaine (use occurring in about one-third of individuals with substance abuse) and amphetamines. Note, however, that both of these studies were executed with clinical populations.

Some researchers have hypothesized that shared impulsivity between bulimic disorders and substance abuse could be a common cause for both disorders, and some time ago Lacey and Evans[58] created the term "multi-impulsive bulimia." Impulsivity in bulimia might also account for other "high risk behaviors" like shoplifting, self-injury, and suicide attempts.[59]

Attention-Deficit Hyperactivity Disorder

Recent studies underline an association between ADHD and eating disorders. In a large prospective case-control study, 123 girls with ADHD and 106 controls were followed into late adolescence. Girls with ADHD were 3.6 times more likely to meet criteria for an eating disorder than control girls and 5.6 times more likely to fulfill criteria for BN.[60] Girls with both disorders also had increased rates of mood, anxiety, and disruptive behavior disorders. A similar result was obtained in a 5-year longitudinal study by Mikami and colleagues.[61] The group of ADHD girls was divided into ADHD-combined and ADHD-inattentive subtypes, each of which was compared with controls. Girls with the combined subtype of ADHD were at the highest risk for bulimic behavior and body image disturbances followed by the inattentive subtype. Childhood impulsivity symptoms best predicted adolescent eating problems.

Thus, girls with ADHD should be monitored for the development of an eating disorder in adolescence. Unfortunately, to the author's knowledge, there are only case reports, but no controlled studies that have investigated women with bulimic behavior for ADHD rates.

Personality Traits and Disorders

As has already been mentioned here, perfectionism, rigidity, and obsessiveness seem to be robust personality traits in AN patients, which are evident both during acute illness and after long-term recovery.[55,62] Some investigators even hypothesize that perfectionism and obsessiveness might be a risk factor in childhood for later AN.[49,63] In addition, anorectic individuals report high levels of anxiety, harm avoidance, and feelings of worthlessness, even after recovering from their eating disorder (data collected at least 1 month after recovery). Accordingly, the most prevalent personality disorders in adult AN patients are cluster-C disorders, which include obsessive-compulsive and avoidant or dependent personality disorder.[53,55]

Perfectionistic traits are also often observed in bulimic patients.[64] As has been mentioned earlier, many bulimic individuals display impulsive or sensation-seeking behavior. Thus, in addition to cluster-C personality disorders, patients with the binge eating/purging subtype of AN and those with BN often receive a cluster-B diagnosis, such as borderline personality disorder.[50]

As with other psychiatric disorders, personality disorders commonly predict a negative long-term course for both eating disorders.[65]

ASSESSMENT

In typical AN, it is easy to make a diagnosis. However, early signs of the illness are sometimes difficult to recognize (**Box 3**). In contrast, diagnosis of BN is more complicated, because many patients feel ashamed of their behavior and deny their symptoms.

At the time a patient is admitted to a mental health or pediatric service, a full medical and psychometric assessment is necessary for diagnosis, treatment planning, and judgment of progress. The patient should always be weighed and should have her height measured. She should be asked about her ideal weight and how she feels about her actual shape. The clinician should obtain information about the highest weight in the past and the extent and rapidity of current weight loss. Frequently, patients do

---

Box 3
Early symptoms of eating disorders

- Growing interest in composition of food and calorie content
- Avoidance or skipping of main meals
- Restriction to healthy food
- Frequent weighing
- Increased energy or physical restlessness
- Discontent with weight and shape
- Increasing achievement motivation and social isolation

Box 4
Medical assessment recommended for eating disorders

- Physical assessment (heart rate, blood pressure, body temperature)
- Complete blood count
- Biochemical profile (sodium, potassium, calcium, chloride, magnesium, phosphate, creatinine, urea, serum proteins, glucose, liver enzymes, amylase)
- ECG
- EEG, MRI, CT (in case of atypical eating disorder eg, men, children, or manifestation of seizures)

---

not seek medical advice for their eating disorder, but complain of hair loss, brittle nails, constipation, headache, or fatigue. The medical care provider or therapist must be patient in obtaining the patient's history of dietary restraint and other eating disorder symptoms, such as vomiting and purging, and menstrual irregularities. A thorough medical examination is recommended (**Box 4**). Some therapists prefer to have an anorectic patient weighed by the family practitioner or some other clinician not engaged in the treatment of the patient. However, restoration of body weight is one of the main targets of treatment, and the act of weighing may convey valuable information about the patient's body image concerns and weight phobia.

Various assessment methods have been developed for the measurement of specific eating disorder psychopathology. Valuable strategies comprise structured or semi-structured clinical interviews, self-report questionnaires, and self-monitoring. Commonly used clinical interviews include the Eating Disorder Examination (EDE[66]) and the Structured Interview for Anorexia and Bulimia Nervosa (SIAB[67]). Probably the most widely used self-report questionnaires are the Eating Disorder Inventory (EDI-2[68]) and the Eating Attitudes Test (EAT[69]). All of these instruments have been translated into different languages and have been validated in several countries and cultures.

In addition to specific eating disorder symptomatology, comorbidity with other mental disorders, especially depression, anxiety, and obsessions (see above), should be assessed carefully at admission and monitored during the process of refeeding.

For most patients, medical and psychologic assessment is the first step to treatment. At this point it is often easier to help the patient recognize the relationship between her eating disordered behavior and medical or psychologic problems than through direct confrontation or challenge. Both patient and family should be informed about the course and nature of the adolescent's eating disorder, including the extent of underweight and its medical consequences. Finally, treatment options have to be discussed in detail. As a rule, the threshold for intervention should be lower in adolescence than in adulthood, because research has clearly demonstrated that outcomes are worse for patients who are severely underweight.[70] A trusting and non-judgmental relationship between the therapist and patient at assessment can set the tone for change and be the beginning of successful treatment.

SUMMARY

In this article diagnostic and classification issues of adolescent eating disorders have been reviewed. Many clinicians have to face the problem of several of their young patients not fitting into the narrowly defined category of AN or BN. More than half of childhood and adolescent eating disorder diagnoses seem to fall under EDNOS, so research on the symptoms, course, and outcome of this "residual" category is urgently needed. Other concerns involve the validity of current AN and BN criteria and an inadequate sensitivity for developmental aspects. Prevalence rates of AN seem to have remained stable during the last decades; however, recent epidemiologic studies indicate that AN is still on the rise in adolescent and adult women. It remains unclear whether there is a true decrease in the incidence of BN or whether this is the result of changes in patients' referral or service use.

Eating disorders are serious, often chronic, and potentially life-threatening disorders. The clinician should be well aware of medical complications in severely underweight or purging adolescents. Significant strides have been made in the past 10 years in elucidating patterns of comorbidity. Anxiety disorders (including OCD) seem to be of special importance, probably even for our knowledge on nosology and prevention.

Special efforts should be made for the appropriate and right in-time identification of childhood and adolescent disorders so that earlier and probably more effective intervention can be applied.

REFERENCES

1. Nicholls D, Viner R. Eating disorders and weight problems. BMJ 2005;330:950–3.
2. Hebebrand J, Muller TD, Holtkamp K, et al. The role of leptin in anorexia nervosa: clinical implications. Mol Psychiatry 2007;12(1):23–35.
3. Steinhausen HC. The outcome of anorexia nervosa in the 20th century. Am J Psychiatry 2002;1284–93.
4. Eddy KT, Keel PK, Dorer DJ, et al. Longitudinal comparison of anorexia nervosa subtypes. Int J Eat Disord 2002;31:191–201.
5. Bulik CM, Hebebrand J, Keski-Rahkonen A, et al. Genetic epidemiology, endophenotypes, and eating disorder classification. Int J Eat Disord 2007;40:52–60.
6. Hebebrand J, Casper R, Treasure J, et al. The need to revise the diagnostic criteria for anorexia nervosa. J Neural Transm 2004;111(7):827–40.
7. Strober M, Freeman R, Morrell W. Atypical anorexia nervosa: separation from typical cases in course and outcome in a long-term prospective study. Int J Eat Disord 1999;25:135–42.
8. Garfinkel PE, Lin E, Goering P, et al. Should amenorrhoea be necessary for the diagnosis of anorexia nervosa? Evidence from a Canadian community sample. Br J Psychiatry 1996;68:500–6.
9. Garfinkel PE, Lin E, Goering P, et al. Bulimia nervosa in a Canadian community sample: prevalence and comparison of subgroups. Am J Psychiatry 1995;152: 1052–8.
10. Keel PK, Mayer SA, Harnden-Fischer JH. Importance of size in defining binge eating episodes in bulimia nervosa. Int J Eat Disord 2001;29(3):294–301.
11. Eddy KT, Dorer DJ, Debra FL, et al. Should bulimia nervosa be subtyped by history of anorexia nervosa? A longitudinal validation. Int J Eat Disord 2007;40: 67–71.
12. Fairburn CG, Cooper Z. Thinking afresh about the classification of eating disorders. Int J Eat Disord 2007;40:107–10.
13. Nicholls D, Chater R, Lask B. Children into DSM don't go: a comparison of classification systems for eating disorders in childhood and early adolescence. Int J Eat Disord 1999;28:317–24.

14. Eddy KT, Doyle AC, Hoste RR, et al. Eating disorder not otherwise specified in adolescents. J Am Acad Child Adolesc Psychiatry 2008;47(2):156–64.
15. Lewinsohn PM, Striegel-Moore RH, Seeley MS. Epidemiology and natural course of eating disorders in young women from adolescence to young adulthood. J Am Ac Chuld Adolesc Psychiatry 2000;39:1284–92.
16. Herpertz-Dahlmann B, Wille N, Ravens-Sieberer U, et al. Eating disordered behavior, associated psychopathology and health-related quality of life—results from the BELLA-study. Eur J Child Adolesc Psychiatry, in press.
17. Workgroup for Classification of Eating Disorders in Children and Adolescents (WCEDCA). Classification of child and adolescent eating disturbances. Int J Eat Disord 2007;40:117–22.
18. Lowinger K, Griffiths RA, Beumont PJ, et al. Fluid restriction in anorexia nervosa: a neglected symptom or new phenomenon. Int J Eat Disord 1999;26: 392–6.
19. Holtkamp K, Herpertz-Dahlmann B, Hebebrand K, et al. Physical activity and restlessness correlate with leptin levels in patients with adolescent anorexia nervosa. Biol Psychiatry 2006;60(3):311–3.
20. Keys A, Brozek J, Henschel A, et al. The biology of human starvation. Minneapolis (MN): University of Minneapolis Press; 1950.
21. Fairburn CG, Welch SL, Doll HA, et al. Risk factors for bulimia nervosa. A community-based control study. Arch Gen Psychiatry 1997;54:509–17.
22. Currin L, Schmidt U, Treasure J, et al. Time trends in eating disorders incidence. Br J Psychiatry 2005;186:132–5.
23. Hoek HW. Incidence, prevalences and mortality of anorexia nervosa and other eating disorders. Curr Opin Psychiatry 2006;19(4):389–94.
24. Machado PP, Machado BC, Goncalves S, et al. The prevalences of eating disorders not otherwise specified. Int J Eat Disord 2007;40(3):212–7.
25. Keski-Rahkonen A, Hoek HW, Susser ES, et al. Epidemiology and course of anorexia nervosa in the community. Am J Psychiatry 2007;164(8):1259–65.
26. Van Son GE, van Hoeken D, Bartelds AI, et al. Time trends in the incidence of eating disorders: a primary care study in the Netherlands. Int J Eat Disord 2006; 39(7):565–9.
27. Keel PK, Heatherton TF, Dorer DJ, et al. Point prevalence of bulimia nervosa in 1982, 1992, and 2002. Psychol Med 2006;36(1):119–27.
28. Fichter M, Quadflieg N. Twelve-year course and outcome of bulimia nervosa. Psychol Med 2004;34:1395–406.
29. Striegel-Moore RH, Leslie D, Petrill SA, et al. One-year use and cost of inpatient and outpatient services among female and male patients with an eating disorder: evidence from a national database of health insurance claims. Int J Eat Disord 2000;27(4):381–9.
30. Krauth C, Buser K, Vogel H. How high are the costs of eating disorders—anorexia nervosa and bulimia nervosa – for German society? Eur J Health Econom 2002;3: 244–50.
31. Mika C, Holtkamp K, Heer M, et al. A 2-year perspective study of bone metabolism and bone mineral density in adolescents with anorexia nervosa. J Neural Transm 2007;114(12):1611–8.
32. Misra M, Klibanski A. Anorexia nervosa and osteoporosis. Rev Endocr Metab Disord 2006;7:91–9.
33. Pollice CP, Kaye WH, Greeno CG, et al. Relationship of depression, anxiety, and obsessionality to state of illness in anorexia nervosa. Int J Eat Disord 1997;21: 367–76.

34. Halmi KA, Eckert E, Marchi P, et al. Comorbidity of psychiatric diagnoses in anorexia nervosa. Arch Gen Psychiatry 1991;712–8.
35. Salbach-Andrae H, Lenz K, Simmendinger N, et al. Psychiatric comorbidities among female adolescents with anorexia nervosa. Child Psychiatry Hum Dev 2008;39:261–72.
36. Herpertz-Dahlmann B, Wewetzer C, Remschmidt H, et al. The predictive value of depression in anorexia nervosa. Acta Psychiatr Scand 1995;91:114–9.
37. Herzog DB, Keller MB, Sacks NR, et al. Psychiatric comorbidity in treatment-seeking anorexics and bulimics. J Am Acad Child Adolesc Psychiatry 1992; 31(5):810–8.
38. Rastam M. Anorexia nervosa in 51 Swedish adolescents: premorbid problems and comorbidity. J Am Acad Child Adolesc Psychiatry 1992;31:819–29.
39. Bushnell JA, Wells JE, McKenzie JM, et al. Bulimia comorbidity in the general population and in the clinic. Psychol Med 1994;24:605–11.
40. Perdereau F, Faucher S, Wallier J, et al. Family history of anxiety and mood disorders in anorexia nervosa: review of the literature. Eat Weight Disord 2008;13(1): 1–13.
41. Wade TD, Bulik CM Neale M, et al. Anorexia nervosa and major depression: shared genetic and environmental risk factors. Am J Psychiatry 2000;157: 469–71.
42. Lilenfeld LR, Kaye WH, Greeno CG, et al. A controlled family study of anorexia nervosa and bulimia nervosa: psychiatric disorders in first-degree relatives and effects of proband comorbidity. Arch Gen Psychiatry 1998;55(7): 603–10.
43. Brewerton TD, Lydiard RB, Herzog DB, et al. Comorbidity of axis I psychiatric disorders in bulimia nervosa. J Clin Psychiatry 1995;56:77–80.
44. Piran N, Kennedy S, Garfinkel PE, et al. Affective disturbance in eating disorders. N Nerv Ment Dis 1985;173:395–400.
45. Herpertz-Dahlmann B. Psychiatrische Erkrankungen im Vorfeld der Anorexia nervosa. Klin Päd 1988;200:108–12.
46. Neufang S, Specht K, Konrad K. et al. Sex differences and the impact of steroid hormones on the developing human brain. Cerebr Cort, in press.
47. Franko DL, Keel PK. Suicidality in eating disorders: occurrence, correlates, and clinical implications. Clin Psychol Rev 2006;26(6):769–82.
48. Bulik CM, Thornton L, Pinheiro AP, et al. Suicide attempts in anorexia nervosa. Psychosom Med 2008; [Epub ahead of print].
49. Kaye WH, Bulik CM, Thornton L, et al. Comorbidity of anxiety disorders with anorexia and bulimia nervosa. Am J Psychiatry 2004;161(12):2215–21.
50. Jordan J, Joyce PR, Carter FA, et al. Specific and nonspecific comorbidity in anorexia nervosa. Int J Eat Disord 2008;41(1):47–56.
51. Godart NT, Flament MF, Lecrubier Y, et al. Anxiety disorders in anorexia nervosa and bulimia nervosa: co-morbidity and chronology of appearance. Eur Psychiatry 2000;15:38–45.
52. Shoebridge P, Gowers SG. Parenteral high concern and adolescent-onset anorexia nervosa. A case-control study to investigate direction of causality. Br J Psychiatry 2000;176:132–7.
53. Swinbourne JM, Touyz SW. The co-morbidity of eating disorders and anxiety disorders: a review. Eur Eat Disord Rev 2007;15(4):253–74.
54. Wentz-Nilsson E, Gillberg C, Gillberg IC, et al. Ten-year follow-up of adolescent-onset anorexia nervosa: personality disorders. J Am Acad Child Adolesc Psychiatry 1999;1389–95.

55. Herpertz-Dahlmann B, Müller B, Herpertz S, et al. Prospective ten-year follow-up in adolescent anorexia nervosa—course, outcome and psychiatric comorbidity. J Child Psychol Psychiatry 2001;42:603–12.

56. Thompson-Brenner H, Eddy KT, Franko DL, et al. Personality pathology and substance abuse in eating disorders: a longitudinal study. Int J Eat Disord 2008; 41(3):203–8.

57. Fischer S, le Grange D. Comorbidity and high-risk behaviors in treatment-seeking adolescents with bulimia nervosa. Int J Eat Disord 2007;40(8):751–3.

58. Lacey JH, Evans CD. The impulsivist: a multi-impulsive personality disorder. Br J Addiction 1986;81:715–23.

59. Stein D, Lilenfeld LR, Wildmann PC, et al. Attempted suicide and self-injury in patients diagnosed with eating disorders. Compr Psychiatry 2004;45:447–51.

60. Biederman J, Ball SW, Monuteaux MC, et al. Are girls with ADHD at risk for eating disorders? Results from a controlled, five-year prospective study. J Dev Behav Pediatr 2007;28:302–7.

61. Mikami AY, Hinshaw SP, Patterson KA, et al. Eating pathology among adolescent girls with attention-deficit/hyperactivity disorder. J Abnorm Psychol 2008;117(1): 225–35.

62. Halmi KA, Sunday SR, Strober M, et al. Perfectionism in anorexia nervosa: variation by clinical subtype, obsessionality, and pathological eating behaviour. Am J Psychiatry 2000;157(11):1799–805.

63. Fairburn CG, Cooper Z, Doll HA, et al. Risk factors for anorexia nervosa: three integrated case-control comparisons. Arch Gen Psychiatry 1999;56:468–76.

64. Lilenfeld LR, Stein D, Bulik CM, et al. Personality traits among currently eating disordered, recovered and never ill first-degree female relatives of bulimic and control woman. Psychol Med 2000;30(6):1399–410.

65. Nilsson K, Sundbom E, Hägglöf B. A longitudinal study of perfectionism in adolescent onset anorexia nervosa-restricting type. Eur Eat Disord Rev 2007; [Epub ahead of print].

66. Cooper Z, Cooper PF, Fairburn CG. The validity of eating disorder examination and its subscales. Br J Psychiatry 1989;154:807–12.

67. Fichter M, Herpertz S, Herpertz-Dahlmann B, et al. Structured interview for anorexia and bulimic disorder. Int J Eat Disord 1998;24:227–49.

68. Garner DM. Eating disorder inventory (EDI-2). 2nd professional manual. Odessa (FL): Psychological Assessment Resources, Inc; 1991.

69. Garner DM. Eating attitude test (EAT). Psychological Medicine 1979;9:273–9.

70. Hebebrand J, Himmelmann GW, Herzog W, et al. Prediction of low body weight at long-term follow-up in acute anorexia nervosa by low body weight at referral. Am J Psychiatry 1997;154:566–9.

Psychological and Psychiatric Aspects of Pediatric Obesity

Johannes Hebebrand, MD[a],*, Beate Herpertz-Dahlmann, MD[b]

KEYWORDS

- Self-awareness • Quality of life • Suicide • Depression
- Eating disorders

A thorough dealing with psychological and psychiatric aspects of obesity requires careful consideration of causal implications. It is nowadays readily comprehensible that obesity can entail psychiatric symptoms, because stigmatization of obese children and adolescents, including teasing and bullying, is a common event. Sources include peers, teachers, parents, and health care providers. It would indeed seem peculiar if this ongoing and intense stigmatization has not already affected mental well-being at a rather early stage of life. Nevertheless, it is important to realize that many obese children may be resilient to the negative social consequences of obesity, similar to observations in children with other physical disabilities.[1] Puhl and Latner[2] have recently published an excellent review of all aspects related to stigmatization—a true must for readers interested in any aspect of this complex issue. It appears that stigmatization has actually increased over time.[3,4] Future research needs to more specifically address potential mediators of poor psychological outcomes that have been associated with pediatric obesity; protective factors entailing resilience warrant additional research efforts.[2]

Apart from stigmatization and the associated victimization, participation of an *extremely* obese child/adolescent in all aspects of everyday life is not possible, potentially also entailing elevated risks for poor outcomes. For example, regular physical activity has recently been shown to be associated with a substantially reduced risk for some mental disorders in adolescents and young adults;[5] obviously, extremely obese children and adolescents might not be able to be as physically active as their normal-weight counterparts. Finally, the coping of a child with obesity can have implications for development of psychiatric disorders and in particular eating disorders. Thus, a child may resort to dieting behavior as an attempt to cope with overweight

[a] Department of Child and Adolescent Psychiatry, University of Duisburg-Essen, Virchowstr. 174, 45147 Essen, Germany
[b] Department of Child and Adolescent Psychiatry, University Clinics, Technical University of Aachen
* Corresponding author.
E-mail address: johannes.hebebrand@uni-due.de (J. Hebebrand).

Child Adolesc Psychiatric Clin N Am 18 (2008) 49–65
doi:10.1016/j.chc.2008.08.002   childpsych.theclinics.com
1056-4993/08/$ – see front matter © 2008 Elsevier Inc. All rights reserved.

and through that very mechanism lay the foundation for the development of binge-eating attacks and binge-eating disorder (BED).

The reverse causality has, however, been invoked earlier on. For example, Bruch considered it essential that therapists deal with parents' unconscious needs and narcissistic drives that they had groomed their obese child to fulfill.[6] More recently, several studies have consistently shown that depressive symptomatology in childhood and adolescence predicts weight gain. Because the complex pathways in body weight regulation have been shown to be intricately linked to other systems, including sleep, mood, anxiety, and cognition, it is necessary to view obesity as a condition that, in theory, can in part be attributed to psychological/psychiatric variables, traits, or symptoms that affect medium- and long-term energy intake and expenditure. Vice versa, obesity could directly, through central nervous system pathways, or indirectly, through stigmatization/victimization and endurance of physical implications and medical complications, affect mental well-being.

A crucial aspect in dealing with psychological and psychiatric aspects of early onset obesity is to consider whether or not the respective findings pertain to patients seeking therapeutic help, most commonly through enlistment in a weight loss program. A considerable bulk of evidence, particularly in adults, clearly indicates that clinically ascertained patients are psychiatrically different from obese individuals in the general population; high rates of mood, anxiety, and eating disorders have consistently been described in clinical patients. The degree of overweight is a potential confounder in such studies, as population-based obese individuals can have a lower body mass index (BMI) than those seeking treatment.

Finally, in epidemiologic studies, the co-assessment of self-perception of weight status has proven to be important, particularly because those adolescents who report being overweight or obese have a lower quality of life and engage in unhealthy behaviors, irrespective of whether or not they are objectively overweight.

An extensive amount of literature pertaining to psychological and psychiatric aspects of pediatric obesity is available, thus requiring a selection of topics. This article begins by assessing whether children (and their parents and health care providers) correctly perceive their weight status. The findings with reference to health-related quality of life (HRQoL) and stigmatization are summarized and psychiatric comorbidity in clinical and epidemiologic samples is dealt with, with a special focus on eating disorders. Findings related to suicide and suicidal behavior warrant particular attention in light of recent findings in adults indicating a protective effect of obesity on suicide rates.

PERCEPTION OF OBESITY AMONG CHILDREN AND ADOLESCENTS, THEIR PARENTS, AND PHYSICIANS

Awareness of childhood overweight/obesity is dependent on many factors including criteria for classification of weight status; sampling strategy; wording of respective questions used in such studies; and age, socioeconomic status, nationality, ethnicity and race of the child. In addition, secular trends for both overweight and obesity need to be considered as well as the extent to which obesity is viewed as a public health problem among the lay public and professionals. In general, awareness of obesity increases with increasing age of the child and increasing degree of obesity; with respect to these variables parents and physicians show a similar bias. Obesity is more readily self-reported by girls than boys. Recent evidence indicates that children and adolescents who live in environments in which parents and schoolmates are overweight/obese may more frequently underestimate their weight status.[7]

Self-Perception

Already, in 5-year-old girls, higher weight status is associated with greater body dissatisfaction. Whereas body dissatisfaction and weight concerns are correlated, no direct relationship was found between girls' weight status and girls' weight concerns.[8,9] According to the longitudinal extension of this study,[10] girls tend to maintain their rank in weight concerns and body dissatisfaction across ages 5 to 9 years. The associations among girls' weight concerns, body dissatisfaction, and weight status increase with age. In addition, positive associations were found between changes in girls' weight concerns, body dissatisfaction, and weight status across ages 7 to 9 years. High weight concerns or high body dissatisfaction across ages 5 to 7 years predicted higher dietary restraint, more maladaptive eating attitudes, and a greater likelihood of dieting at age 9 years, independent of the weight status. Apparently, young girls are aware of what is considered physically attractive and judge their own bodies accordingly.

In adolescents, self-reported anthropometric data correlate highly (r >0.9) with measured data,[11] thus paralleling observations among adults. Adolescent females underreport weight to a greater extent than males (1.02 versus 0.19 kg). According to data obtained in the National Longitudinal Study of Adolescent Health, self-reported BMI (based on self-reported height and weight) was higher (0.03 kg/m^2) than BMI based on measurements in boys; the reverse was true for the adolescent girls (−0.27 kg/m^2). In contrast to the quite accurate self-reported BMI data, both the adolescents and their parents were poor informants with respect to subjective obesity: They failed to identify those adolescents who were obese and incorrectly classified non-obese as obese (for specificity and sensitivity see),[11] thus implying that obese adolescents may not be seeking needed treatment and that non-obese adolescents may be receiving inappropriate treatment or are suffering distorted body image. Although both groups did poorly with respect to subjective assessment of obesity, parents were more accurate than the adolescents themselves.

Reports of 12- to 16-year-old adolescents enrolled in the National Health and Nutrition Examination Survey III of whether they considered themselves overweight or normal weight correlated poorly with medical definitions of overweight: 52% of girls who considered themselves overweight were normal weight (BMI, ≤85th percentile), whereas only 25% of boys who considered themselves overweight were normal weight. Dieting behavior was associated with whether adolescents viewed themselves as overweight, independent of whether they actually were overweight.[12] The perception of being overweight during adolescence has recently been shown to be a risk factor for depression in young adult men and women. Accordingly, the perception of being overweight during adolescence should be considered a possible target for prevention intervention.[13]

Parental Perception

Mothers have a good perception of their own body weight, but do rather poorly when asked to judge the weight of their young children. According to a study conducted in 1998/1999 in Kentucky and Ohio,[14] only 21% of the mothers correctly perceived their child as overweight as defined with a weight-for-height percentile ≥90th percentile; the percentage was higher in mothers with a higher level of education. In an Australian study[15] conducted in 1997 and representative for primary schools in Victoria, based on data for 2,863 children aged 5 to 13 years, of whom 17% were overweight and 5.7% obese, 42% and 81% of parents with obese and overweight children did not report concern about their child's weight. A higher proportion of parents of underweight than overweight children expressed weight concerns (approximately 30% versus 19%); among parents of obese children concerns were greater if the child was female (approximately 70% versus 50%). Concern was, however, not significantly related to child gender, parental BMI, or parental education after controlling for child BMI.

Primary Health Care Providers

The authors briefly point out that parental perception is not altogether different from that of health care providers: In late 2001 and early 2002, 2,515 visits of children aged 3 months to 16 years to US health care providers were analyzed retrospectively.[16] About 9.7% of the patients were classified as obese; providers documented obesity in their assessments for only 53% of these patients. Obesity identification was lowest among preschool children (31%) and highest among adolescent patients (76%); milder forms of obesity were less likely to be detected. For primary health care specialists, the availability of reference data on weight adjusted for height and age and, in particular, BMI age centiles and their implementation in daily routine clinical work are essential.

QUALITY OF LIFE AND SELF-ESTEEM

Health-related quality of life provides an assessment of well-being measured along different dimensions, including physical, functional, psychological, and social well-being. In studies pertaining to obese children and adolescents, the degree of adiposity needs to be considered in addition to the sampling procedure (clinical or population based); furthermore, the additional subjective experience of being overweight merits consideration. In this context, the finding that HRQoL of a clinical sample of severely obese children and adolescents was exceedingly poor and comparable to that of young cancer patients[17] is potentially the result of enrichment of the sample for these 3 factors. In this well-known study, 106 children and adolescents (age range, 5–18 years; mean age, 12.1 years) with a mean BMI of 34.7 ± 9.3 kg/m^2 scored 67 ± 16.3 in comparison with 83 ± 14.8 for controls on a pediatric HRQoL inventory (range, 0–100); cases were 5.5 times more likely to have impaired HRQoL.

Epidemiologic studies are suited to address the degree of impairment representatively; however, similar to the situation on assessment of psychiatric comorbidity, the size of a population-based sample is crucial in that only large samples enable the ascertainment of a sufficiently large sample of extremely obese probands (see discussion later). In addition, the formation of subgroups within even large samples can entail loss of power precluding the detection of existing effects.

Based on a subsample (n = 4827) of the National Longitudinal Study of Adolescent Health, assessed in 1995/1996, 6 dichotomous outcomes were considered, including general health, functional limitations, illness symptoms, depression, self-esteem, and school/social functioning. Adolescents who were either overweight or obese were significantly more likely to report poor general health than adolescents with normal BMI. Overweight and obese adolescents—as well as underweight adolescents—were also more likely to report 1 or more functional limitations. However, no differences between overweight/obese and non-overweight individuals in the 4 other outcomes were detected; this even applied to the group of the most overweight adolescents defined as a BMI category at or above the 97th CDC percentile plus 2 BMI units. In age-stratified analyses, only the youngest age group (12- to 14-year-olds) was more likely to be depressed when overweight/obese: Similarly, this young overweight subgroup also reported lowered self-esteem and poor school and social functioning.[18]

In Australia, a community-based study (n = 1456) included 294 (20.2%) overweight and 63 (4.3%) obese children of a mean age of 10.4 years. Both parent-proxy and child self-reported HRQoL scores decreased with increasing child weight. At the subscale level, physical and social functioning for obese children was lower than those for children who were not overweight (all P<0.001). Similar to the US data on adolescents, decreases in emotional and school functioning scores by weight category were not significant. The authors concluded that the effects of child overweight and obesity on HRQoL were smaller in this community-based sample than in clinical samples.[19]

A recent nationally representative German study based on 6,669 adolescents aged 11 to 17 years revealed a slightly reduced HRQoL score for the overweight/obese (17.7% of the sample) as compared with the normal weight probands. However, self-perception of being overweight or obese (55.4% of the girls, 35.6% of the boys) was associated with a much more reduced score.[20]

Self-Esteem

Self-esteem specific to physical appearance was shown to be inversely associated with BMI in both male and female US adolescents. The magnitude of the association, however, was modest. In the respective study, low self-esteem did not predict the development of obesity over time.[21] According to a longitudinal study based on 1,520 9- to 10-year-old children, ascertained through their mothers, participating in the National Longitudinal Survey of Youth, scholastic and global self-esteem scores were not significantly different among 9- to 10-year-old obese and non-obese children. However, over the 4-year follow-up period, obese Hispanic and white girls showed significantly decreased levels of global self-esteem compared with non-obese females; mild decreases in self-esteem were also observed in obese boys compared with non-obese boys. Decreasing levels of self-esteem in obese children were associated with significantly increased rates of sadness, loneliness, nervousness, smoking, and drinking compared with obese children whose self-esteem increased or remained unchanged.[22]

In an Australian community-based longitudinal study, overweight/obese children had lower self-esteem scores than non-overweight children at baseline (ages, 5 through 10 years) and even more so at follow-up 4 years later. After accounting for baseline self-esteem, higher baseline BMI z score predicted poorer self-esteem at follow-up. Vice versa, after accounting for baseline BMI z score, poorer baseline self-esteem did not predict higher BMI z score. Whereas non-overweight children with low baseline self-esteem were twice as likely to develop overweight/obesity, this accounted for only a small proportion of the incidence of overweight during the 4-year period.[23] Both the US and Australian studies suggest a causal relationship between overweight and development of lowered self-esteem. If during the transition from childhood to adolescence an obese proband develops lower self-esteem, this potentially predicts other mental health problems.

SUICIDE AND SUICIDAL BEHAVIOR

Recent large-scale studies have convincingly shown that obesity is protective of suicide in adults. The first such study was based on nearly 1.3 million Swedish male teens whose BMI was assessed at age 18 to 19 years on conscription between 1968 and 1999 and who were followed-up to a maximum of 31 years. For each 5 kg/m^2 increase in BMI, the risk of suicide during the follow-up period decreased by 15%.[24] This inverse relationship between BMI and suicide rates has subsequently been confirmed.[25–27] Thus, US data from the combined 1986 to 1994 National Health Interview Surveys linked to the 1986 to 2002 Multiple Cause of Death file through the National Death Index quite similarly revealed that for each 5-kg/m^2 increase in BMI, the risk of suicide decreased by 18% for men; the same relationship was found to apply to females, too, who showed a 24% decreased risk for each 5-kg/m^2 increment.[26] In a Norwegian study based on a total of 74,332 males and females, 44,396 of whom also filled out the Hospital Anxiety and Depression Rating Scale (HADS), the hazard ratio per standard deviation increase in BMI was 0.82 on adjustment for psychological, social, and lifestyle factors. Interestingly, in fully adjusted models the odds ratio (OR) for depression (Hospital Anxiety and Depression Rating Scale score > 8) per standard deviation in BMI was 1.11. Thus, seemingly paradoxically higher BMI was associated with elevated depression but lower suicide rates.[27]

The authors are not aware of a study showing a correlation between actual suicide rates and BMI in adolescents, be it positive or negative. However, several studies have revealed that suicide ideation and suicide attempts are associated with adolescent overweight and obesity.[28–30] Data of the 2001 Youth Risk Behavior Survey, a school-based survey administered to a nationally representative sample of 13,601 US students in grades 9 through 12, revealed that both underweight (OR compared with normal weight students, 1.4) and overweight (OR, 1.3) predicted suicide ideation and suicide attempts; ethnic and racial differences were apparent in that, for example, the latter relationship did not apply to black students. However, on inclusion of perceived body weight, these relationships were no longer significant.[30] Compared with those who perceive themselves as having about the right weight, students who perceived themselves as very underweight (OR, 2.29), slightly underweight (OR, 1.36), slightly overweight (OR, 1.33), and very overweight (OR, 2.50) had greater adjusted odds of suicide ideation. Among white students, suicide attempts were also more common among those who perceived themselves as very underweight (OR, 3.04) or very overweight (OR, 2.74;).[30] Several clinical and general population studies have found that adolescents with unhealthy weight control practices are at increased risk for suicide ideation, suicide attempts, and death by suicide (for literature see);[30] this relationship persisted after controlling for depression.[31] Eaton and coworkers showed that the association of BMI and suicidal behavior persisted on controlling for weight control practices.

Weight-based teasing is possibly the major mediator of the association between overweight/obesity and suicide ideation in adolescents. Thus, this form of teasing has been shown to account for the elevated suicide ideation in male and female adolescents.[32] Eisenberg and colleagues, in this issue, found that suicide ideation was twice as frequent among girls who experienced weight-based teasing (51%) in comparison to those who did not report this experience (25%). Weight teasing potentially predicts other negative outcomes. Thus, it has longitudinally been shown to increase the risk of developing disordered eating behaviors.[33] Furthermore, lower self-esteem, lower body image, and higher depressive symptoms have also been attributed to weight teasing.[34]

DEPRESSION PREDICTS WEIGHT GAIN

Short-term influences of, for instance, stress, mood, or anxiety on appetite and physical activity levels are a common experience; however, comparatively little is known about their influence on medium- and long-term regulation of body weight in humans. Alterations of appetite and/or body weight represent symptoms of single psychiatric disorders apart from eating disorders. For example, significant weight loss or gain (or failure to make expected weight gains in childhood) and/or decrease or increase in appetite represent symptoms used for diagnosing a major depressive episode.[35]

Based on findings obtained in children and adolescents, elevated depression scores have repeatedly been inferred to result in weight gain. The respective longitudinal studies have revealed a predictive value of depressive symptoms in childhood and adolescence for obesity in later childhood, adolescence, and adulthood;[36–41] these findings remained stable after adjustment for potential confounders. Whereas both the design and results of these studies differed, the findings linking "depression" to subsequent weight gain are remarkably consistent. In a large study encompassing 9,374 adolescents in grades 7 through 9, depressed mood assessed with a depression scale was not related to baseline BMI.[37] The OR for obesity at the 1 year follow-up for those with a depressed mood was approximately 2 after controlling for BMI at baseline, age, race, gender, parental obesity, number of parents in the home, socioeconomic status, smoking, physical activity, conduct disorder, self-esteem, and delinquent behavior. Causality is implied by the fact that the duration of depression between childhood and adulthood also emerged as a predictor of adult BMI;[36] even among children with obesity at baseline, the depression scale score predicted BMI 1 year later.[37] These studies suggest that rates of obesity can potentially be reduced by successful treatment of depression in children and adolescents. A word of caution is, however, warranted: It cannot be excluded that the repeatedly described predictive effect of depressive symptoms is causally related to a different factor. Indeed, Stice and colleagues[41] confirm the effect in a univariate analysis; however, a significant effect of depressive symptoms was not discernible in the multivariate model investigating the unique effects of the risk factors that showed significant univariate effects while controlling for the effects of the other risk factors. In this model, only dietary restraint and perceived parental obesity remained significant predictors.

PSYCHIATRIC COMORBIDITY
Comorbidity Apart from Eating Disorders

Single studies have assessed psychiatric symptomatology in obese children and adolescents using both dimensional and categorical diagnostic evaluations. For an appropriate understanding of the respective results, it is again crucial to distinguish between clinical and population-based samples. Furthermore, differences in age, gender, the severity of obesity, psychiatric classification schemes (Diagnostic and Statistical Manual Of Mental Disorders 4th edition [DSM] versus ICD-10 Classification of Behavioural and Mental Disorders), interviews, questionnaires, and rating scales need to be taken into account. Because eating disorders are of special relevance in this issue, the association of pediatric obesity with eating disorders is separately dealt with (see discussion later).

In clinical samples, that is, among children and adolescents who seek weight reduction, higher rates of anxiety and mood disorders have repeatedly been reported.[42,43] In a clinical study encompassing 54 children and adolescents with a mean age of 12.1 years, who participated in a weight management program, 32% of the study group fell in the depressed group, as defined by a score of ≥ 13 on the Children's Depression Inventory (CDI).[44] Within the study group no correlation was found between Children's Depression Inventory [CDI] score and BMI. About 42.6% of the participants were classified as mildly obese (BMI between 20 and 30), 44.4% as moderately obese (BMI between 30 and 39), and 13% as severely obese (BMI >40 kg/m^2). In a clinical study group of 47 (30 female) extremely obese adolescents with a mean BMI of

42.4 kg/m^2, only 14 (29.8%) did not receive a lifetime DSM-IV diagnosis; 16 (34%) fulfilled criteria for 3 or more diagnoses.[42] Lifetime rates for mood, anxiety, substance abuse/dependence, somatoform, and eating disorders were 42.6%, 40.4%, 36.2%, 14.9%, and 17.0%, respectively. Most of these patients retrospectively predated their obesity to the development of their psychiatric disorders.

In contrast, epidemiologically based studies have not revealed an elevated rate of psychopathology in obese children and adolescents. For example, a study of 393 10th-grade female adolescents (mean age, 15.8 ± 0.3 years) revealed no differences in anxiety (State-Trait Anxiety Inventory) and depression (Children's Depression Inventory [CDI]) between underweight, average, and overweight females.[45] The 47 most obese adolescents (mean BMI, 29.8 kg/m^2) of a representative sample of 1,655 adolescents did not show elevated rates of psychiatric disorders.[42] These 47 adolescents formed a subgroup of 3,021 German subjects aged 14 to 21 years in whom obesity was also not associated with increased rates of psychiatric disorders.[46]

Recent and, in comparison to the aforementioned epidemiologic study based on adolescents and young adults,[46] considerably larger epidemiologic studies in adults have revealed that obesity entails slightly elevated risks for mood and anxiety disorders,[47–49] with 1 study also indicating elevated risks for specific personality disorders (antisocial, avoidant, schizoid, paranoid, and obsessive-compulsive).[49] Whereas Simon and colleagues[47] found a lower risk for substance use disorders, Petry and colleagues detected an increased risk for alcohol use disorder. For those disorders found to be associated with obesity, ORs calculated in the respective studies were mostly below 2. Modest associations (ORs generally in the range of 1.2–1.5) were observed between obesity and depressive disorders, and between obesity and anxiety disorders, in pooled data across different countries. These associations were concentrated among those with severe obesity and among females.[50]

The elevated rates of psychopathology of obese children and adolescents seeking weight reduction are reminiscent of findings in adults.[51] Alternatively, or additionally, treatment-seeking young obese patients might have higher BMIs than obese children and adolescents detected in school- or population-based surveys.[42] A large population-based sample would, for instance, be required to ascertain a sufficient number of adolescents with a BMI ≥ 40 kg/m^2. Irrespective of these considerations, current data imply that psychiatric screening of obese children and adolescents seeking weight reduction, and of young subjects with extreme obesity, should be part of their diagnostic assessment.

Eating Disorders

In contrast to previous assumptions, eating disorder issues are not exclusively found in underweight females, but are also found in overweight and obese children and adolescents of both sexes. In a national US survey of more than 6,500 male and female adolescents between 5th and 12th grades, a strong positive association was found between BMI and disordered eating (Commonwealth Fund Survey).[52] The prevalence of disordered eating (binge-purge cycling) was highest in obese and overweight girls, with rates of 20% and 17%, respectively, in comparison to "only" 9% in underweight girls (BMI <15th percentile). Lundstedt and colleagues,[53] at the Karolinska University Hospital in Stockholm, demonstrated that adolescent obese girls were comparable to DSM-IV eating disorder-diagnosed girls on the majority of the subscales of the Eating Disorder Inventory,[54] a well-known detailed instrument for assessing eating disorders in adolescence (for further information see the article by Herpertz-Dahlmann, elsewhere in this issue). In a nationally representative sample of 1,900 German adolescents aged 11 to 17 years, more than one-third of the overweight and more than half of the obese participants reported disordered eating behavior assessed by the SCOFF,[55] an instrument consisting of 5 questions originally developed to screen for eating disorders in clinical settings (for a more detailed description of the distribution of eating-disordered behavior in different body weight categories according to the German (BELLA-study)[56] see **Fig. 1**) Most of the eating-disordered obese or overweight probands confirmed loss of control (LOC) over eating.

In general, 2 kinds of eating-disordered behavior—in most cases to be classified in the residual category of DSM-IV "eating disorder not otherwise specified"—can be distinguished in overweight youth:

1. Inappropriate or unhealthy weight control behavior
2. Binge eating

Additionally, almost all overweight children and adolescents with eating-disordered behavior complain of body dissatisfaction as well as shape and weight concerns.

Inappropriate weight control behavior
The term "weight control behavior" refers to a spectrum of modest to extreme behaviors aimed at influencing one's shape and weight.[57] These strategies range from (1) *moderate* dieting and exercising to (2) *unhealthy* practices, such as skipping meals, using food substrates, fasting, smoking more cigarettes, and finally (3) *extreme* (harmful) behavior, such as abuse of laxatives and diuretics, intake of diet pills, and vomiting.[58]

In a population-based study on eating patterns and weight concerns of more than 4,500 adolescents from Minnesota public middle and high schools, 69% of the overweight (BMI 85th to <95th percentile) and 76% of the obese girls (≥95th percentile) pursued unhealthy weight control behaviors. Extreme weight control behavior was reported by 16% and 18% of the overweight and obese girls, respectively (Project Eating Among Teens [EAT],[58] similar results were obtained in other studies).[59] More than half of the sample studied by Neumark-Sztainer and colleagues[60] could be

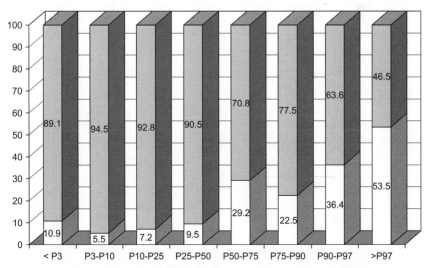

Fig. 1. Prevalence of disordered eating (defined by a SCOFF score ≥2) in different weight categories. BELLA-study, Germany. (*Data from* Herpertz-Dahlmann B, Wille N, Ravens-Sieberer et al. Disordered eating behaviour and attitudes, associated psychopathology and health-related quality of life—results from the BELLA study. Eur J Child Adolesc Psychiatry, in press.)

followed up after 5 years; there was a steep increase in the use of *unhealthy* weight control behaviors in females between early to middle adolescence from half of the sample to nearly 60%, and between middle to late adolescence, *extreme* weight control behaviors increased from 15% to 24%. The authors reported that one-fifth of females were taking diet pills in late adolescence.

Generally, most of the studies indicate that overweight girls are at greater risk than boys for resorting to unhealthy or harmful weight control behavior. Youth of minority populations are at a similar risk as those of the white population.[61]

Binge eating

The syndrome of BED has not yet achieved official diagnostic recognition and is still included in the research criteria section of the DSM-IV-TR. Patients currently fulfilling criteria for this disorder would technically fall under "eating disorder not otherwise specified" in the DSM or ICD 10 (for a review see).[62]

Although primarily conceptualized as a disorder of adulthood, there is growing evidence that BED is also prominent in childhood and adolescence. Diagnostic criteria of BED in children and adolescents are often controversial. The definition of eating a large amount of food (criterion A/1) is even more ambiguous in children than in adults. In addition, it is not clear whether the amount of the ingested food is associated with any change in mood or other psychopathology, whereas LOC over eating (criterion A/2) is nearly always linked to distress. Modulating strong affective states by consuming food and eating in the absence of hunger (criterion B/3) also seem to be correlates of BED in children.[63]

Several authors[64,65] have suggested using broader and more flexible criteria for defining eating disorders in childhood and adolescence (see also the article by Herpertz-Dahlmann elsewhere in this issue). Based on empiric studies, Marcus and Kalarchian conceptualized provisional criteria for diagnosing BED in children (**Table 1**).

Taking these criteria into account, Shapiro and colleagues[66] designed a short interviewer-based assessment instrument for subthreshold and full-blown BEDs in children aged 5 to 13 years (children's binge eating disorder scale, C-BEDS), which might be helpful for clinicians in identifying binge eating early in the development of obesity and eating disorders.

Table 1
Provisional BED research criteria for children
A. Recurrent episodes of binge eating. An episode of binge eating is characterized by both of the following:
1. Food seeking in the absence of hunger (eg, after a full meal)
2. A sense of lack of control over eating (eg, endorse that "When I start to eat, I just can't stop")
B. Binge episodes are associated with one or more of the following:
1. Food seeking in response to negative affect (eg, sadness, boredom, restlessness)
2. Food seeking as a reward
3. Sneaking or hiding food
C. Symptoms persist over a period of 3 mo
D. Eating is not associated with the regular use of inappropriate compensatory behaviors (eg, purging, fasting, and excessive exercise) and does not occur exclusively during the course of anorexia nervosa or bulimia nervosa

Abbreviation: BED, binge-eating disorder.

In a recent article, Tanofsky-Kraff and colleagues[67] proposed a revision of the criteria by Marcus and Kalarchian by focusing even more on LOC of eating (LOC eating) in children aged 12 years or younger. LOC eating is defined as eating with the associated experience of being unable to control the amount of eating independent of whether the size of the meal is objectively large. However, further research involving the clinical significance of diagnostic criteria in BED in childhood is urgently needed.

In the school-based sample described here (EAT project), 3.1% of all girls and 0.9% of all boys fulfilled DSM-IV research criteria for BED.[68] In addition, the authors found that 7.5% of girls and 1.6% of boys had a sub-clinical level of binge eating. In another study investigating only obese children and adolescents seeking residential care, 36.5% of the subjects reported binge-eating episodes without fulfilling all DSM-IV research criteria.[65] Other studies also report a high prevalence of binge eating in treatment-seeking obese youth, with estimates ranging from 20% to 30%.[69-71] In our own field study in the city of Aachen, Germany, 6.3% of 5- to 6-year-old children with a body weight equal to or above the 90th percentile reported binge-eating episodes.[72]

In contrast to inappropriate weight control behavior, binge eating seems to be equally distributed between both sexes in childhood,[70] with a higher proportion of girls demonstrating this behavior during adolescence.[73]

The co-occurrence of binge-eating episodes with psychiatric symptoms in overweight youth is much higher than that estimated by chance. However, as clarified here, it is crucial to distinguish between clinical and population-based samples. Binge-eating episodes and the full-blown disorder are more prevalent in clinical than in epidemiologic overweight samples. Moreover, most studies found an association between binge eating, negative mood, and anxiety in treatment-seeking youth.[71,74,75] Obese adolescents presenting for a weight loss program with high weight and shape concerns reported greater impairments in mental and physical health as well as in emotional and social functioning than those with low-weight-and shape-related concerns.[76] One of the possible reasons for a more severe psychiatric symptomatology in clinical samples is that these patients may have even higher BMIs than those detected at school or in population-based studies.[42]

Sequelae of eating-disordered behavior in overweight youth

In previous studies, binge eating and LOC have been associated with higher prevalence rates of overweight and obesity, greater severity of obesity, and greater amounts of body fat.[68,77,78] In a cross-sectional school-based survey of 31,000 pupils from grades 7 to 12, overweight probands were significantly more likely to engage in chronic weight control behavior and binge eating than their non-overweight counterparts.[79] In addition, there is prospective evidence that binge eating in childhood and adolescence increases the likelihood for obesity later in life.[80] In the prospective study mentioned here, adolescents with unhealthy weight control strategies increased their BMI by about 1 unit more than adolescents not practicing weight control behavior.[60] Furthermore, their risk of being overweight 5 years later was approximately 3 times higher in comparison to that of adolescents without unhealthy weight strategies.

Subthreshold eating disorder and obesity in childhood are both prominent risk factors for developing a full-blown eating disorder,[60,81] especially BED or bulimia nervosa.[82] Thus, it is relatively likely that the combination of eating-disordered behavior and obesity, with a high risk of each disorder for somatic and psychiatric comorbidity, even potentiates the risk for a full eating disorder syndrome or psychiatric disorder.

SUMMARY

Obese children and adolescents are typically not concerned with the long-term implications of their elevated body weight despite the fact that diverse risk factors for the development of comorbid disorders can frequently be detected early on. Such children and adolescents do, however, intensely experience the effects of stigmatization, including teasing and victimization. Young individuals with extreme obesity can additionally suffer due to their incapability of pursuing specific everyday life activities. As such, the psychosocial impact of being obese represents the major concern at this stage of life. The mere feeling of being obese entails a reduced quality of life and a lowered self-esteem; it is also known that mood and anxiety disorders are common in adolescents seeking weight reduction. What further differentiates obese children and adolescents with and without the feeling of being obese?

Recent research has shown that elevated depression scores at baseline predict above average weight gain in the future. What are the mediators of this relationship? Is eating behavior the relevant mediator? Longitudinal studies are also required to assess what if any other psychological/psychiatric variables predict excess weight gain. Similar to the longitudinal studies pertaining to depressed mood, it is necessary to analyze if elevated anxiety, impulsivity, inattention, and hyperactivity entail above average weight gain. Such studies are important because they will lay a solid foundation for the determination of the relevance of psychological factors in weight regulation. For example, if depression indeed predicts obesity, are there joint genetic risk factors underlying both disorders? The success of genome-wide association studies in the elucidation of polygenes predisposing to complex disorders should make it possible to address the potential overlap of such findings between obesity and mood disorders.

In clinical and more practical terms, future research on psychological and psychiatric aspects in childhood and adolescent obesity would profit from a careful delineation of the respective ascertainment procedure. Is the study sample representative of obese subjects or is it enriched with individuals who feel obese and/or seek treatment? Furthermore, the degree of adiposity needs to be made transparent by referring, for example, to BMI percentiles or BMI-standard deviation score values (mean, range) in addition to provision of absolute BMI and age. This will make it easier to assess to what extent these items have an influence on the respective results.

APPENDIX 1: PSYCHIATRIC ASPECTS OF EATING-DISORDERED BEHAVIOR

Although most studies have assessed the association between overweight/obesity and mental disorder symptoms, few studies have examined the relationship between disordered eating behavior (apart from BMI) and behavioral problems, although many adolescents are affected by subthreshold disorders of eating.

In a Minnesota school-based survey with more than 80,000 participants, 56% of 9th-grade girls and 28% of 9th-grade boys reported disordered eating behaviors, such as fasting, vomiting, or binge eating; in 12th-grade girls and boys, slightly higher rates of 57% and 31%, respectively, were found (Minnesota Student Survey).[61] In a North Italian study, 28% of 15- to 19-year-old female high school adolescents reported unhealthy eating behaviors as described above.[83] One author's (B.H.-D.) recent study with 1,900 German adolescents (BELLA-study) established eating-disordered behavior and attitudes in about one-third of the girls and 15% of the boys.[56]

In sum, girls report more disordered eating and body image concerns than boys, and youngsters in higher grades are more vulnerable to such concerns than those in lower grades.

Disordered eating symptoms are associated with a wide range of psychopathological and psychosocial concerns. In the Commonwealth Fund Survey, strong correlates of dieting and eating-disordered behavior were low self-esteem, depression, and suicidal ideation.[52] Similar results were obtained in the population-based German investigation (BELLA-study).[56] Even after controlling for BMI, probands who reported disordered eating had significantly higher levels of depression and anxiety. This was reported not only by the adolescents, but also by their parents. Similar to the results of the Neumark-Sztainer group, the authors observed significantly more suicidal ideation and suicidal behavior in adolescents who screened positive for disordered eating than in those who screened negative. In another investigation by the Neumark-Sztainer research team, severity of depression in youth was positively associated with weight concerns, perceived barriers to healthy eating, and unhealthy weight control behaviors.[84] In the prospective study mentioned above (EAT project), body dissatisfaction predicted depressive mood and low self-esteem 5 years later.[85]

In contrast to the many studies examining internalizing problems in eating-disordered adolescents, there are only a few studies that have investigated the coincidence of disturbed eating behavior and externalizing symptoms. In a longitudinal investigation of externalizing behavior and disordered eating attitudes at 11, 14, and 17 years of age, externalizing behavior predicted increases in weight preoccupation, body dissatisfaction, and the use of inappropriate compensatory weight control behaviors. The reverse sequence was also true: earlier use of inappropriate compensatory weight control behavior predicted increases in externalizing behavior disorders.[86] In our study, parents described significantly more externalizing problems in their sons and daughters with disordered eating behavior than did parents of children without such problems, even after adjustment for BMI.[56]

Results of the Commonwealth Fund Survey demonstrated a direct and significant association between alcohol and drug use with both dieting and disordered eating, which also remained statistically significant after controlling for BMI and sociodemographic status.[52]

In conclusion, disordered eating behavior, whether or not in combination with overweight or obesity, is linked to a wide range of psychopathologies and to psychosocial burden. Thus, youngsters with severe shape and weight concerns, or those engaging in unhealthy weight control practices or bingeing, should be examined for other serious mental or social problems.

REFERENCES

1. Wardle J, Cooke L. The impact of obesity on psychological well-being. Best Pract Res Clin Endocrinol Metab 2005;19:421–40.
2. Puhl RM, Latner JD. Stigma, obesity, and the health of the nation's children. Psychol Bull 2007;133:557–80.
3. Hebebrand J, Wulftange H, Goerg T, et al. Epidemic obesity: are genetic factors involved via increased rates of assortative mating? Int J Obes Relat Metab Disord 2000;24(3):345–53.
4. Latner JD, Stunkard AJ. Getting worse: the stigmatization of obese children. Obes Res 2003;11:452–6.
5. Ströhle A, Höfler M, Pfister H, et al. Physical activity and prevalence and incidence of mental disorders in adolescents and young adults. Psychol Med 2007;37(11):1657–66.
6. Bruch H. Eating disorders: obesity, anorexia nervosa and the person within. New York: Basic Books, Inc.; 1973.

7. Maximova K, McGrath JJ, Barnett T, et al. Do you see what I see? Weight status misperception and exposure to obesity among children and adolescents. Int J Obes 2008;32:1008–15.
8. Davison KK, Markey CN, Birch LL, et al. Etiology of body dissatisfaction and weight concerns among 5-year-old girls. Appetite 2000;35:143–51.
9. Davison KK, Birch LL. Weight status, parent reaction, and self-concept in five-year-old girls. Pediatrics 2001;107:46–53.
10. Davison KK, Markey CN, Birch LL. A longitudinal examination of patterns in girls' weight concerns and body dissatisfaction from ages 5 to 9 years. Int J Eat Disord 2003;33:320–32.
11. Goodman E, Hinden BR, Khandelwal S. Accuracy of teen and parental reports of obesity and body mass index. Pediatrics 2000;106:52–8.
12. Strauss RS. Self-reported weight status and dieting in a cross-sectional sample of young adolescents: National Health and Nutrition Examination Survey III. Arch Pediatr Adolesc Med 1999;153(7):741–7.
13. Al Mamun A, Cramb S, McDermott BM, et al. Adolescents' perceived weight associated with depression in young adulthood: a longitudinal study. Obesity (Silver Spring) 2007;15(12):3097–105.
14. Baughcum AE, Chamberlin LA, Deeks CM, et al. Maternal perceptions of overweight preschool children. Pediatrics 2000;106(6):1380–6.
15. Wake M, Salmon L, Waters E, et al. Parent-reported health status of overweight and obese Australian primary school children: a cross-sectional population survey. Int J Obes Relat Metab Disord 2002;26:717–24.
16. O'Brien SH, Holubkov R, Reis EC. Identification, evaluation, and management of obesity in an academic primary care center. Pediatrics 2004;114(2):e154–9.
17. Schwimmer JB, Burwinkle TM, Varni JW. Health-related quality of life of severely obese children and adolescents. JAMA 2003;289:1813–9.
18. Swallen KC, Reither EN, Haas SA, et al. Overweight, obesity, and health-related quality of life among adolescents: the National Longitudinal Study of Adolescent Health. Pediatrics 2005;115:340–7.
19. Williams J, Wake M, Hesketh K, et al. Health-related quality of life of overweight and obese children. JAMA 2005;293(1):70–6.
20. Kurth B-M, Ellert U. [Perceived or true obesity: which causes more suffering in adolescents?]. Dtsch Arztebl 2008;105(23):406–12 [German].
21. French SA, Perry CL, Leon GR, et al. Self-esteem and change in body mass index over 3 years in a cohort of adolescents. Obes Res 1996;4:21–7.
22. Strauss RS. Childhood obesity and self-esteem. Pediatrics 2000;105(1):e15.
23. Hesketh K, Wake M, Waters E. Body mass index and parent-reported self-esteem in elementary school children: evidence for a causal relationship. Int J Obes Relat Metab Disord 2004;28(10):1233–7.
24. Magnusson PK, Rasmussen F, Lawlor DA, et al. Association of body mass index with suicide mortality: a prospective cohort study of more than one million men. Am J Epidemiol 2006;163(1):1–8.
25. Mukamal KJ, Kawachi I, Miller M, et al. Body mass index and risk of suicide among men. Arch Intern Med 2007;167(5):468–75.
26. Kaplan MS, McFarland BH, Huguet N. The relationship of body weight to suicide risk among men and women: results from the US National Health Interview Survey Linked Mortality File. J Nerv Ment Dis 2007;195:948–51.
27. Bjerkeset O, Romundstad P, Evans J, et al. Association of adult body mass index and height with anxiety, depression, and suicide in the general population: the HUNT study. Am J Epidemiol 2008;167:193–202.

28. Neumark-Sztainer D, Story M, French SA, et al. Psychosocial concerns and health-compromising behaviors among overweight and nonoverweight adolescents. Obes Res 1997;5:237–49.

29. Falkner NH, Nuemark-Sztainer D, Story M, et al. Social, educational, and psychological correlates of weight status in adolescents. Obes Res 2001;9:32–42.

30. Eaton DK, Lowry R, Brener ND, et al. Associations of body mass index and perceived weight with suicide ideation and suicide attempts among US high school students. Arch Pediatr Adolesc Med 2005;159:513–9.

31. Crow S, Eisenberg ME, Story M, et al. Suicidal behavior in adolescents: relationship to weight status, weight control behaviors, and body dissatisfaction. Int J Eat Disord 2008;41:82–7.

32. Eisenberg ME, Neumark-Stainer D, Story M. Associations of weight-based teasing and emotional well-being among adolescents. Arch Pediatr Adolesc Med 2003;157:733–8.

33. Haines J, Neumark-Sztainer D, Eisenberg ME, et al. Weight teasing and disordered eating behaviors in adolescents: longitudinal findings from Project EAT (Eating Among Teens). Pediatrics 2006;117(2):e209–15.

34. Eisenberg ME, Neumark-Sztainer D, Haines J, et al. Weight-teasing and emotional well-being in adolescents: longitudinal findings from Project EAT. J Adolesc Health 2006;38(6):675–83.

35. American Psychiatric Association. Diagnostic and Statistical Manual of Mental Disorders (DSM-IV), 4th edition. Washington, DC: American Psychiatric Association; 1994 .

36. Pine DS, Goldstein RB, Wolk S, et al. The association between childhood depression and adulthood body mass index. Pediatrics 2001;107:1049–57.

37. Goodman E, Whitaker RC. A prospective study of the role of depression in the development and persistence of adolescent obesity. Pediatrics 2002;110:497–504.

38. Richardson LP, Davis R, Poulton R, et al. A longitudinal evaluation of adolescent depression and adult obesity. Arch Pediatr Adolesc Med 2003;157:739–45.

39. Hasler G, Pine DS, Klaghofer R, et al. The associations between psychopathology and being overweight: a 20-year prospective community study. Psychol Med 2004;34:1047–57.

40. Franko DL, Striegel-Moore RH, Thompson D, et al. Does adolescent depression predict obesity in black and white young adult women? Psychol Med 2005;35:1505–13.

41. Stice E, Presnell K, Shaw H, et al. Psychological and behavioral risk factors for obesity in adolescent girls: a prospective study. J Consult Clin Psychol 2005; 73:195–202.

42. Britz B, Siegfried M, Ziegler A, et al. Rates of psychiatric disorders in a clinical study group of adolescents with extreme obesity and in obese adolescents ascertained via a population based study. Int J Obes 2000;24:1707–14.

43. Vila G, Zipper E, Dabbas M, et al. Mental disorders in obese children and adolescents. Psychosom Med 2004;66:387–94.

44. Wallace W, Sheslow D, Hassink S. Obesity in children: a risk for depression. Ann N Y Acad Sci 1993;699:301–3.

45. Wadden TA, Foster GD, Stunkard AJ, et al. Dissatisfaction with weight and figure in obese girls: discontent but not depression. Int J Obes 1989;13:89–97.

46. Lamertz CM, Jacobi C, Yassouridis A, et al. Are obese adolescents and young adults at higher risk for mental disorders? A community survey. Obes Res 2002;10:1152–60.

47. Simon GE, Von Korff M, Saunders K, et al. Association between obesity and psychiatric disorders in the US adult population. Arch Gen Psychiatry 2006;63(7): 824–30.

48. Scott KM, Bruffaerts R, Simon GE, et al. Obesity and mental disorders in the general population: results from the world mental health surveys. Int J Obes 2008;32(1):192–200.

49. Petry NM, Barry D, Pietrzak RH, et al. Overweight and obesity are associated with psychiatric disorders: results from the National Epidemiologic Survey on Alcohol and Related Conditions. Psychosom Med 2008;70(3):288–97.

50. Scott KM, McGee MA, Wells JE, et al. Obesity and mental disorders in the adult general population. J Psychosom Res 2008;64(1):97–105.

51. Friedman MA, Brownell KD. Psychological correlates of obesity: moving to the next research generation. Psychol Bull 1995;117:3–20.

52. Neumark-Sztainer D, Hannan J. Weight-related behaviors among adolescent girls and boys. Arch Pediatr Adolesc Med 2000;54:569–77.

53. Lundstedt G, Edlund B, Engström I, et al. Eating disorder traits in obese children and adolescents. Eat Weight Disord 2006;11:45–50.

54. Garner DM. Eating Disorder Inventory (EDI-2). 2nd Professional Manual. Odessa (FL): Psychological Assessment Resources; Inc.; 1991. PO Box 998.

55. Morgan JF, Reid F, Lacey JH. The SCOFF questionnaire: assessment of a new screening tool for eating disorders. BMJ 2003;319:1467–8.

56. Herpertz-Dahlmann B, Wille N, Ravens-Sieberer et al. Disordered eating behaviour and attitudes, associated psychopathology and health-related quality of life—results from the BELLA study. Eur J Child Adolesc Psychiatry, in press.

57. Goldschmidt AB, Aspen VP, Sinton MM, et al. Disordered eating attitudes and behaviors in overweight youth. Obesity 2008;16:257–64.

58. Neumark-Sztainer D, Story M, Hannan PJ, et al. Weight-related concerns and behaviors among overweight and nonoverweight adolescents. Arch Pediatr Adolesc Med 2002;156:171–8.

59. Boutelle K, Neumark-Sztainer D, Story M, et al. Weight control behaviors among obese, overweight, and nonoverweight adolescents. J Pediatr Psychol 2002;27:531–40.

60. Neumark-Sztainer D, Wall M, Eisenberg ME, et al. Overweight status and weight control behaviors in adolescents: longitudinal and secular trends from 1999 to 2004. Prev Med 2006;43:52–9.

61. Croll J, Neumark-Sztainer D, Story M, et al. Prevalence and risk and protective factors related to disordered eating behaviors among adolescents: relationship to gender and ethnicity. J Adolesc Health 2002;31:166–75.

62. Bulik CM, Brownley KA, Shapiro JR. Diagnosis and management of binge eating disorder. World Psychiatry 2007;6:142–8.

63. Marcus MD, Kalarchian MA. Binge eating in children and adolescents. Int J Eat Disord 2003;34:S47–57.

64. Nicholls D, Chater R, Lask B. Children into DSM don't go; a comparison of classification systems for eating disorders in childhood and early adolescence. Int J Eat Disord 2000;28:317–24.

65. Decaluwe V, Braet C, Fairburn CG. Binge eating in obese children and adolescents. Int J Eat Disord 2003;33:78–84.

66. Shapiro JR, Woolson W, Hamer RM, et al. Evaluation binge eating in children: development of the Children's Binge Eating Scale (C-BEDS). Int J Eat Disord 2007;40:82–9.

67. Tanofsky-Kraff M, Marcus MD, Yanovski SZ, et al. Loss of control eating disorder in children aged 12 years and younger: proposed research criteria. Eat Behav 2008;9:360–5.

68. Ackard DM, Neumark-Sztainer D, Story M, et al. Overeating among adolescents: prevalence and associations with weight-related characteristics and psychological health. Pediatrics 2003;111:67–74.

69. Isnard P, Michel G, Frelut ML, et al. Binge eating and psychopathology in severely obese adolescents. Int J Eat Disord 2003;34:235–43.

70. Tanofsky-Kraff M, Faden D, Yanovski SZ, et al. The perceived onset of dieting and loss of control eating behaviors in overweight children. Int J Eat Disord 2005;38. 122–22.

71. Eddy KT, Tanofsky-Kraff M, Thompson-Brenner H, et al. Eating disorder pathology among overweight treatment-seeking youth: clinical correlates and cross-sectional risk modeling. Behav Res Ther 2007;45:2360–71.

72. Lamerz A, Kuepper-Nybelen J, Bruning N, et al. Prevalence of obesity, binge eating, and night eating in a cross-sectional field survey of 6-year-old children and their parents in a German urban population. J Child Psychol Psychiatry 2005;46:385–93.

73. Neumark-Sztainer D, Falkner N, Story M, et al. Weight-teasing among adolescents: Correlations with weight status and disordered eating behaviors. Int J Obes 2002;26:123–31.

74. Glasofer DR, Tanofsky-Kraff M, Eddy KT, et al. Binge eating in overweight treatment-seeking adolescents. Ped Psychology 2007;32:95–105.

75. Goossens L, Braet C, Dacaluwe V. Loss of control over eating in obese youngsters. Behav Res Ther 2007;45:1–9.

76. Doyle AC, le Grange D, Goldschmidt A, et al. Psychosocial and physical impairment in overweight adolescents at high risk for eating disorders. Obesity 2007; 15:145–54.

77. Morgan CM, Yanovski SZ, Ngyuen TT, et al. Loss of control over eating, adiposity, and psychopathology in overweight children. Int J Eat Disord 2002;31:430–41.

78. Tanofsky-Kraff M, Cohen ML, Yanovski SZ, et al. A prospective study of psychological predictors of body fat gain among children at high risk for adult obesity. Pediatrics 2006;117:1203–9.

79. Neumark-Sztainer D, Story M, French SA, et al. Psychosocial correlates of health compromising behaviors among adolescents. Health Educ Res 1997;12:37–52.

80. Stice E, Cameron RP, Killen JD, et al. Naturalistic weight-reduction efforts prospectively predict growth in relative weight and onset of obesity among female adolescents. J Consult Clin Psychol 1999;67:967–74.

81. Childress AC, Brewerton TD, Hodges EL, et al. The kid's eating disorders survey (KEDS): a study of middle school students. J Am Acad Child Adolesc Psychiatry 1993;32:843–50.

82. Fairburn CG, Welch SL, Doll HA, et al. Risk factors for bulimia nervosa: a community-based, case-control study. Arch Gen Psychiatry 1997;54:509–17.

83. Toselli AL, Villani S, Ferro AM, et al. Eating disorders and their correlates in high school adolescents of Northern Italy. Epidemiol Psichiatr Soc 2005;14:91–9.

84. Fulkerson JA, Sherwood NE, Perry CL, et al. Depressive symptoms and adolescents eating and health behaviors: a multifaceted view in a population-based sample. Prev Med 2004;38:865–75.

85. Neumark-Sztainer D, Wall M, Guo J, et al. Obesity, disordered eating, and eating disorders in a longitudinal study of adolescents: how do dieters fare 5 years later? J Am Diet Assoc 2006;106:559–68.

86. Marmorstein NR, von Ranson KM, Iacono WG, et al. Longitudinal associations between externalizing behaviour and dysfunctional eating attitudes and behaviors: a community-based study. J Clin Child Adolesc Psychol 2007;36:87–94.

Environmental and Genetic Risk Factors for Eating Disorders: What the Clinician Needs to Know

Suzanne E. Mazzeo, PhD[a], Cynthia M. Bulik, PhD[b],*

KEYWORDS

- Anorexia nervosa • Bulimia nervosa • Binge eating disorder
- Genetic • Environment • Risk

The significant role genetic factors play in the development of eating disorders is becoming increasingly clear.[1–3] Family studies of anorexia nervosa and bulimia nervosa have consistently found a higher lifetime prevalence of eating disorders among relatives of eating disorder probands than among relatives of controls.[4–6] Further, numerous twin studies[3,7–10] suggest that liability to anorexia and bulimia nervosa is significantly influenced by additive genetic factors. Although somewhat less developed, family and twin studies point toward binge eating disorder (BED) being both familial[11] and influenced by additive genetic factors.[12,13] Of note, although many molecular genetic studies have been conducted, they have yet to yield an unambiguous replicated finding (see references[14–16] for reviews). The emergence of powerful and novel approaches, such as genome-wide association studies, could bring significant advances to the field. Given that the effect size of single gene variants is likely to be small, large collaborative investigations are required to identify risk alleles. The authors propose that advances in genetic research will assist us not only with identification of risk alleles, but will unlock new methodological approaches to help identify differential risk to environmental risk factors dependent on genotype.

This research was supported by the National Institutes of Health Grant MH-068520 (Mazzeo).

[a] Departments of Psychology and Pediatrics, Virginia Commonwealth University, 806 West Franklin Street, Richmond, VA 23284-2018, USA

[b] Department of Psychiatry and Nutrition, University of North Carolina at Chapel Hill, 101 Manning Drive, Chapel Hill, NC 27516, USA

* Corresponding author. CB #6170, 101 Manning Drive, Department of Psychiatry, University of North Carolina at Chapel Hill, Chapel Hill, NC 27599.

E-mail address: cbulik@med.unc.edu (C.M. Bulik).

Child Adolesc Psychiatric Clin N Am 18 (2008) 67–82
doi:10.1016/j.chc.2008.07.003
1056-4993/08/$ – see front matter © 2008 Elsevier Inc. All rights reserved.

childpsych.theclinics.com

Although genetic epidemiology of eating disorders has emerged with force in the past decade, environmental risk factors have received the bulk of research and clinical attention.[17–19] In particular, sociocultural influences, such as unrealistically thin media images, have been hypothesized to promote disordered eating and body dissatisfaction[20,21] on the causal pathway to eating disorders. However, it is clear that although virtually all women are exposed to these sociocultural influences, only a small proportion develop clinical eating disorders.[22]

Ultimately, the elucidation of causal models for eating disorders will no doubt include various types of genetic and environmental interplay. One of these is gene–environment correlation (or r_{GE}), which has been described as occurring "when the exposure to positive or negative environmental influences is not randomly distributed with respect to genetic differences."[1] Three types of G-E correlations have been described in the literature:[1,23] passive, evocative, and active. Passive gene-environment (G-E) correlations occur because children receive genes from the same individuals who create their family environment (unless they are adopted). Thus, the same parents who may be passing down genes that influence liability to eating disorders may also be modeling eating disordered behaviors (eg, restriction, compulsive exercise) and attitudes (eg, body dissatisfaction, drive for thinness) to their children. Children in these circumstances could be receiving a "double-dose" of eating disorder risk, as a result of both genetic and environmental exposures.

G-E correlations may also be evocative or evoked by the individual with a genetic predisposition to a given disorder.[1] For example, an individual with a genetic predisposition to an eating disorder may disproportionately seek out appearance-related comments from parents or peers. These comments may be positive or negative; what is particularly important about them is that they reinforce the individual's tendency to overvalue appearance and may promote the initiation or maintenance of eating disordered behaviors. Therefore, for example, a young girl who is dissatisfied with her body may constantly ask her parents for reassurance that she does not look fat. The resultant environment may seem very appearance focused, but that emphasis may actually be evoked by this reassurance-seeking behavior.

Finally, active G-E correlations occur when an individual with genetic vulnerability to an eating disorder seeks out environments that reinforce a strong emphasis on appearance, such as modeling or gymnastics.[1] Thus, the preponderance of disordered eating in ballet companies (eg, references [24,25]) may not only be caused by the influence of ballet on disordered eating, but may also reflect the fact that individuals prone to eating disorders select themselves into that high-risk environment.

A second type of G-E interplay is gene × environment (G × E) interaction. Unlike r_{GE}, in which an individual's genotype influences the *likelihood of exposure* to environmental risk factors, G × E interaction occurs when an individual's genotype influences his or her *vulnerability or response to environmental risk factors*.[26,27] For example, the influence of a weight-preoccupied coach on the eating disordered behaviors of the athletes he or she coaches is likely to vary as a function of the athletes' genotype.

The analysis of G–E interplay is complex, and as Klump and colleagues[23] have noted, our ability to unravel the nature of G × E interplay will be enhanced once we have identified true risk alleles for eating disorders. Ultimately, genetic research may prove to be the key to unlocking our understanding of environmental risk factors for eating disorders by helping us enhance our specificity in identifying *which risk factors* affect *which individuals*, resulting in *which eating disordered behaviors*.

Although genetic research in eating disorders is frankly in its infancy, patients, families, and clinicians are aware of this research and face challenges in incorporating this knowledge into either their personal conceptions of their (or their family member's) illness, or in the case of clinicians, helping patients and their families to understand the implications of this knowledge. Simplistic nature versus nurture dichotomies are easy to understand, yet rarely capture the complexity of reality and definitely fail to do so in the case of eating disorders. Clinicians and researchers must become educated in the nuances of G × E interplay and avoid perpetuating purely environmental or purely genetic conceptualizations of eating disorder etiology.[23]

Many excellent reviews of environmental risk factors[17,18,28,29] for eating disorders and genetic influences on eating disorders[14–16] exist. The interested reader is directed to those sources for comprehensive treatments of each. In this article, the authors do not duplicate these excellent efforts, but highlight what is known about risk factors for eating disorders within the conceptual framework of gene and environment interplay. In addition, the authors discuss the clinical implications of these correlations and interactions, including ways of incorporating this knowledge into practice and directions for future treatment and prevention efforts.

A PLAUSIBLE SCENARIO OF HOW GENES MIGHT INFLUENCE EATING DISORDERS

A question commonly posed by clinicians, families, and patients alike is, how do genes work in influencing risk for eating disorders? The lay conception of genetics tends to overemphasize the deterministic aspect of genetic risk. Modeled after mendelian 1 gene–1 disorder examples (eg, Huntington's chorea), the misperception emerges that there is 1 gene for anorexia nervosa and if you have that gene you are destined to develop the condition. Clinicians are well positioned to dispel these myths and offer more realistic, albeit complicated, explanations for complex inheritance patterns. By definition, eating disorders are complex traits. That means that their inheritance pattern in families does not follow traditional mendelian patterns, and that they are influenced by multiple genetic and environmental factors of small to moderate effect. There is not 1 gene for anorexia nervosa or 1 gene for bulimia nervosa. More likely there are several genes that code for proteins that influence traits that index vulnerability to these disorders. Complicating the risk picture even further, these genes exist in concert with other genetic factors that may confer protection against eating disorders, along with main effects of risk and protective environments, and G × E interplay as discussed in the following section.

INTEGRATING RISK FACTOR RESEARCH WITH A GENETIC EPIDEMIOLOGIC PERSPECTIVE ON EATING DISORDERS
Gene-Environment Relationships Potentially Influencing Eating Disorder Etiology

For decades, parenting styles have been unrightfully blamed for causing eating disorders. Considerable care must be taken when discussing G × E interplay not to convey the message that somehow parenting is to blame for these pernicious illnesses. Conversely, a purely genetic explanation should not be taken to mean that parents need not examine their parenting style and the influence it might have on their children. The context for the following discussion is that parenting does matter. Moreover, parenting style is in part influenced by the parents' genes, and the effect of parenting style is similarly influenced by the offsprings' genotype. For an example outside of the eating disorders world, alcoholism has a known genetic component. An alcoholic father's erratic and authoritarian parenting is in part influenced by his genetic predisposition to alcoholism. His 2 children may be differentially influenced by that parenting style owing to their own genetically influenced constitution—one may be vulnerable and sensitive to rejection and verbal abuse whereas the other may remain effectively impervious to rejecting parenting. The authors now explore some of the identified risk factors for eating disorders through this complex lens.

Parental role modeling of eating disordered behavior

In the clinic, it is not uncommon to see either frank eating disorders or shadows of disordered eating, appearance focus, exercise obsession, body preoccupation, or personality traits associated with eating disorders, such as perfectionism or obsessionality in parents of individuals with eating disorders. Of course, this is not always the case, and there are many examples of families in which these traits are not evident. Through their relationships with food and their own bodies, parental role modeling of unhealthy eating behaviors and attitudes likely represents an example of passive G-E correlation. The literature suggests that such modeling has an effect on offspring, as case studies indicate that children indeed imitate their mothers' purging and restricting behaviors.[30–32] Studies conducted in non–treatment-seeking samples have found similarities between mothers' and daughters' restraint and dieting behaviors among children as young as 10-years old.[33] Mothers' comments about their own weight and appearance are associated with the body esteem of their fourth and fifth grade daughters and sons,[34] and mothers who complain about their own weight are more likely to have daughters who are weight concerned. Moreover, maternal drive for thinness and restraint are associated with the development of overeating behaviors among children in their first 5 years of life.[35] Thus, although not solely causal, the principle of children being more likely to "do as you do" rather than "do as you say" renders parental role modeling of healthy eating and weight behaviors important to the task of creating a protective environment—especially in genetically vulnerable offspring.

Problematic feeding behaviors

A second area where parental genotype and environment intersect dramatically is in the feeding behaviors of children. Mothers tend to retain primary responsibility for nurturing their offspring. For most mothers this is a joyous part of motherhood; however, for women with eating disorders this can represent an emotionally charged and highly challenging part of the job. Clinicians working with mothers with eating disorders should be keenly aware of the potential difficulties they may encounter in what should be this very natural mother–child interaction. Studies have shown that mothers with eating disorders are more likely to use food for nonnutritive purposes, such as rewarding, comforting, or punishing their children.[36,37] One retrospective study found that adults whose parents used food in this manner were more likely to exhibit disordered eating behaviors than those who did not recall such parenting behaviors, even when factors, such as current body mass index (BMI), childhood weight status, ethnicity, and age, were controlled.[38]

Mothers' own eating restraint and disinhibition also appear to influence their approach to feeding their children. In 2 studies of 5-year-old girls, mothers' restraint and weight concerns were positively associated with the degree of restriction they imposed on their daughters' eating.[39,40] Maternal disinhibition of eating was also related to children's eating behavior. For example, Johnson and Birch[41] found that parental disinhibition was inversely associated with children's ability to self-regulate energy intake. For both sexes, a tendency to overeat in the presence of food-related cues may be transmitted across generations.

Parental overemphasis on child weight and shape

In addition to having concerns about their own shape and weight, women with eating disorders may similarly be overconcerned about their children's weight, even when it is well within normal limits.[30,36,37] One study[36] found that 15% of mothers with a history of bulimia nervosa had attempted to "slim down" their normal weight infants. Similarly, Waugh and Bulik[42] found that 20% of the mothers with eating disorder histories in their sample tried to change their children's appearance. Maternal restriction of children's eating is a concern, as previous research[41] suggests that maternal control of children's eating interferes with the development of dietary self-regulation. These effects have been found among children as young as 2 years of age.[41]

In another example of how genes and environment may interact, mothers' disordered eating attitudes appear to influence their perceptions of their children's appearance. For example, Stein and colleagues[43] found that mothers' satisfaction with their children's size was inversely related to the severity of their own eating disorder symptomatology. Further, other research has found that mothers' comments about their children's weight were associated with children's body esteem and the frequency of children's weight loss attempts.[44]

The influence of maternal perceptions on daughters' eating disordered behavior seems to continue into adolescence and young adulthood. For example, mothers whose daughters engaged in eating disordered behavior were more likely to view their daughters as overweight[45,46] than were mothers of non-eating disordered daughters (controlling for weight differences between groups). Further, this appearance pressure is not necessarily limited to weight, as mothers of daughters with eating disorder symptomatology also rated their daughters as less attractive than the daughters rated themselves.[46] These results are concerning, as they suggest that daughters who engage in eating disordered behaviors may not only lack a maternal role model of healthy eating, but also feel maternal pressure to lose weight and enhance their appearance. This of course could reflect several complex intergenerational processes. On one hand, mothers may harbor threshold or subthreshold eating disturbances themselves, and their comments or behaviors could reflect their underlying pathology. Alternatively or complementarily, the daughters' pathology could render them more sensitive to maternal comments that in other situations may be perceived as culturally normative. These environmental experiences could facilitate the expression of an existing genetic predisposition for eating disorder symptomatology.

Life events and distress tolerance

Historically, research on parenting and its relation to eating disorders has focused on family/parent characteristics, an important component of which is termed "shared environment" in twin research. Shared environment refers to those familial experiences that act to increase similarity amongst family members. However, genetic epidemiologic research has suggested that most of the environmental variance in eating disordered symptomatology is influenced by "unique environment" or environmental factors experienced by only one member of a twin pair or family.[23,47] Unique environmental influences act to increase dissimilarity amongst family members. However, even the definitions and existence of shared and unique environmental factors are disputed. For example, adverse life events, such as abuse experiences to which only 1 member of a twin pair was subjected, might exemplify unique environmental factors salient to the development of an eating disorder. Yet, it has been posited that the frequency and intensity of defining unique environmental events[48] and the impact of these unique life experiences are at least partially under genetic control.[49] For example, Klump and colleagues[23] (p123) stated, "Genetic differences … may provide the mechanisms by which nonshared environment exerts its influence." Thus, it seems appropriate to review research on adverse life events and their association with eating disorder etiology from a genetic epidemiologic perspective.

As noted above, adverse life events may be one significant way in which the unique environment can act to increase eating disorder risk. The association between negative life events and the onset of eating disorders has received significant clinical and research attention.[23,50–52] However, as Schmidt and colleagues[51] have noted, most of the studies in this area have used case reports to identify life events and did not include non-eating disordered comparison groups. However, 1 case–control study[52] found that some adverse experiences were more common among women with bulimia nervosa in the year before illness onset (eg, a major move, illness, pregnancy, physical abuse, and sexual abuse). Further, the more life events an individual experienced in the last year, the more likely she was to have bulimia nervosa. However, the frequency of several other life events (eg, bereavement, illness of a close relative, friend or partner, and beginning or end of a new romantic relationship) did not differentiate women with and without the disorder. In addition, nearly one-third of women with bulimia nervosa did not experience any of the life events assessed in the previous year. Thus, although there seems to be some association between experiences of adverse life events and bulimia onset, there is also significant variability among affected individuals with respect to recent experiences.

The impact of recent life events on the development of BED was investigated by Pike and colleagues[50] using a case–control sample. Women with BED experienced more adverse life events in the year before the onset of their eating disorder (than nonclinical and psychiatric controls), and the likelihood of BED was positively associated with the frequency of negative events. Compared with both the nonclinical and psychiatric control groups, women with BED more frequently reported major changes in life circumstances and relationships. Physical abuse, perceived risk for physical abuse, safety concerns, stress, and experiences of weight- and shape-related criticism were also more common in the BED group (versus nonclinical controls).

The impact of stressful life events is obviously at least partially dependent on how individuals perceive or think about these experiences, and how they attempt to cope with them. Thus, studies on the impact of life events on eating disorder etiology should also be considered in light of the significant body of research supporting the influence of cognitive appraisal on psychologic outcomes.[53,54] According to appraisal theory, the impact of life events depends on how they are appraised by the individual.[53,54] The appraisal process involves both determining if a given situation is threatening to the individual (primary appraisal) and if so, evaluating whether his/her resources are sufficient to manage this threat (secondary appraisal). It seems plausible that both genetically influenced traits (eg, trait anxiety, fearfulness) and environmental factors (social support, socioeconomic status [SES]) would influence primary and secondary appraisal. This hypothesis is supported by the results of a twin study,[55] which found that specific coping behaviors (turning to others and problem solving) were significantly influenced by genetic factors.

Distress tolerance is another construct related to appraisal and coping processes. The degree to which a given individual possesses the ability to tolerate distress is also likely influenced by a complex combination of genetic and environmental factors. According to Corstorphine and colleagues,[56] distress tolerance is "the ability to endure and accept negative affect, so that problem-solving can take place ... [and it] manifests as high emotional vulnerability and an inability to regulate emotion". Although no extant research has investigated the heritability of the specific construct of distress tolerance, related variables, such as neuroticism, have been found to be strongly familial[57,58] and to predict the later development of anorexia nervosa.[59] Further, emotion regulation difficulties have been found in women with eating disorders of all subtypes (eg, references[60,61]). A recent study[56] found that eating disordered attitudes were associated with scores on 2 components of a distress tolerance measure: high avoidance of affect and low acceptance and management of problems.

Research in other clinical areas has indicated that distress tolerance skills can be improved with the implementation of a specific cognitive-behavioral intervention (eg, dialectical behavioral therapy [DBT] for borderline personality disorder[62]). Thus, interventions aimed at individuals at high risk for eating disorders (and thus potentially genetically prone to low distress tolerance) should perhaps include elements of DBT focusing on affect regulation and coping skills training. Thus, in this manner, an environmental intervention could directly address genetic vulnerabilities. Future studies of G-E correlations should include the construct of distress tolerance, to evaluate its interaction with life events and specific genetic vulnerabilities.

Evocative Gene-Environment Correlations Potentially Influencing Eating Disorder Etiology

Interaction of temperamental style and environment

Genes may also influence the risk for eating disorders through the way in which one's genotype evokes certain responses from the environment. For example, considerable work has explored temperamental style in individuals with eating disorders. In the current context, the authors are interested not only in how temperament may be associated with eating disorders risk, but also in the various ways that temperament influences interactions with the environment. As suggested here, personality characteristics (such as neuroticism) can make us more or less vulnerable to environmental insults; but these traits can also influence our tendency to evoke certain responses from the environment.

Recent work on temperamental factors influencing eating disorder etiology indicates that anorexia nervosa is associated with a temperamental style characterized by perfectionism, a need for order and exactness, harm avoidance, and sensitivity to praise and reward.[63–66] Bulimia nervosa shares many of these same characteristics, but commonly coupled with features of novelty seeking and impulsivity.[64,65,67] These temperamental traits have been shown to be influenced by genetic factors.[68,69] However, these temperamental characteristics also influence how individuals interface with their environment. Thus, it is plausible that individuals genetically susceptible to eating disorders owing (to some degree) to their temperament may hold themselves to extremely high standards and through their own actions, actively seek out praise or evaluation of their efforts from others. Comments evoked from others, even if positive, may in turn reinforce perfectionist tendencies, including those relevant to eating disordered behavior.

On the other hand, parents may treat even identical (or monozygotic, MZ) twins differently, which could also influence eating disorder susceptibility. For example, in a study of MZ twins discordant for bulimia nervosa, Wade and colleagues[70] found that affected twins reported higher parental expectations than their unaffected co-twins. It is not possible from this study to determine if parents actually did hold 1 twin to higher standards or if this finding reflects the retrospectively recalled experience of the affected twin. That is, the answers may reflect the affected twin's attempt to make sense of her childhood experiences and current symptomatology. Longitudinal studies are needed to clarify the role of parental expectations (both actual and perceived) in eating disorders etiology.

Teasing and weight- and shape-related criticism

Another environmental issue relevant to eating disorders risk is weight-related teasing and critical comments about weight (particularly those made by parents), which have been identified as risk factors for a range of eating disordered behaviors (eg, see references[18,50,70,71]), although not all studies have identified this association (eg, see reference[19]). The association between teasing and risk for eating disorders is unlikely to be a simple one and a complete understanding of risk mechanisms needs to consider G × E relationships.

Klump and colleagues[23] suggested that weight-related teasing may reflect an evocative G-E correlation relevant to eating disorders. For example, teasing experienced by an overweight adolescent may be in part evoked by his or her simply being overweight. Thus, in this case, a trait significantly influenced by genetic factors (ie, BMI) influences the comments an individual is exposed to in the environment.

Another possible way in which genetic and environmental factors may interact to influence teasing-related risk is that teasing experiences may be appraised more negatively among individuals with different genetically influenced temperaments. Individuals genetically predisposed to eating disorders and neuroticism, for example, may be particularly prone to ruminate about weight-related teasing or critical comments about weight, thereby exacerbating the negative effects of these occurrences. Supporting this observation, clinicians report that many individuals with eating disorders recall triggering events that prompted their eating disorder. Although highly salient and even defining to these individuals, many of these events fall within normative experience and could easily be brushed off by individuals less sensitive to their salience. As in the case with the overweight teen mentioned earlier eliciting comments about weight, it is also possible that individuals genetically vulnerable to eating disorders may elicit comments about their appearance through their frequent seeking of reassurance (and these comments may, in some cases, be critical). These evoked responses may reinforce their eating disordered tendencies or behaviors.

Further, it should also be considered that, as noted above, even MZ twins may be treated differently by their parents, particularly with respect to appearance. Research on MZ twins discordant for anorexia and bulimia nervosa found that affected twins report receiving more critical comments regarding their weight than their non-affected co-twins.[70] As these twins are virtually identical genetically, this finding may represent a true nonshared environmental difference. Nonetheless, specific genetic vulnerabilities (eg, to a higher-than average BMI or sensitivity to praise) may still influence the etiology of eating disorders in this case. It is also possible that these findings are influenced by recall bias, as participants were not surveyed about their childhood experiences until they were already adults. Thus, perhaps affected twins were more likely to view parent comments regarding weight as salient to their current functioning.

Active Gene-Environment Correlations Potentially Influencing Eating Disorder Etiology

Media

One potential pitfall of genetic research on eating disorders is the misinterpretation that environmental factors, such as the media, do not matter. Western media's idealization of an ultrathin female body type has long been viewed as an important sociocultural risk factor for eating disorders.[72,73] However, given the ubiquity of this influence in Western cultures, other factors must influence vulnerability to the thin cultural ideal. As Bulik[1] suggests, genetically vulnerable individuals might seek out experiences, such as exposure to thin-ideal media images, which reinforce their negative body image. This hypothesis is supported by a longitudinal study that found that adolescent girls whose eating disorder symptomatology increased over a 16-month period also reported significantly greater fashion magazine reading at time 2 than time 1.[74]

Peer group selection

Similarly, individuals genetically predisposed to eating disorder symptomatology, such as thin-ideal internalization, might also actively choose to affiliate with peers who place a similar high value on weight and appearance.[23] One potential example of this form of active selection could be the decision to join a sorority (particularly for European-American women). European-American sorority members report high levels of eating disorder symptomatology, including weight preoccupation, drive for thinness, and body dissatisfaction.[75] A longitudinal study[76] found that sorority and nonsorority members did not differ on three measures of disordered eating (drive for thinness, body dissatisfaction, and bulimia) at time 1 and time 2 (first and second year of undergraduate study, respectively). However, by time 3 (third year of under-graduate study), nonmembers' drive for thinness scores had decreased, whereas members' scores on this measure remained roughly the same, and this difference was statistically significant. Thus, the investigators concluded that characteristics of the sorority environment could contribute to the persistence of a higher degree of drive for thinness. Although this study did not include a measure of actual or putative ge-netic vulnerability to eating disorders, it is plausible to speculate that an environment that promotes the maintenance of eating disordered characteristics would be partic-ularly problematic for a genetically vulnerable individual.

Potential Environmental Buffering Effects for High-Risk Groups

The authors have focused primarily on environmental risk factors and how they could plausibly interact with various facets of genetic vulnerability to increase the risk for eat-ing disorders. Given our inability to modify genetic risk at this point in time, it is critical to present a balanced picture of the environment. Just as both risk and protective genetic factors can exist, so can both risk and protective environmental factors. In addition, protective factors may function differentially depending on the genotype of the exposed individual. Given the field's focus on pathology, much less is known about differential effects of buffering environmental factors based on genetic differences.

Family meals and breakfast eating

One fascinating and modifiable environmental factor that has emerged as a possible buffer against the development of eating disorders in adolescent girls is family meals.[77] Likewise, breakfast eating may also play a role in preventing the development of eating problems. For example, Fernández-Aranda and colleagues[78] found that women with eating disorders were less likely to have eaten breakfast regularly during childhood than non-eating disordered controls. Although retrospective, these findings are consistent with those of a large (n = 2216), longitudinal study that found that breakfast-eating frequency was inversely associated with dieting and weight-control behaviors and positively related to dietary quality and physical activity in adoles-cents.[79] Overall, these studies offer preliminary insight into potential buffers against eating disorders; however, research in this area has not yet progressed to assess the differential effect of these protective factors in individuals at high risk for eating dis-orders versus the general population.

Distress tolerance/anxiety management

Another factor that offers promise as a potential buffer against the development of eating disorders is the enhancement of emotion regulation skills. As noted above, in-dividuals with eating disorders experience high levels of perceived stress and difficul-ties regulating emotion.[56,61] Thus, interventions aimed at enhancing emotion regulation skills might be of particular benefit to high-risk groups. However, research incorporating mindfulness techniques has not specifically targeted high-risk groups.

For example, a recent study investigated the effectiveness of a primary prevention program incorporating elements of mindfulness (eg, yoga), targeting fifth-grade girls.[80] This program integrated mindfulness into an empirically based curriculum, which also included other elements, such as media literacy and the promotion of dissonance regarding idealization of an ultraslim body type. Compared with a control group, girls in the intervention reported lower body dissatisfaction and uncontrolled eating and higher social self-concept at post-testing. However, there were no significant changes on other variables assessed, including drive for thinness, perceived stress, physical self-concept, and perceived competence. Nonetheless, these outcomes do provide some support for the inclusion of mindfulness-based activities in prevention. In contrast, a study with undergraduate women[81] did not find any differences between participants in a yoga program and a control group on eating disorder symptoms at post-testing. Future studies should target high-risk groups to evaluate the efficacy of mindfulness-based techniques within this specific sample.

Reducing weight- and shape-related attentional biases
Previous studies have found that individuals with eating disorders manifest attentional biases (or selective attention) toward weight- and shape-related information.[82,83] These biases are likely influenced by both genetic and environmental factors. However, a recent study[83] found that these biases were reduced in women with eating disorders following completion of a specific form of cognitive-behavioral therapy. Future research should investigate the effectiveness of incorporating some of these specific cognitive-behavioral techniques into prevention programs targeting high-risk individuals.

In summary, simplistic nature versus nurture explanations could never suffice to capture the many ways in which genes and environment may interact to influence eating disorder risk. Moreover, many of these processes are likely to be operative over time in any given individual and risk may be cumulative. The critical message for the clinician working with eating disorders is not necessarily to educate patients and parents about all potential forms of G × E interplay, but definitely to guard against simplistic explanations that lead to inaccurate conclusions and inappropriate solutions.

Clinical Implications

After reviewing the various and complex ways that genes and environment can interact and correlate, the clinician, although enlightened, will want to know how best to incorporate this knowledge into clinical practice. Given the state of the science of treatment for eating disorders—especially in the absence of any effective medications for anorexia nervosa—the question remains how best to work with the patient and family to bolster protective environmental influences, reduce evoked environmental exposures, and develop strategies in the patient to minimize the deleterious effects that sensitivity to the environment can create.

Focus on the parents
One prong in the approach to incorporating genetics into clinical work focuses on the parents of individuals with eating disorders. Whether the parents are involved in parent training, traditional family therapy, or other types of supportive interventions, they can be educated about genetic factors influencing eating disorders. A sensitive explanation that incorporates knowledge about complex genetic etiology (not the 1 gene–1 disease model) and about how genes and environment interact can serve to relieve guilt in parents who have been blamed for creating the illness in their offspring (or

alternatively erroneously assumed that their parenting was to blame). A genetic and biological explanation can help parents understand that their child's resistance is not just stubbornness or deviousness, but that in his or her recovery, their child is fighting an uphill battle against his or her biology. This knowledge can empower parents to understand and can decrease frustration. Care should be taken that parents do not transform this knowledge into a new form of guilt (ie, feeling guilty for passing on risk genes), as the roll of the genetic dice is one thing over which we have no control. Likewise, care should be taken not to allow the genetic information to impart complete absolution on parents, as parenting can always improve and positive parenting changes should also be prescribed as part of treatment. Finally, symptomatic parents should be referred for treatment. Although few data exist, clinically, it is an uphill battle for offspring to recover from an eating disorder if they are faced on a day-to-day basis with a parent who is actively suffering from the illness.

Focus on the next generation
Intervention with mothers with eating disorders can be viewed as a form of targeted prevention. Eating disorder prevention is a complicated endeavor. Although primary prevention deserves additional research attention, interventions targeting individuals at risk for developing eating disorders may be a particularly promising focus of prevention efforts.[84,85] Such intervention could serve to improve maternal efficacy and confidence in feeding their children, increase modeling of healthy eating behaviors and attitudes, decrease mothers' anxiety regarding parenting behaviors, and increase self-efficacy and confidence in general parenting skills. In the long term, this type of intervention may assist mothers with developing a healthy buffering environment, which minimizes modeling of behaviors and attitudes associated with disordered eating.

Results from focus groups[86] and clinical case studies[87] suggest that mothers with eating disorders are eager to learn about how best to care for their children, especially with respect to feeding. However, they report that the level of assistance they desire is not routinely offered by their health care providers. In one of the only published interventions conducted with this population, Stein and colleagues[88] studied 80 mothers with eating disorders and their 4- to 6-month-old infants to test whether a 13-session intervention of video-feedback treatment in conjunction with cognitive behavioral self-help was more effective than cognitive behavioral self-help alone in reducing mealtime conflict and other aspects of maternal–child interaction. Mothers in the video-feedback group exhibited significantly less conflict than control mothers and significant improvements in infant autonomy and several other interaction measures. In addition, maternal eating psychopathology was reduced across both groups. Such interventions could help break the "cycle of risk" associated with eating disorders,[16] by providing parents with useful buffering strategies.

Focus on the patient
Patients read enormous amounts about their illness and are often aware of the genetic research on eating disorders yet they struggle to understand what the data mean for them and the challenges they face every day during recovery. Helping patients to understand the genetic literature is a first step. Although they might not initially see its relevance to their situation, helping them map how disordered eating and temperamental traits track in their families by using techniques, such as labeling family trees, can provide a useful context for understanding genetic and environmental contributions to their current situation. An understanding of genetic and environmental interplay can provide them with an explanatory model for not only their illness, but also

for understanding their sensitivity to the environment. It can help provide them with the motivation to acquire skills that may help buffer them from the environment and combat their biology most effectively.

SUMMARY

Although several decades ago there was significant debate about the influence of "nature" versus "nurture" on the development of psychological traits and outcomes, it is now generally accepted that both genes and environment interact to influence personality and behavior. However, in the clinical setting, genetic influences on clients' presentation of their personal histories, including characteristics of their family-of-origin environment, their perceptions of stressful life events, and their experiences within their social network, are not generally viewed from a genetic–epidemiologic perspective. Similarly, risk factor research typically includes a broad range of individuals with varying genetic vulnerability to eating disorders. Thus, it is not possible to determine from the results of these large-scale studies *what risk factors* are particularly potent for *which individuals* with *what specific genetic vulnerability* to eating disorders. Moreover, given the low base rate of clinical eating disorders in the population,[22] it is possible that some potent environmental risk factors may be overlooked if they are not associated with eating disorder symptomatology in the general population. Thus, although genetic research has not yet progressed to a point where it can be informative for either treatment or prevention, it is time to develop interventions aimed at promoting buffering rather than predisposing environments. Such interventions could help families transform a double disadvantage into a single disadvantage. Given the current state of knowledge in the genetics and eating disorder fields, such interventions may be the best approach to reducing risks for these pernicious and devastating disorders.

REFERENCES

1. Bulik CM. Genetic and biological risk factors. In: Thompson JK, editor. Handbook of eating disorders and obesity. Hoboken (NJ): John Wiley & Sons, Inc.; 2004. p. 3–16.
2. Bulik CM. Exploring the gene-environment nexus in eating disorders. J Psychiatry Neurosci 2005;30:335–8.
3. Bulik CM, Sullivan PF, Kendler KS. Heritability of binge-eating and broadly defined bulimia nervosa. Biol Psychiatry 1998;44:1210–8.
4. Hudson JI, Pope HG, Jonas JM, et al. A controlled family study of bulimia. Psychol Med 1987;17:883–91.
5. Lilenfeld L, Kaye W, Greeno C, et al. A controlled family study of restricting anorexia and bulimia nervosa: comorbidity in probands and disorders in first-degree relatives. Arch Gen Psychiatry 1998;55:603–10.
6. Strober M, Freeman R, Lampert C, et al. Controlled family study of anorexia nervosa and bulimia nervosa: evidence of shared liability and transmission of partial syndromes. Am J Psychiatry 2000;157:393–401.
7. Kendler KS, MacLean C, Neale M, et al. The genetic epidemiology of bulimia nervosa. Am J Psychiatry 1991;148:1627–37.
8. Klump KL, Miller KB, Keel PK, et al. Genetic and environmental influences on anorexia nervosa syndromes in a population-based twin sample. Psychol Med 2001;31:737–40.

9. Wade T, Martin NG, Tiggemann M. Genetic and environmental risk factors for the weight and shape concerns characteristic of bulimia nervosa. Psychol Med 1998; 28:761–71.

10. Wade TD, Bulik CM, Neale M, et al. Anorexia nervosa and major depression: shared genetic and environmental risk factors. Am J Psychiatry 2000;157: 469–71.

11. Hudson JI, Lalonde JK, Berry JM, et al. Binge-eating disorder as a distinct familial phenotype in obese individuals. Arch Gen Psychiatry 2006;63:313–9.

12. Javaras KN, Laird NM, Reichborn-Kjennerud T, et al. Familiality and heritability of binge eating disorder: results of a case-control family study and a twin study. Int J Eat Disord 2008;41:174.

13. Reichborn-Kjennerud T, Bulik CM, Kendler KS, et al. Gender differences in binge-eating: a population-based twin study. Acta Psychiatr Scand 2003;108:196–202.

14. Bulik CM, Slof-Op't Landt MC, van Furth EF, et al. The genetics of anorexia nervosa. Annu Rev Nutr 2007;27:263–75.

15. Hinney A, Friedel S, Remschmidt H, et al. Genetic risk factors in eating disorders. Am J Pharmacogenomics 2004;4:209–33.

16. Slof-Op 't Landt MC, VanFurth EF, Meulenbelt I, et al. Eating disorders: from twin studies to candidate genes and beyond. Twin Res Hum Genet 2005;8:467–82.

17. Jacobi C, Hayward C, de Zwaan M, et al. Coming to terms with risk factors for eating disorder: application of risk terminology and suggestions for a general taxonomy. Psychol Bull 2004;130:19–65.

18. Neumark-Sztainer DR, Wall MM, Haines JI, et al. Shared risk and protective factors for overweight and disordered eating in adolescents. Am J Prev Med 2007;33:359–69.

19. Stice E, Whitenton K. Risk factors for body dissatisfaction in adolescent girls: a longitudinal investigation. Dev Psychol 2002;38:669–78.

20. Stice E, Spangler D, Agras WS. Exposure to media-portrayed thin-ideal images adversely affects vulnerable girls: a longitudinal experiment. J Soc Clin Psychol 2001;20:270–88.

21. Striegel-Moore RH, Silberstein LR, Rodin J. Toward an understanding of risk factors for bulimia. Am Psychol 1986;41:246–63.

22. Hudson JI, Hiripi E, Pope HG Jr, et al. The prevalence and correlates of eating disorders in the National Comorbidity Survey Replication. Biol Psychiatry 2007; 61:348–58.

23. Klump KL, Wonderlich S, Lehoux P, et al. Does environment matter? A review of nonshared environment and eating disorders. Int J Eat Disord 2002;31:118.

24. Ringham R, Klump K, Kaye W, et al. Eating disorder symptomatology among ballet dancers. Int J Eat Disord 2006;39:503–8.

25. Thomas JJ, Keel PK, Heatherton TF. Disordered eating attitudes and behaviors in ballet students: examination of environmental and individual risk factors. Int J Eat Disord 2005;38:263–8.

26. Hardin E, Adinoff B. Family history of alcoholism does not influence adrenocortical hyporesponsiveness in abstinent alcohol-dependent men. Am J Drug Alcohol Abuse 2008;34:151–60.

27. Johnson W. Genetic and environmental influences on behavior: capturing all the interplay. Psychol Rev 2007;114:423–40.

28. Polivy J, Herman CP. Causes of eating disorders. Annu Rev Psychol 2002;53: 187–213.

29. Stice E. Risk and maintenance factors for eating pathology: a meta-analytic review. Psychol Bull 2002;128:825–48.

30. Russell GFM, Treasure J, Eisler I. Mothers with anorexia who underfeed their children: their recognition and management. Psychol Med 1998;28:93–108.
31. Franzen U, Gerlinghoff M. Parenting by patients with eating disorders: experiences with a mother-child group. Eat Disord 1997;5:5–14.
32. Timini S, Robinson P. Disturbances in children of patients with eating disorders. Eur Eat Disord Rev 1996;4:183–8.
33. Hill AJ, Weaver C, Blundell JE. Dieting concerns of 10-year old girls and their mothers. Br J Clin Psychol 1990;29:346–8.
34. Smolak L, Levine MP, Schermer F. Parental input and weight concerns among elementary school children. Int J Eat Disord 1999;25:263–71.
35. Stice E, Agras WS, Hammer LD. Risk factors for the emergence of childhood eating disturbances: a five-year prospective study. Int J Eat Disord 1999;25:375–87.
36. Lacey JH, Smith G. Bulimia nervosa: the impact of pregnancy on mother and baby. Br J Psychiatry 1987;150:777–81.
37. Agras S, Hammer L, McNicholas F. A prospective study of the influence of eating-disordered mothers on their children. Int J Eat Disord 1999;25:253–63.
38. Puhl RM, Schwartz MB. If you are good you can have a cookie: how memories of childhood food rules link to adult eating behaviors. Eat Behav 2003;4:283–93.
39. Francis LA, Hofer SM, Birch LL. Predictors of maternal-child feeding style: maternal and child characteristics. Appetite 2001;37:231–43.
40. Birch LL, Fisher JO. Mothers' child-feeding practices influence daughters' eating and weight. Am J Clin Nutr 2000;71:1054–61.
41. Johnson SL, Birch LL. Parents' and children's adiposity and eating style. Pediatrics 1994;94:653–61.
42. Waugh E, Bulik CM. Offspring of women with eating disorders. Int J Eat Disord 1999;25:123–33.
43. Stein A, Murray L, Cooper P, et al. Infant growth in the context of maternal eating disorders and maternal depression: a comparative study. Psychol Med 1996;26: 569–74.
44. Striegel-Moore RH, Kearney-Cooke A. Exploring parents' attitudes and behaviors about their children's physical appearance. Int J Eat Disord 1994;15:377–85.
45. Moreno A, Thelen MH. Parental factors related to bulimia nervosa. Addict Behav 1993;18:681–9.
46. Pike KM, Rodin J. Mothers, daughters, and disordered eating. J Abnorm Psychol 1991;100:198–204.
47. Bulik CM, Sullivan PF, Wade TD, et al. Twin studies of eating disorders: a review. Int J Eat Disord 2000;27:1–20.
48. Bolinskey P, Neale MC, Jacobson KC, et al. Sources of individual differences in stressful life event exposure in male and female twins. Twin Res 2004;7:33–8.
49. Kendler KS, Karkowski-Shuman L. Stressful life events and genetic liability to major depression: genetic control of exposure to the environment? Psychol Med 1997;27:539–47.
50. Pike KM, Wilfley D, Hilbert A, et al. Antecedent life events of binge-eating disorder. Psychiatry Res 2006;142:19–29.
51. Schmidt UH, Troop N, Treasure JL. Events and the onset of eating disorders: correcting an "age old" myth. Int J Eat Disord 1999;25:83–8.
52. Welch S, Doll H, Fairburn C. Life events and the onset of bulimia nervosa: a controlled study. Psychol Med 1997;27:515–22.
53. Folkman S, Lazarus RS, Dunkel-Schetter C, et al. Dynamics of a stressful encounter: cognitive appraisal, coping, and encounter outcomes. J Pers Soc Psychol 1986; 50:992–1003.

54. Folkman S, Lazarus RS, Gruen RJ, et al. Appraisal, coping, health status, and psychological symptoms. J Pers Soc Psychol 1986;50:571–9.

55. Kendler K, Kessler R, Heath A, et al. Coping: a genetic epidemiological investigation. Psychol Med 1991;21:337–46.

56. Corstorphine E, Mountford V, Tomlinson S, et al. Distress tolerance in the eating disorders. Eat Behav 2007;8:91–7.

57. Flint J. The genetic basis of neuroticism. Neurosci Biobehav Rev 2004;28:307–16.

58. Fullerton J, Cubin M, Tiwari H, et al. Linkage analysis of extremely discordant and concordant sibling pairs identifies quantitative-trait loci that influence variation in the human personality trait neuroticism. Am J Hum Genet 2003;72:879–90.

59. Bulik CM, Sullivan PF, Tozzi F, et al. Prevalence, heritability, and prospective risk factors for anorexia nervosa. Arch Gen Psychiatry 2006;63:305–12.

60. Heatherton TF, Baumeister RF. Binge eating as escape from self-awareness. Psychol Bull 1991;110:86–108.

61. deZwaan M, Biener D, Bach M, et al. Pain sensitivity, alexithymia, and depression in patients with eating disorders: are they related? J Psychosom Res 1996;41:65–70.

62. Linehan M. Cognitive-behavioural treatment of borderline personality disorders. New York: Guilford; 1993.

63. Cassin S, von Ranson KM. Personality and eating disorders: a decade in review. Clin Psychol Rev 2005;25:895–916.

64. Fassino S, Abbate-Daga G, Amianto F, et al. Temperament and character profile of eating disorders: a controlled study with the Temperament and Character Inventory. Int J Eat Disord 2002;32:412–25.

65. Klump KL, Strober M, Bulik CM, et al. Personality characteristics of women before and after recovery from an eating disorder. Psychol Med 2004;34:1407–18.

66. Wade T, Tiggemann M, Bulik C, et al. Shared temperament risk factors for anorexia nervosa: a twin study. Psychosom Med 2008;70:239–44.

67. Bulik C, Sullivan PF, Joyce PR, et al. Temperament, character, and personality disorder in bulimia nervosa. J Nerv Ment Dis 1995;183:593–8.

68. Goldsmith H, Buss K, Lemery K. Toddler and childhood temperament: expanded content, stronger genetic evidence, new evidence for the importance of environment. Dev Psychol 1997;33:891–905.

69. Saudino K. Behavioral genetics and child temperament. J Dev Behav Pediatr 2005;26:214–23.

70. Wade T, Gillespie N, Martin NG. A comparison of early family life events amongst monozygotic twin women with lifetime anorexia nervosa, bulimia nervosa, or major depression. Int J Eat Disord 2007;40:679–286

71. Fairburn C, Doll HA, Welch SL, et al. Risk factors for binge eating disorder: a community-based, case-control study. Arch Gen Psychiatry 1998;55:425–32.

72. Levine M, Harrison K. Media's role in the perpetuation and prevention of negative body image and disordered eating. In: Thompson JK, editor. Handbook of eating disorders and obesity. Hoboken (NJ): John Wiley & Sons, Inc; 2004. p. 695–717.

73. Stice E, Schupak-Neuberg E, Shaw H, et al. Relation of media exposure to eating disorder symptomatology: an examination of mediating mechanisms. J Abnorm Psychol 1994;103:836–40.

74. Vaughn K, Fouts G. Changes in television and magazine exposure and eating disorder symptomatology. Sex Roles 2003;49:313–20.

75. Schulken E, Pinciaro PJ, Sawyer RG, et al. Sorority women's body size perceptions and their weight-related attitudes and behaviors. J Am Coll Health 1997;46:69–74.

76. Allison KC, Park CL. A prospective study of disordered eating among sorority and nonsorority women. Int J Eat Disord 2004;35:354–8.
77. Neumark-Sztainer D, Eisenberg ME, Fulkerson JA, et al. Family meals and disordered eating in adolescents: longitudinal findings from project EAT. Arch Pediatr Adolesc Med 2008;162:17–22.
78. Fernández-Aranda F, Krug I, Granero R, et al. Individual and family eating patterns during childhood and early adolescence: an analysis of associated eating disorder factors. Appetite 2007;49:476–85.
79. Timlin M, Pereira MA, Story M, et al. Breakfast eating and weight change in a 5-year prospective analysis of adolescents: Project EAT (Eating Among Teens). Pediatrics 2008;121:e638–45.
80. Scime M, Cook-Cottone C. Primary prevention of eating disorders: a constructivist integration of mind and body strategies. Int J Eat Disord 2008;41:134–42.
81. Mitchell K, Mazzeo S, Rausch S, et al. Innovative interventions for disordered eating: evaluating dissonance-based and yoga interventions. Int J Eat Disord 2007; 40:120–8.
82. Dobson K, Dozois D. Attentional biases in eating disorders: a meta-analytic review of Stroop performance. Clin Psychol Rev 2004;23:1001–22.
83. Shafran R, Lee M, Cooper Z, et al. Effect of psychological treatment on attentional bias in eating disorders. Int J Eat Disord 2008;41:348–54.
84. Pearson J, Goldklang D, Streigel-Moore R. Prevention of eating disorders: challenges and opportunities. Int J Eat Disord 2002;31:233–9.
85. Mann T, Nolen-Hoeksema S, Huang K, et al. Are two interventions worse than none? Joint primary and secondary prevention of eating disorders in college females. Health Psychol 1997;16:215–25.
86. Mazzeo SE, Zucker NL, Gerke CK, et al. Parenting concerns of women with a history of eating disorders: development of a targeted intervention. Int J Eat Disord 2005;37:S77–9.
87. Hodes M, Timini S, Robinson P. Children of mothers with eating disorders: a preliminary study. Eur Eat Disord Rev 1997;5:11–24.
88. Stein A, Woolley H, Senior R, et al. Treating disturbances in the relationship between mothers with bulimic eating disorders and their infants: a randomized, controlled trial of video feedback. Am J Psychiatry 2006;163:899–906.

Environmental and Genetic Risk Factors in Obesity

Johannes Hebebrand, MD*, Anke Hinney, PhD

KEYWORDS

- Monogenic • Polygenic • Socioeconomic status • Television

Over the past 100 years, the etiology of childhood obesity has been perceived differently; the pendulum has swung from biological to psychological explanations and back. In the beginning of the 20th century, dysfunction of the pituitary/hypothalamic system was assumed to underlie obesity.[1] Later, from the 1940s through the 1970s, psychological and psychodynamic aspects were thought to play the most prominent role.[2,3] In 1956 Prader, Labhart, and Willi delineated the first syndromal form of obesity. As of the 1970s the relevance of (psycho)social factors has been discussed.[4–7] At the end of the 1980s and 1990s milestone twin and adoption studies substantiated that genetic factors play a prominent role in body weight regulation.[8–10]

The cloning of the leptin gene in 1994[11] led to a virtual explosion of biomedical research and marked the introduction of large-scale molecular genetic studies. The detection of leptin deficiency[12] in children and successful treatment with recombinant leptin[13] for the first time proved that mutations in a single gene can lead to hyperphagia and obesity in individuals of normal intelligence. Genetic, biological, physiologic, and pharmacologic research over the past 15 years has tremendously broadened our understanding of the mechanisms involved in body weight regulation. It has become evident that body weight is tightly regulated by way of peripheral and central mechanisms; numerous hormones, including leptin and ghrelin, anorexigenic and orexigenic neuropeptides, their respective receptors, and intracellular signaling pathways, underlie this regulation.[14,15] One of the main functions of these pathways is to enable adaptation to semi-starvation (see the article by Müller and colleagues, elsewhere in this issue).

The most recent years have viewed a strengthening of the hypothesis that obesity is a neuroendocrine and metabolic disorder, which results if "obesogenic" environmental factors and a polygenic predisposition act in concert. Put simplistically, "the genetic background loads the gun, but the environment pulls the trigger."[16] The genetic predisposition is thought to affect metabolic and behavioral features. Obesity

---

Department of Child and Adolescent Psychiatry, Rheinische Kliniken Essen, University of Duisburg-Essen, Virchowstr, 174, D-45147 Essen, Germany
* Corresponding author.
E-mail address: Johannes.Hebebrand@uni-duisburg-essen.de (J. Hebebrand).

Child Adolesc Psychiatric Clin N Am 18 (2008) 83–94
doi:10.1016/j.chc.2008.07.006
1056-4993/08/$ – see front matter © 2008 Elsevier Inc. All rights reserved.

is thus a truly complex disorder that is caused by several genetic and nongenetic risk factors.

Public interest in obesity has also witnessed an unparalleled boom over the past 20 years—reflecting the obesity epidemic, the discovery of novel pathways involved in body weight regulation, greater health concerns, the perception of social inequality, and a stronger awareness of the societal norms for body weight.

FORMAL GENETIC ASPECTS

There is a general consensus that parental obesity is by far the strongest risk factor for childhood and adolescent obesity. The degree of parental obesity influences this risk, which is further elevated if both parents are obese.[17,18] According to several studies, offspring BMI is somewhat more strongly correlated with maternal than paternal BMI,[19] suggesting intrauterine influences, imprinting effects, an influence of mitochondrial genes, or a rearing effect. Formal genetic studies have led to the conclusion that the strong predictive value of the parental BMI mainly stems from genetic rather than environmental factors.[20] Accordingly, older studies that failed to include parental weight as a variable are seriously flawed. For example, the well-known finding that parental neglect during childhood predicts obesity in young adulthood[5] was not controlled for parental obesity.

Twin studies have produced the most consistent and highest heritability estimates, in the range of 0.6 to 0.9 for BMI.[20,21] These high estimates apply to both twins reared together or apart. However, only single and comparatively small studies exist for twins reared apart, in contrast to the vast amount of studies pertaining to twins reared together, some of which included thousands of twin pairs. Additionally, a substantial number of reared-apart twin pairs were not separated immediately after birth.

Except for the newborn period, for which a lower heritability (approximately 0.4) has been calculated,[22] age does not affect heritability estimates of body weight to a substantial degree. The influence of the intrauterine environment on birth weight is strong; it is well known that particularly in monozygotic (MZ) twins, other anthropometric measurements, such as body height, also correlate less well in infancy. Genetic factors are subsequently able to exert their influence; in school-aged children, high heritability of BMI already applies. Possibly, the heritability of BMI is maximal (≈ 0.9) during late childhood and adolescence.[23]

Adoption and family studies have mostly derived considerably lower heritability estimates for BMI ranging from 0.25 to 0.7.[20,24] Twin studies have the advantage of a better control for age effects on BMI. They are more valid if non-additive genetic factors play a relevant role in body weight regulation. It is worth pointing out that direct and indirect genetic effects are subsumed under the genetic component. If for example infant twins of an MZ pair are frequently irritable because of a biologically driven hunger (direct genetic effect), frequent feedings by the caretaker ensue (indirect genetic effect); even if the twins are separated at birth, the respective caretakers can be expected to respond similarly.

Another interesting and important aspect of formal genetic studies has been the frequent observation that non-shared environment explains considerably more variance of the quantitative phenotype (BMI) than shared environment. In the large twin study of Stunkard and coworkers,[10] which comprised adult twin pairs reared together or apart, shared environment did not explain variance at all; instead non-shared environment totally explained the environmental component (approximately 30%). Accordingly, only genetic factors would account for a familial loading with obesity. However, studies that are more recent indicate that the shared environment might play a more substantial role after all, particularly in school-aged children.[24] Past research may have underestimated common environmental effects on BMI because the designs lacked the power or ability to detect them. Finally, the environment of modern day societies (easy access to a large variety of cheap and tasty foods, a lifestyle promoting physical inactivity) is quite similar for all children, irrespective of the family in which they grow up.

The complexity of the genetic basis of obesity applies from different perspectives:[24] Metabolic phenotypes, including resting energy expenditure, are partially under genetic control.[25] Behavioral genetic research has convincingly demonstrated that approximately 50% of the variance of diverse complex quantitative behaviors is genetically determined.[26] Macronutrient intake[27] and activity levels[28] have been shown to be genetically codetermined. For restrained eating, drive for thinness, and other eating behaviors, heritability estimates range from 20% to 55%.[24] It seems that TV viewing may also have a heritable component, albeit a small one.[29]

Because the gene pool of a population cannot have changed within the past generation, environmental changes affecting energy intake and expenditure are assumed to underlie the obesity epidemic.[30] These changes are presumed to have a major impact because, according to the thrifty genotype hypothesis,[31] many common genotypes render humans obesity prone. Gene variants facilitating energy deposition as fat have accumulated over time in different species to enhance survival during periods of famine.

A small genetic contribution to the obesity epidemic cannot be dismissed. For one, overweight women have more children.[32] Secondly, the recent increase in social stigmatization (Hebebrand and colleagues, this issue) of obese individuals might actually have led to an increase in assortative mating.[21] This mechanism could conceivably contribute to epidemic obesity, particularly by affecting the uppermost tail of the BMI distribution through genetic and environmental factors.

Epigenetic phenomena have also been invoked to contribute to the obesity epidemic. Indeed, it is conceivable that modern-day living might affect methylation patterns of specific genes, which in turn increase the risk for obesity. In line with these considerations young monozygous twins are epigenetically indistinguishable from each other during the early years of life, whereas remarkable differences in their overall content and genomic distribution of 5-methylcytosine DNA and histone acetylation with an effect on gene expression become evident with increasing age.[33] Such environmentally induced changes could have an influence on BMI. However, the contribution of epigenetic factors to human obesity has not been proven as of today.

MOLECULAR GENETIC FINDINGS
Syndromal Obesity

The Prader–Willi syndrome (PWS) is caused by the deficiency of one or more paternally expressed imprinted transcripts within chromosome 15q11-q13, including SNURF-SNRPN and multiple small nucleolar RNAs (snoRNAs). Recently, a microdeletion of the HBII-85 snoRNAs in a child with the typical features of the PWS provided conclusive evidence that deficiency of HBII-85 snoRNAs causes the key characteristics of the PWS phenotype.[34] The pleiotropic Bardet–Biedel syndrome, of which obesity is a feature, has been shown to have an oligogenic basis.[35]

Monogenic Obesity

Over the past 15 years, mutations in the genes for leptin, leptin receptor, prohormone convertase 1 (PC1), and pro-opiomelanocortin (POMC)[24,35] have been shown to lead to autosomal recessive forms of obesity in humans. All of these mutations are rare and lead to early-onset extreme obesity induced by an increased energy intake. Additional phenotypic manifestations, including adrenal insufficiency (POMC), red hair (POMC), reduced or impaired fertility (PC1, leptin, and leptin receptor), and impaired immunity (leptin), are observed in the mutation carriers.

As of 1998, over 90 functionally relevant mutations have been detected in the melanocortin-4 receptor gene (MC4R),[36] which result in a codominantly inherited form of obesity. About 2% to 6% of extremely obese children and adolescents harbor such mutations. Relevant mutations lead to a reduced or total loss of receptor function; the endogenous ligand α-melanocyte stimulating hormone (α-MSH) is not able to induce its satiating effect. Adult male and female mutation carriers are 15 and 30 kg heavier than their sex-matched wild-type relatives;[37] estimates for children are not available. The effect sizes of these mutations are lower than those of the leptin or leptin receptor gene mutations. Phenotypic effects of MC4R mutations other than obesity have been shown to encompass hyperinsulinemia, elevated growth rate, and higher bone density.[38] In contrast to the original report,[39] MC4R mutations seemingly do not induce binge eating.[40,41] Children with MC4R mutations have been shown to eat more at a test meal than obese controls.[38]

Polygenic Obesity

A large number of association and linkage studies have been performed in "normal" obesity.[24] Whereas many associations have been reported, it is largely unclear which of these represent truly positive findings. Presumably, the power of many of these studies is too low to detect minor genes; false-positive findings can result from a lack of correction for multiple testing. More than 40 genome-wide linkage scans pertaining to obesity and related phenotypes have been performed; as yet unequivocal evidence for the contribution of a specific gene to one of these peaks has not been provided. The region on chromosome 16 harboring the currently most relevant polygene FTO ("fat mass and obesity associated" gene, see later discussion) was detected in a meta-analysis of 37 genome-wide linkage studies comprising data on more than 31,000 individuals from over 10,000 families. However, the combined analysis of these genome-wide linkage studies revealed that despite having substantial statistical power, specific chromosomal regions for BMI or obesity were not unequivocally detected.[42] This most likely indicates that the effect sizes of genes influencing adiposity are small to very small, and, in addition, suggests substantial genetic heterogeneity and variable dependence on environmental factors.

Presumably, the effect sizes of most gene variants predisposing to obesity are small (polygenic inheritance). The MC4R can also be considered as a polygene: The minor alleles of the 2 (Val103Ile = rs2229616; Ile251Leu) MC4R polymorphisms are negatively associated with obesity.[43–46] Adult carriers of the minor alleles are on average 0.5 kg/m^2 less heavy than wild-type carriers; the Ile103 variant also exerts an as-yet-unquantified small effect in children.

Genome-wide association studies (GWA) have become feasible through major improvements in high-throughput chip technologies, which can process hundreds of thousands of SNPs quickly and affordably. The power of GWAs for the detection of genes/alleles for different complex disorders was recently proved.[47,48] The first GWA, based on approximately 100,000 SNPs analyzed in families of the Framingham study, identified the association of a single nucleotide polymorphism (SNP) in the proximity of the insulin-induced gene 2 (INSIG2; rs7566605) with obesity. Approximately 10% of the analyzed individuals harbored the CC genotype that, according to this study, predisposes to obesity.[49] Several attempts to replicate the INSIG2 finding have been or are currently being undertaken. Confirmations[50] and negative findings[51–53] have been reported. Currently, data are being compiled for a large-scale meta-analysis, which will in the near future help to clarify whether *INSIG2* is a real poly-gene. It was recently shown that CC homozygotes for the relevant *INSIG2* SNP (rs7566605) lost less weight in a 1-year lifestyle intervention program than individuals with the 2 other genotypes. This finding further implicates a role for this polymorphism in weight regulation.[54]

One of the genes picked up in GWA studies for type 2 diabetes mellitus (T2DM) was *FTO (fat mass and obesity associated* gene).[55,56] Frayling and colleagues[55] statistically adjusted for BMI and thus found that the association to T2DM was actually due to the higher BMI of diabetic cases in comparison to nondiabetic controls. Confirmation of this effect on body weight was obtained in a total of 38,759 individuals. A meta-analysis showed that the A allele of SNP rs9939609 was associated with a 31% increased risk to develop obesity. About 16% of adults who were homozygous for the risk allele on average weighed about 3 kg more and had 1.67-fold increased odds for obesity when compared with those not carrying a risk allele. A subsequent confirmation in a total of 25,508 European individuals substantiated *FTO* as an important polygene for obesity.[57,58]

The first GWA for early-onset extreme obesity was recently performed. Six SNPs in *FTO* showed the strongest evidence for association with obesity.[59] The finding could be confirmed in independent obesity families based on at least 1 young obese index patient. Hence, this first obesity GWA represents a further proof of concept for GWAs to detect genes relevant to highly complex phenotypes, such as obesity, and demonstrates the power of carefully selected patient samples.

Most recently and in the currently largest study, a GWA based on combined data of 7 studies (total n = 16,876) identified an SNP (rs17782313) 188 kb downstream of *MC4R*, which predisposes to obesity. The location of rs17782313 indicates that the effect on weight regulation is likely to be mediated through effects on *MC4R* expression.[60] The finding was confirmed in a further 60,352 adults and 5,988 children and 660 nuclear families encompassing 1 or more obese offspring and both parents. Amongst the adults, each copy of the rs17782313 C allele was associated with a difference in BMI of approximately +0.22 kg/m^2; a copy of the C allele also resulted in a higher mean height (0.21 cm) and weight (760 g), suggesting that this SNP (or the functionally relevant SNP[s] in linkage disequilibrium) influences overall adult size. A copy of the allele resulted in an 8% and 12% increased odds ratio for overweight and obesity, respectively; no significant gender differences were detected.

Genotyping of almost 6,000 children revealed that the effect of the C allele was not detectable in children before age 7 years. However, in children aged 7 to 11 years the effect size of a copy of the C allele was twice the amount observed in adults; no effect was observed for body height. The effect on weight was disproportionately due to fat mass. Finally, Loos and colleagues[60] showed that *FTO* and the novel *MC4R* alleles have additive effects.

ENVIRONMENTAL FACTORS

Secular changes in energy intake and expenditure are assumed to underlie the obesity epidemic.[30] However, attempts to unequivocally pinpoint the relevant mechanisms, even within a single country or society, have been largely futile. Controversy exists as to the proportional contribution of an elevated energy intake in comparison to a reduced energy expenditure due to the modern-day sedentary lifestyle. In England, energy intake counterintuitively seemingly declined between 1970 and 1990;[61]

however, during the same time period, the physically active labor force declined, too. Daily calories provided by the US food supply increased from 3300 to 3800 per capita between 1970 and the late 1990s; how much of this 500-calorie surplus is actually consumed is unknown. In addition, self-reported calorie intake also increased from 1800 to 2000 between the 1970s and 1996.[62] As pointed out by Swinburn, (elsewhere in this issue), an increased energy intake has potentially made a greater contribution to the obesity epidemic than a reduced energy expenditure.

Decreased Physical Activity

The relationship between excessive TV viewing and obesity has been studied repeatedly in cross-sectional studies. Several, but by no means all, studies have shown a clear-cut association in the expected direction; however, only single longitudinal studies have been performed that allow a causal inference. Gortmaker and colleagues[63] observed a dose-dependent effect of the daily hours spent watching TV on obesity rates; a 5-fold higher rate applied to those children and adolescents who watched TV for more than 5 hours/day than those who watched for less than 2 hours. Over the 4-year study period, 60% of the obesity incidence was attributed to watching TV. More recently, a longitudinal study of 980 children followed up biannually from age 3 to 15 years and at ages 21 and 26 years, revealed that the population attributable fraction for overweight at age 26 years due to viewing between ages 5 and 15 years was 17% after adjustment for potential confounders.[64]

Inactivity is prominent among children and adolescents of industrialized countries. According to a Scottish study[65] the mean time spent in sedentary behavior was 79% and 76% of monitored hours of children at ages 3 and 5 years, respectively. Children spent only 2% of their time pursuing moderate to vigorous activity. According to a representative survey conducted in 2002, 61.5% of US children aged 9 to 13 years did not participate in any organized physical activity during non–school hours.[66] Overweight and obesity are associated with a poorer body gross motor development and endurance performance.[67] Comparisons of motor skills, such as a 6-minute long run, a 50-m sprint, and the number of push-ups within 30 seconds using the same test procedure in German children, who were 10 years old in 1976 and 1996, revealed a significantly poorer performance in the latter study group.[68]

Inactivity of children has increased due to several reasons apart from TV, video, and personal computer use. The walk or cycle ride to the neighborhood friend or school has become increasingly infrequent due to increased traffic and fear of crime. In addition, in some countries and regions, the birth rate has declined substantially entailing the requirement to absolve longer distances by car to meet a friend. Children seem to have more time constraints than in previous times, entailing the necessity to use public transportation or the family car. Finally, physical education at school in many countries does not figure as prominently as 20 to 30 years ago.

Increased Energy Intake

As stated earlier, US data indicate an increase in daily calorie consumption. Portion sizes have increased substantially over the past decades. The energy content of a McDonald's menu item increased from 984 (medium) to 1150 (large) to 1258 (supersize) calories between 1990 and 2000; in 1955 a regular soft drink roughly contained 0.2 L; nowadays, children receive 0.35 L, the large serving contains 0.47 L, and the supersize soft drink filled 1.24 L. Food prices have declined, particularly for fast food products. Advertisements are frequently based on the motto "eat more, pay less." In energy terms eating an apple (125 calories) for 50 cents is a poor deal in comparison with a same-priced chocolate bar (500 calories).

Most of the implicated dietary factors are nevertheless viewed controversially, and unequivocal data causally linking the obesity epidemic to any one of them are virtually absent. Apart from increased portion sizes and energy intake,[69,70] elevations in fat or carbohydrate intake,[71] reduced intake of fruits and vegetables, and increased consumption of soft drinks[72,73] have all been implicated in the obesity epidemic. Consumer trends and food marketing strategies, including advertisement, have also been deemed important.[62,74,75]

Other Factors

The relationship between socioeconomic status and obesity has been subject to change over time in cross-sectional studies. In more recent years, most studies have reported an inverse relationship, and, in contrast to former times, a positive association was not detected in any study.[76] Parental education seems to be the major factor underlying the relationship between low socioeconomic status (SES) and elevated childhood obesity rates.[77,78] Complex interactions between SES and parental overweight on BMI of 5- to 7-year-old offspring have been reported: SES has no impact on offspring BMI if none of the parents are overweight. However, if both parents are overweight, SES roughly explains variance of one BMI unit.[78] Because low SES and low parental education are associated with a host of unhealthy behaviors, it has proven difficult to pinpoint the exact mechanisms underlying the elevated risk for obesity in such families.

Maternal smoking during pregnancy is associated with an increased risk for childhood obesity.[17,79] A minor protective effect of breast feeding has been observed repeatedly, which according to some studies is still detectable in adolescence.[80] However, as-yet-undetected confounding variables cannot be excluded as underlying the associations.[81] Cross-sectional studies have revealed that a shorter duration of sleep is associated with obesity during childhood[17,82] and adulthood.[83] In adults with a short sleep duration, serum levels of the anorexigenic hormone leptin were reduced, whereas those of the orexigenic hormone ghrelin were elevated, thus suggesting a mechanism for the elevated BMI.[83]

It is an everyday experience that psychological traits, cognitions, and social factors, such as mood, anxiety, stress, loneliness, and the perception of boredom, influence our short-term eating behavior. However, long-term effects on body weight have not been uncovered with one exception: an elevated depression score has repeatedly and largely consistently been shown to predict a higher body weight at follow-up in children and adolescents (Hebebrand and colleagues, this issue).

Medications

Several different kinds of medication can induce weight gain; for psychiatrists it is important to realize that this side effect is particularly common and potentially prominent with atypical antipsychotics, lithium, and valproate.[84,85] In adults, clozapine and olanzapine have been associated with the greatest weight gain, the individual extent of which is apparently genetically codetermined.[86] In children and adolescents weight gain, obesity, and related metabolic complications can ensue on use of atypical neuroleptics.[86–89] Overeating and in some cases binge eating attacks have been observed in adolescent patients receiving clozapine or olanzapine.[87,90]

SUMMARY

Disentangling the diverse mechanisms underlying variation of BMI and, in particular, overweight and obesity is proving exceedingly difficult. The advent of GWA will continue to enable the detection of polygenes. DNA of tens of thousands individuals is required to validate an initial finding, thus illustrating the small effect sizes. Complex interactions between genes and environmental factors can be assumed to occur.

Treatment of obesity is difficult in both children and adults. Whereas weight gain is comparatively easy to achieve, weight regain sets in over time; body weight is defended through renewed exposure to risk factors or inherent physiologic mechanisms. Current prevention strategies have frequently not proven successful in reducing BMI and obesity prevalence and incidence rates.

The following (preliminary) conclusions can be drawn from the current status of risk factor research: (1) The total number of risk factors is likely to be large. (2) Many if not most of the risk factors have small effect sizes. Accordingly, removal of a risk factor with a small effect size will have a small individual impact. Nevertheless, on the population level its removal will entail a sizeable reduction of the obesity prevalence rate. (3) Future treatment or prevention efforts tailored to the set of risk factors of a single individual seem unlikely as a complete overlap of risk factors between two obese individuals seems unlikely. From an economical perspective, it thus would appear rather expensive to devise and carry out individual risk-based interventions. However, interventions aimed at common combinations of different risk factors harbor the potential to improve the currently dire outcomes of treatment and prevention programs.

REFERENCES

1. Fröhlich A. Ein fall von tumor der hypophysis cerebri ohne akromegalie. Wiener Klinische Rundschau 1901;15:833–6 906–8. [German].
2. Bruch H. Obesity in childhood and personality development. 1941. Obes Res 1997;5(2):157–61.
3. Bruch H. Psychological aspects of overeating and obesity. Psychosomatics 1964; 5:269–74.
4. Garn SM, Clark D. Nutrition, growth, development, and maturation: findings of the Ten State Nutritional Survey of 1968–70. Pediatrics 1975;56(2):306–19.
5. Lissau I, Sörensen TIA. Parental neglect during childhood and increased risk of obesity in young adulthood. Lancet 1994;343(8893):324–7.
6. Sobal J, Stunkard AJ. Socioeconomic status and obesity: a review of the literature. Psychol Bull 1989;105(2):260–75.
7. Strauss RS, Knight J. Influence of the home environment on the development of obesity in children. Pediatrics 1999;103(6):e85.
8. Bouchard C, Tremblay A, Despres JP, et al. The response to long-term overfeeding in identical twins. N Engl J Med 1990;322(21):1477–82.
9. Stunkard AJ, Sorensen TI, Hanis C, et al. An adoption study of human obesity. N Engl J Med 1986;314(4):193–8.
10. Stunkard AJ, Harris JR, Pedersen NL, et al. The body mass index of twins who have been reared apart. N Engl J Med 1990;322(21):1483–7.
11. Zhang Y, Proenca R, Maffei M, et al. Positional cloning of the mouse obese gene and its human homologue. Nature 1994;372(6505):425–32.
12. Montague CT, Farooqi IS, Whitehead JP, et al. Congenital leptin deficiency is associated with severe early-onset obesity in humans. Nature 1997;387(6636): 903–8.
13. Farooqi IS, Jebb SA, Langmack G, et al. Effects of recombinant leptin therapy in a child with congenital leptin deficiency. N Engl J Med 1999;341(12):879–84.
14. Friedman JM. A war on obesity, not the obese. Science 2003;299(5608):856–8.

15. Friedman JM. Modern science versus the stigma of obesity. Nat Med 2004;10(6): 563–9.
16. Bray GA. The epidemic of obesity and changes in food intake: the fluoride hypothesis. Physiol Behav 2004;82(1):115–21.
17. Reilly JJ, Armstrong J, Dorosty AR, et al. Early life risk factors for obesity in childhood: cohort study. BMJ 2005;330(7504):1357.
18. Whitaker RC. Predicting preschooler obesity at birth: the role of maternal obesity in early pregnancy. Pediatrics 2004;114(1):e29–36.
19. Magnusson PK, Rasmussen F. Familial resemblance of body mass index and familial risk of high and low body mass index. A study of young men in Sweden. Int J Obes Relat Metab Disord 2002;26(9):1225–31.
20. Maes HH, Neale MC, Eaves LJ. Genetic and environmental factors in relative body weight and human adiposity. Behav Genet 1997;27(4):325–51.
21. Hebebrand J, Wulftange H, Görg T, et al. Epidemic obesity: are genetic factors involved via increased rates of assortative mating? Int J Obes Relat Metab Disord 2000;24(3):345–53.
22. Vlietinck R, Derom R, Neale MC, et al. Genetic and environmental variation in the birth weight of twins. Behav Genet 1989;19(1):151–61.
23. Pietilainen KH, Kaprio J, Rissanen A, et al. Distribution and heritability of BMI in Finnish adolescents aged 16 y and 17 y: a study of 4884 twins and 2509 singletons. Int J Obes Relat Metab Disord 1999;23(2):107–15.
24. Hebebrand J, Wemter A, Hinney A. Genetic aspects. In: Kiess W, Marcus C, Wabitsch M, editors. Obesity in childhood and adolescence, vol. 9. Basel (Switzerland): Karger; 2004. p. 80–90.
25. Bosy-Westphal A, Wolf A, Bührens F, et al. Familial influences and obesity-associated metabolic risk factors contribute to the variation in resting energy expenditure: the Kiel Obesity Prevention Study. Am J Clin Nutr 2008;87(6):1695–701.
26. Plomin R, DeFries JC, McClearn GE, et al. Behavioral genetics. New York: Freeman WH; 1997.
27. Reed DR, Bachmanov AA, Beauchamp GK, et al. Heritable variation in food preferences and their contribution to obesity. Behav Genet 1997;27(4):373–87.
28. Pérusse L, Tremblay A, Leblanc C, et al. Genetic and environmental influences on level of habitual physical activity and exercise participation. Am J Epidemiol 1989;129(5):1012–22.
29. Plomin R, Corley R, Carey G, et al. Individual differences in television viewing in early childhood: nature as well as nurture. Psychol Sci 1990;1:371–7.
30. Taubes G. As obesity rates rise, experts struggle to explain why. Science 1998; 280(5368):1367–8.
31. Neel JV, Weder AB, Julius S. Type II diabetes, essential hypertension, and obesity as "syndromes of impaired genetic homeostasis": the "thrifty genotype" hypothesis enters the 21st century. Perspect Biol Med 1998;42(1):44–74.
32. Ellis L, Haman D. Population increases in obesity appear to be partly due to genetics. J Biosoc Sci 2004;36(5):547–59.
33. Fraga MF, Ballestar E, Paz MF, et al. Epigenetic differences arise during the lifetime of monozygotic twins. Proc Natl Acad Sci U S A 2005;102(30):10604–9.
34. Sahoo T, del Gaudio D, German JR, et al. Prader-Willi phenotype caused by paternal deficiency for the HBII-85 C/D box small nucleolar RNA cluster. Nat Genet 2008;40(6):719–21.
35. Farooqi IS, ÓRahilly S. Monogenic obesity in humans. Annu Rev Med 2005;56: 443–58.

36. Hinney A, Bettecken T, Tarnow P, et al. Prevalence, spectrum, and functional characterization of melanocortin-4 receptor gene mutations in a representative population-based sample and obese adults from Germany. J Clin Endocrinol Metab 2006;91(5):1761–9.
37. Dempfle A, Hinney A, Heinzel-Gutenbrunner M, et al. Large quantitative effect of melanocortin-4 receptor gene mutations on body mass index. J Med Genet 2004; 41(10):795–800.
38. Farooqi IS, Yeo GS, Keogh JM, et al. Dominant and recessive inheritance of morbid obesity associated with melanocortin 4 receptor deficiency. J Clin Invest 2000;106(2):271–9.
39. Branson R, Potoczna N, Kral JG, et al. Binge eating as a major phenotype of melanocortin 4 receptor gene mutations. N Engl J Med 2003;348(12):1096–103.
40. Herpertz S, Siffert W, Hebebrand J. Binge eating as a phenotype of melanocortin 4 receptor gene mutations. N Engl J Med 2003;349(6):606–9.
41. Hebebrand J, Geller F, Dempfle A, et al. Binge-eating episodes are not characteristic of carriers of melanocortin-4 receptor gene mutations. Mol Psychiatry 2004;9(8):796–800.
42. Saunders CL, Chiodini BD, Sham P, et al. Meta-analysis of genome-wide linkage studies in BMI and obesity. Obesity (Silver Spring) 2007;15(9):2263–75.
43. Geller F, Reichwald K, Dempfle A, et al. Melanocortin-4 receptor gene variant I103 is negatively associated with obesity. Am J Hum Genet 2004;74(3):572–81.
44. Heid IM, Vollmert C, Hinney A, et al. Association of the 103I MC4R allele with decreased body mass in 7937 participants of two population based surveys. J Med Genet 2005;42(4):e21.
45. Young EH, Wareham NJ, Farooqi S, et al. The V103I polymorphism of the MC4R gene and obesity: population based studies and meta-analysis of 29 563 individuals. Int J Obes (Lond) 2007;31(9):1437–41.
46. Stutzmann F, Vatin V, Cauchi S, et al. Non-synonymous polymorphisms in melanocortin-4 receptor protect against obesity: the two facets of a Janus obesity gene. Hum Mol Genet 2007;16(15):1837–44.
47. Wellcome Trust Case Control Consortium. Genome-wide association study of 14,000 cases of seven common diseases and 3,000 shared controls. Nature 2007;447(7145):661–78.
48. Christensen K, Murray JC. What genome-wide association studies can do for medicine. N Engl J Med 2007;356(11):1094–7.
49. Herbert A, Gerry NP, McQueen MB, et al. A common genetic variant is associated with adult and childhood obesity. Science 2006;312(5771):279–83.
50. Lyon HN, Emilsson V, Hinney A, et al. The association of a SNP upstream of INSIG2 with body mass index is reproduced in several but not all cohorts. PLoS Genet 2007;3(4):e61.
51. Dina C, Meyre D, Samson C, et al. Comment on "A common genetic variant is associated with adult and childhood obesity". Science 2007;315(5809):187.
52. Loos RJ, Barroso I, O'Rahilly S, et al. Comment on "A common genetic variant is associated with adult and childhood obesity". Science 2007;315(5809):187.
53. Rosskopf D, Bornhorst A, Rimmbach C, et al. Comment on "A common genetic variant is associated with adult and childhood obesity". Science 2007; 315(5809):187.
54. Reinehr T, Hinney A, Nguyen TT, et al. Evidence of an influence of a polymorphism near the INSIG2 on weight loss during a lifestyle intervention in obese children and adolescents. Diabetes 2008;57(3):623–6.

55. Frayling TM, Timpson NJ, Weedon MN, et al. A common variant in the FTO gene is associated with body mass index and predisposes to childhood and adult obesity. Science 2007;316(5826):889–94.
56. Scott LJ, Mohlke KL, Bonnycastle LL, et al. A genome-wide association study of type 2 diabetes in Finns detects multiple susceptibility variants. Science 2007; 316(5829):1341–5.
57. Dina C, Meyre D, Gallina S, et al. Variation in FTO contributes to childhood obesity and severe adult obesity. Nat Genet 2007;39(6):724–6.
58. Andreasen CH, Stender-Petersen KL, Mogensen MS, et al. Low physical activity accentuates the effect of the FTO rs9939609 polymorphism on body fat accumulation. Diabetes 2008;57(1):95–101.
59. Hinney A, Nguyen TT, Scherag A, et al. Genome-wide scan for early onset extreme obesity supports the role of fat mass and obesity associated gene (FTO) variants. PLoS ONE 2007;2(12):e1361.
60. Loos RJF, Lindgren CM, Li S, et al. Association studies involving over 90,000 samples demonstrate that common variants near to MC4R influence fat mass, weight and risk of obesity. Nat Genet 2008;40(6):768–75.
61. Prentice AM, Jebb SA. Obesity in Britain: gluttony or sloth? BMJ 1995;311(7002): 437–9.
62. Nestle M. Food politics. Berkely, CA: University of California Press; 2003.
63. Gortmaker SL, Must A, Sobol AM, et al. Television viewing as a cause of increasing obesity among children in the United States, 1986–1990. Arch Pediatr Adolesc Med 1996;150(4):356–62.
64. Hancox RJ, Milne BJ, Poulton R. Association between child and adolescent television viewing and adult health: a longitudinal birth cohort study. Lancet 2004; 364(9430):257–62.
65. Reilly JJ, Jackson DM, Montgomery C, et al. Total energy expenditure and physical activity in young Scottish children: mixed longitudinal study. Lancet 2004; 363(9404):211–2.
66. CDC(Centers for Disease Control and Prevention). Physical activity levels among children aged 9–13 years—United States, 2002. MMWR Morb Mortal Wkly Rep 2003;52(33):785–8.
67. Graf C, Koch B, Kretschmann-Kandel E, et al. Correlation between BMI, leisure habits and motor abilities in childhood (CHILT-project). Int J Obes Relat Metab Disord 2004;28(1):22–6.
68. Hebebrand J, Boes K. Umgebungsfaktoren—körperliche aktivität. In: Wabitsch M, Zwieauer K, Hebebrand J, et al, editors. Adipositas bei kindern und jugendlichen. Berlin: Springer; 2005. p. 50–60 [German].
69. Nielsen SJ, Siega-Riz AM, Popkin BM. Trends in energy intake in US between 1977 and 1996: similar shifts seen across age groups. Obes Res 2002;10(5):370–8.
70. Nielsen SJ, Popkin BM. Patterns and trends in food portion sizes, 1977–1998. JAMA 2003;289(4):450–3.
71. Slyper AH. The pediatric obesity epidemic: causes and controversies. J Clin Endocrinol Metab 2004;89(6):2540–7.
72. Ludwig DS, Peterson KE, Gortmaker SL. Relation between the consumption of sugar sweetened drinks and childhood obesity: a prospective, observational analysis. Lancet 2001;358(9255):505–8.
73. O'Connor TM, Yang SJ, Nicklas TA. Beverage intake among preschool children and its effect on weight status. Pediatrics 2006;118(4):e1010–8.
74. Schlosser E. Fast food nation. Boston, MA: Houghton Mifflin Books; 2001.

75. Lobstein T, Dibb S. Evidence of a possible link between obesogenic food advertising and child overweight. Obes Rev 2005;6(3):203–8.

76. Shrewsbury V, Wardle J. Socioeconomic status and adiposity in childhood: a systematic review of cross-sectional studies 1990–2005. Obesity (Silver Spring) 2008;16(2):275–84.

77. Lamerz A, Kuepper-Nybelen J, Wehle C, et al. Social class, parental education, and obesity prevalence in a study of six-year-old children in Germany. Int J Obes (Lond) 2005;29(4):373–80.

78. Langnäse K, Mast M, Müller MJ. Social class differences in overweight of prepubertal children in northwest Germany. Int J Obes Relat Metab Disord 2002;26(4):566–72.

79. Toschke AM, Koletzko B, Slikker W Jr, et al. Childhood obesity is associated with maternal smoking in pregnancy. Eur J Pediatr 2002;161(8):445–8.

80. Arenz S, Ruckerl R, Koletzko B, et al. Breast feeding and childhood obesity—a systematic review. Int J Obes Relat Metab Disord 2004;28(10):1247–56.

81. Nelson MC, Gordon-Larsen P, Adair LS. Are adolescents who were breast-fed less likely to be overweight? Analyses of sibling pairs to reduce confounding. Epidemiology 2005;16(2):247–53.

82. Von Kries R, Toschke AM, Wurmser H, et al. Reduced risk for overweight and obesity in 5- and 6-y-old children by duration of sleep—a cross- sectional study. Int J Obes Relat Metab Dis 2002;26(5):710–6.

83. Taheri S, Lin L, Austin D, et al. Short sleep duration is associated with reduced leptin, elevated ghrelin, and increased body mass index. PLOS Med 2004;1(3):e62.

84. Schwartz TL, Nihalani N, Jindal S, et al. Psychiatric medication-induced obesity: a review. Obes Rev 2004;5(4):115–21.

85. Zimmermann U, Kraus T, Himmerich H, et al. Epidemiology, implications and mechanisms underlying drug-induced weight gain in psychiatric patients. J Psychiatr Res 2003;37(3):193–220.

86. Theisen FM, Linden A, Geller F, et al. Prevalence of obesity in adolescent and young adult patients with and without schizophrenia and in relationship to antipsychotic medication. J Psychiatr Res 2001;35(6):339–45.

87. Gothelf D, Falk B, Singer P, et al. Weight gain associated with increased food intake and low habitual activity levels in male adolescent schizophrenic inpatients treated with olanzapine. Am J Psychiatry 2002;59(6):1055–7.

88. Martin A, Scahill L, Anderson GM, et al. Weight and leptin changes among risperidone-treated youths with autism: 6-month prospective data. Am J Psychiatry 2004;161(6):1125–7.

89. McConville BJ, Sorter MT. Treatment challenges and safety considerations for antipsychotic use in children and adolescents with psychoses. J Clin Psychiatry 2004;65(Suppl 6):20–9.

90. Theisen FM, Linden A, Konig IR, et al. Spectrum of binge eating symptomatology in patients treated with clozapine and olanzapine. J Neural Transm 2003;110(1):111–21.

Neuroimaging in Eating Disorders and Obesity: Implications for Research

Frederique Van den Eynde, MD[a], Janet Treasure[b,*]

KEYWORDS

- Neuroimaging • Eating disorders • Anorexia nervosa
- Bulimia nervosa • Obesity • fMRI

Medicine and psychiatry have benefited from developments in investigational techniques. Neuroimaging is one such domain that has technically progressed enormously in recent years, resulting in, for example, higher temporal and spatial resolution. Neuroimaging techniques have been widely used in a range of psychiatric disorders, providing new insights into neural brain circuits and neuroreceptor functions in vivo. This allows researchers to study not only the configuration of brain structures but also aspects of normal and anomalous human behavior more accurately.

Throughout evolution, food intake has been, in essence, an instinctive survival strategy, but paradoxically humans' relationship with food has become conflicted in cultures where food is abundantly available. We have reached an age where weight control has been turned away from an instinctual, highly regulated system, to a process requiring considerable cognitive effort.[1] Worldwide, there are increasing numbers of people with abnormal eating patterns as part of or resulting in physical and mental health problems. This spectrum of disorders ranging from extreme underweight to morbid obesity puts an enormous demand on health services. Eating disorders such as anorexia nervosa (AN) and bulimia nervosa (BN) have gained growing media attention and have become—along with what is referred to as the obesity epidemic—a global health concern, not least due to the high medical comorbidity. It remains a matter of debate whether to classify obesity as primarily a somatic or a mental health issue because evidence shows a role for both biological and psychological factors contributing to overeating and binge eating.

Current therapeutic interventions still have modest success rates, with relapse rates being relatively high. Better understanding of pathophysiologic mechanisms that are

[a] Institute of Psychiatry, Section of Eating Disorders PO59, De Crespigny Park, SE5 8AF, London, UK
[b] Department of Psychiatry, 5th Floor, Thomas Guy House, Guy's Hospital, London SE1 9RT, UK
* Corresponding author.
E-mail address: j.treasure@iop.kcl.ac.uk (J. Treasure).

Child Adolesc Psychiatric Clin N Am 18 (2008) 95–115
doi:10.1016/j.chc.2008.07.016
1056-4993/08/$ – see front matter © 2008 Elsevier Inc. All rights reserved.
childpsych.theclinics.com

present in, and contribute to, the chronicity of eating disorders and obesity is expected to improve psychotherapeutic and drug treatment strategies.

In this review, we summarize the findings of brain imaging procedures in eating disorders and obesity. We aim to highlight the potential contribution of brain imaging to the conceptual framework of the etiology and pathophysiology in eating disorders.

BIOLOGY OF EATING BEHAVIOR

The central control of eating behavior is held by two interdependent systems, a homeostatic and a hedonic system (**Fig. 1**).[2] The homeostatic component or "nutrostat" links somatic and metabolic signals with autonomic nervous activity and the regulation of food intake. The hypothalamus is deemed to be the central key factor of this system. The discovery of leptin as the missing link in the homeostatic control of eating contributed substantially to the unfolding of the cascade of central mechanisms within the hypothalamus and beyond.

In the hedonic system, two components can be distinguished, both contributing to the reward associated with food intake: "wanting" and "liking." Although these processes are assumed not to be structurally embodied in a neural substrate, it is believed that distinct underlying neurochemical pathways can separately influence these concepts. The incentive component (wanting, desire, or at the extreme, craving for food) involves dopaminergic pathways. The incentive component is moderated by homeostatic factors and is shaped by experiences with the environment.

Contrastingly, the consummatory pleasure or "liking" network involves opiate and cannabinoid systems. The hedonic system does not merely subserve appetite for food, but is considered to be part of a global organizational unit governing behavioral

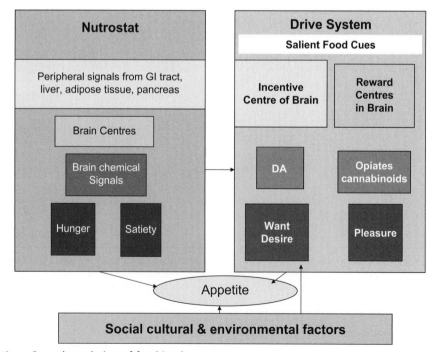

Fig. 1. Central regulation of food intake.

choice. Decisions are made on the basis of reward and pleasure to be gained and the time frame in which they are expected.

In recent years, the distinction between implicit and explicit "wanting" and "liking" has been advocated to enhance understanding of the expression of food reward.[3] Exploration of this notion suggests that implicit wanting is not systematically downregulated by the physiologic consequences of food consumption in the same way as hunger and, therefore, may be largely independent of homeostatic processes influencing intake, whereas explicit wanting and explicit liking are. Because of this, implicit wanting might constitute an independent risk factor for overconsumption.[4]

NEUROIMAGING

Imaging techniques are classically divided into structural (eg, computed tomography or CT; magnetic resonance imaging or MRI) and functional imaging techniques (eg, single photon emission [computed] tomography or SPECT/SPET; positron emission tomography or PET; functional magnetic resonance imaging or fMRI). However, newly developed methods such as magnetic resonance spectroscopy (MRS) and diffusion tensor imaging (DTI) combine both modalities.

STRUCTURAL BRAIN FINDINGS IN THE ACUTE PHASE OF EATING DISORDERS
General

Since Phineas Gage's case there has been a growing interest in brain lesion studies, because they can provide key information about the localization of brain areas involved in certain aspects of human behavior.[5] Anomalies, either congenital or posttraumatic, in the prefrontal, temporal, mesiotemporal cortices and the thalamus, predominantly on the right-hand side, are associated with pathologic eating patterns, including abnormal food intake.[6]

In addition, there is ample evidence that changes in the brain structure take place in the acute phase of an eating disorder. The most consistent alteration is the brain mass reduction found during the ill state of AN. This was first suggested by postmortem findings of reduced cerebral mass with prominent sulci and small gyri[7,8] and later confirmed in vivo in several CT studies that additionally demonstrated enlarged ventricles.[9–11] Along with enlarged ventricles,[12,13] MRI in underweight AN subjects has also shown large cerebrospinal fluid volumes[14,15] in association with deficits in both total gray matter and total white matter volumes.[14,16] However, there is variability in the findings. Some studies found white matter abnormalities with normal gray matter volumes[15] and again others showed gray matter deficits (mainly in the temporal and parietal lobes) without white matter abnormalities.[17]

Abnormalities in ill BN individuals are less pronounced,[18] although they also have decreased cortical mass.[19–21]

Region-Specific Changes?

Few studies have focused on the issue of whether the changes are global or region-specific. Region-specific gray matter loss has been reported in the right anterior cingulate cortex (ACC) in underweight AN patients.[22] Furthermore, reduced pituitary gland volume[23] and amygdala-hippocampal formation[24] reductions have been reported.

Are Structural Changes in Eating Disorders Reversible?

A crucial question is whether cerebral tissue loss and increased cerebrospinal fluid (CSF) volumes, which are thought to be caused by the disorder, are state-dependent.

Data regarding the reversibility of these abnormalities are conflicting. White and gray matter seem to behave differently in this regard. Postmortem examination of brain tissue after weight gain indicates gray matter deficits in recovered AN patients.[25] Longitudinal neuroimaging research also revealed gray matter loss to be persistent, whereas CSF and white matter volumes normalized after weight gain.[16,26] Swayze and colleagues[15] and Castro-Fornieles and colleagues[17] found significant increases in global white and gray matter after weight restoration. In the adolescent AN patients in the Castro-Fornieles and colleagues'[17] study gray matter deficits, both global and region-specific, that is, temporal and parietal, were found in the underfed state. Global gray matter volume was restored, but regionally, some parts in the right temporal and both supplementary motor areas were still smaller.[17] A recent study focused on the volume of the ACC and demonstrated that right dorsal ACC volume reductions in the acute phase normalized with weight restoration. Furthermore, the degree of right dorsal ACC normalization during treatment was related to outcome.[22]

Study of Recovered Patients

Evidence from recent cross-sectional studies in recovered AN patients is somewhat inconsistent. Some studies report on normal brain tissue volumes compared with control subjects,[27] whereas others found global gray (but not white) matter volume decreases of approximately 1%.[28] This loss of gray matter volume was significantly lowered specifically bilaterally in the ACC. Region-specific gray matter loss in the ACC related directly to the severity of the illness (lowest ever body mass index [BMI]), indicating an important role of this area in the pathophysiology of the disorder. Apart from a lack of power in negative studies, a possible explanation for the discrepancy in the findings in recovered AN patients might be the duration of recovery. In the sample with the longest time in recovery, no abnormalities were found,[27] suggesting that brain tissue normalization might lag behind clinical improvement. Patients who recover may be somewhat different from the total eating disorders group, and thus longitudinal studies are of great value.

Mechanism of Structural Changes

The literature seems to suggest that there is brain matter loss, given time. This supports the notion that brain matter loss in the acute phase of an eating disorder is a kind of "pseudoatrophy" and probably a consequence of acute metabolic disruption. The latter may be the consequence of starvation or stress or a combination of both.

Because white matter is principally constituted of myelinated axons with myelin consisting of lipids, it could be argued that reversibility of white matter loss after weight gain is because of the restoration of the lipid/myelin level in the brain.

The actual cause of the structural changes in eating disorders remains unknown. One plausible pathophysiologic pathway is the hyperactivity of the hypothalamus-pituitary-adrenal (HPA) axis in eating disorders, which might contribute to decreased volumes of the amygdala-hippocampal formation in eating disorders,[23,24] because this area is a main target for glucocorticoid effects during stress (for a review of this system in relation to feeding see Peters and colleagues).[29]

Further evidence of HPA axis involvement in structural brain changes comes from findings in adolescent AN patients in whom HPA axis activity was found to positively correlate with CSF volume and negatively with gray matter volume.[14] In addition, the increase in gray matter after weight restoration has been associated with a decrease in cortisol.[22]

Changes in metabolism may also, partially, explain brain matter loss.

MAGNETIC RESONANCE SPECTROSCOPY IN EATING DISORDERS

Neuronal degeneration as a result of starvation may explain the brain shrinkage observed in AN patients, and this may be associated with changes in the metabolic profile, which can be observed with MRS. Metabolic changes in white matter have been reported in the thalamus and the parieto-occipital lobe[30] and in frontal lobe areas.[31,32] Some investigators found no evidence for neuronal degeneration,[30] whereas others observed abnormal metabolite level signals in frontal gray matter,[33,34] occipital gray matter,[31] and the cerebellum.[31] It is of note that the Roser study (1999) pooled both AN and BN subjects.

What is the Underlying Pathophysiology?

These metabolic changes may reflect changes in membrane turnover in the white matter.[30] Metabolic changes are related to the subjects' BMI[31] and reverse with recovery.[32,34] Castro-Fornieles and colleagues[34] referred to the metabolites that were found in anomalous concentrations in their adolescent AN sample as markers of neuronal functionality, energy metabolism, and osmoregulation. In addition, these findings may result from neuronal damage caused by the stress response, because improved metabolic findings are associated with a decrease in cortisol levels.[34]

Structure/Function Associations

Few studies have addressed the relevance of these findings for brain function. Ohrmann and colleagues[33] investigated the relationship between cognitive impairment and cerebral metabolites in the left prefrontal cortex in AN patients. Poor performance on a divided attention task was related with some metabolite levels in the dorsolateral prefrontal cortex, whereas executive functioning and depressive symptomatology were associated with metabolite abnormalities in the ACC. Castro-Fornieles and colleagues[34] also linked markers of neuronal activity with some cognitive parameters (eg, general intelligence).

Deficits in perceptual organization and conceptual reasoning were associated with reduced right dorsal ACC volume.[22] However, no detectable impairment in memory function was found even though structural abnormalities were found in the hippocampus.[24] Low power and poor sensitivity of the assessment tools may explain this discrepancy. This area needs further investigation.

STRUCTURAL IMAGING AND MRS IN OBESITY

The literature on structural abnormalities associated with excess body fat is limited and inconsistent, though alterations of brain morphology have been described in overweight and obese young adults.[35,36] Both gray and white matter changes appear to be associated with increased adiposity. Pannacciulli and colleagues[35] demonstrated focal gray matter volume reductions in several brain areas (post-central gyrus, frontal operculum, putamen, and middle frontal gyrus), accompanied by enlarged orbitofrontal white matter volumes. Haltia and colleagues[36] found only increased white matter volumes in several basal brain regions in obese subjects, which positively correlated with the waist-to-hip ratio. Thus, white matter expansion was partially reversed by dieting. Gray matter abnormalities were not observed, nor was gray matter volume affected by dieting.

These structural alterations may either precede obesity, representing a neural marker of increased propensity to gaining weight, or occur as a consequence of obesity, indicating that the brain is also affected by increased adiposity.

Dramatic weight loss following leptin replacement therapy in 3 subjects with a recessive mutation in the ob gene, producing leptin deficiency and morbid obesity, co-occurred with increases in gray matter concentration in the ACC, the inferior parietal lobule, and the cerebellum.[37]

FUNCTIONAL IMAGING

Functional neuroimaging methods provide information on the integration and interaction of brain regions in spatially distinct neural networks during cognitive or behavioral challenges or in response to physiologic stimuli.[38,39] The development of ligands relating to neurotransmitter/neuroreceptor systems has increased the specificity of SPECT and PET over that obtained by the measurement of blood flow alone. Meanwhile, fMRI has emerged as an advanced means to examine cerebral functioning, with an enormous improvement in spatial and temporal resolution. The different imaging modalities each have their own advantages and disadvantages and their abilities should be considered to be complementary. Further developments such as perfusion MRI—a reliable technique to assess rest-state functional connectivity[40]—are increasingly applied in psychiatry and are expected to be initiated in eating disorder research, too.[39]

From a methodological perspective, a major breakthrough in imaging was the introduction of statistical software packages for data analysis, allowing mathematical analysis instead of visual interpretation of images. Due to the rather small sample sizes that characterize SPECT studies, the reader should interpret the findings of these studies with caution. Ethical considerations have at times hampered the recruitment of control subjects in nuclear imaging studies because of the exposure to radiation.

When describing functional imaging data, it is crucial to distinguish between resting state findings, whereby no specific instruction or task is given to the subject in the scanner, and findings based on scanning paradigms including the presentation of a stimulus. The latter is often aimed at provoking symptoms, though other aspects of psychopathology or pathophysiology might also be the target.

THE RESTING STATE (PET AND SPECT)
Anorexia Nervosa

Globally reduced metabolism
Since the first PET data obtained from eating disorders,[41] the field has expanded considerably. Overall, underweight AN patients were found to have a reduced global and regional cerebral glucose metabolism (rCMRGlu) in the acute state, and this increases with recovery. Most studies found the decrease in global metabolism to be related to weight loss[42–44] and BMI and glucose values.[42,43]

Regional metabolism and blood flow abnormalities
A consistent finding in AN is a hypometabolism in frontal and parietal cortices.[42,43,45,46] Specific areas of reduced metabolism have been found in the anterior cingulate,[47–49] the medial prefrontal cortex,[48] left-sided[50] and right-sided[47] parietal areas, the occipital and insula cortex,[47] the anterior temporal cortex and caudate,[51] the subcallosal gyrus (SCG), posterior cingulated gyrus, and the midbrain.[52] Most of the children and young adolescents with AN were shown to have temporal lobe hypoperfusion and left/right temporal asymmetry.[53,54]

However, an increased level of cerebral perfusion has been reported in the thalamus and the amygdala-hippocampus complex.[48] Increased cortical metabolism was observed not only in the inferior frontal cortex[46] and temporal cortex[41,55] but also in striatal structures, such as the caudate nucleus[41,42,44,46,56] and putamen.[46] Comorbid low mood symptoms could not explain the basal ganglia hypermetabolism.[42]

Is the restricting type different from binge-purging type?

Differentiation between restricting-type anorexia nervosa (RAN) and anorexia nervosa-binge-purging (AN-BP) based on resting state data remains dubious. Yonezawa and colleagues[52] were unable to replicate earlier findings of lower frontal perfusion (especially in the ACC) in the restricting subgroup compared with the binge-purging type.[49]

Do abnormalities in the basal state persist?

In cross-sectional studies with patients who have recovered, no abnormalities in global and regional resting state metabolism[46] or perfusion[57] are found. Longitudinal research has also shown that after weight gain in RAN patients, the abnormal perfusion is reversed in most areas (ie, an increase in the right parietal area and a decrease in the cerebellum and basal ganglia).[47] In 1 study, low-dose physiologic androgen replacement in AN patients with low androgen levels attenuated the hypometabolism in the posterior cingulate gyrus.[58]

Is resting state metabolism related to psychopathology and neurocognition?

Some investigators have attempted to correlate the basal blood flow in people with eating disorders with aspects of their psychopathology. Goethals and colleagues[59] reported that the level of body dissatisfaction in eating disorders correlated with blood flow in the left ventromedial prefrontal cortex and right medial parietal areas, and the subjective sense of ineffectiveness correlated with flow in the lateral ventral prefrontal cortex and left medial parietal areas.[59]

Bulimia Nervosa

Global cerebral functioning

There is less conclusive evidence for abnormal blood flow in BN patients in the ill state.[60] Delvenne and colleagues[44] found reduced cortical metabolism although this was not supported in other reports.

Regional anomalies

Regional cerebral perfusion abnormalities in BN include changes in cerebral functional lateralization, for instance, the loss of a right-greater-than-left asymmetry in frontal regions and the presence of left-greater-than-right asymmetry in temporal lobes.[61,62]

Mood as alternative explanation?

The potential role of mood problems in the interpretation of these results remains unclear, and these are inconsistent findings.[61,63]

State or trait?

Frank and colleagues[64] recruited long-term recovered BN patients and could not demonstrate regional cerebral blood flow (rCBF) abnormalities. This is in favor with the notion that alterations in rCBF reported in the ill state of BN may be state-related phenomena that remit with recovery.[64]

STIMULUS PROVOCATION

Several technical issues need to be considered before interpreting the response of the brain to salient eating disorder cues. The key areas relating to the hedonic response to food may be subject to susceptibility artifacts (eg, the orbitofrontal cortex might be difficult to visualize due to the proximity of the sinuses). Further, the baseline physiology, hunger, and blood glucose level, and so on, may vary between groups and act as significant confounders. Several studies have examined the response to food in both the hungry and satiated state in which the response to satiation typically follows the experimental paradigm in the hungry state. This fixed repetition of the experiment within a short time period is not controlled for. Also, if meals are given, these are often adjusted for body weight and so vary in size.

A diverse range of paradigms have been used including tasting or eating food or presenting pictures of food. The instructions and the required response to the cues can have a profound effect on the results.

Food as Stimulus

Nuclear imaging techniques: An increase in flow in the right frontal and parietal lobe occurred when food was presented to individuals with the bingeing rather than the restricting form of AN.[65] The presentation of high in contrast to low-caloric food increased the blood flow (PET) in the associative visual cortex in patients with AN.[55] The ingestion of food was followed by increased frontal flow in AN[50,66] and decreased flow in BN.[50]

Anorexia Nervosa

The visual presentation of food/drinks
In response to pictures of labeled high- (in contrast to low-) caloric drinks, activation of limbic structures of the fear network, including the amygdala and insula regions, was observed in AN.[67]

Two studies from our research group have reported consistent results.[68,69] In 1 study, the presentation of food images led to greater activation in the left medial orbitofrontal cortex and ACC and less activation in the lateral prefrontal cortex, inferior parietal lobule, and cerebellum in a group of subjects with AN and BN, relative to the comparison group. The BN subgroup had less activation in the lateral and apical prefrontal cortex, relative to the comparison group. Thus, a medial prefrontal response to food stimuli was identified as a common feature of AN and BN and supports the conceptualization of eating disorders as being transdiagnostic at the neural level. In contrast, no differences between AN patients and healthy controls were found when standard emotional/aversive stimuli (fear and disgust) were used.[68] This emphasizes the specificity of the response rather than it being a consequence of anxiety.

High-calorie food images in AN patients was associated with less activation in left inferior parietal region in the satiated state and less activation in the occipital regions in the hungry state.[70]

Food taste
In response to tastants (sucrose versus water) delivered to the tongue, people with a past history of AN showed lowered neural activation in primary and secondary taste cortical regions, such as the insula, and ventral and dorsal striatum.[71]

Bulimia Nervosa

As in other domains, BN has been less well studied than AN. Uher and colleagues[68] found that in addition to a medial prefrontal activation—common with AN—BN patients were specifically characterized by lower levels of activation to food cues in the lateral prefrontal cortex.[68] This brain region is involved in cognitive inhibition and suppression of undesirable behavior;[72] thus, this finding has been interpreted as corresponding to the lack of control overeating.

In response to tastants (glucose) delivered to the tongue, people with BN had less activation in the right ACC and left occipital cortex (cuneus).[73]

Body Image

Abnormalities in the perception and evaluation of body shape are a hallmark of eating disorders and often persist and pose a risk for relapse even after weight recovery. Therefore, there has been interest in examining this aspect of the psychopathology. A variety of different experimental paradigms have been used.

The areas of interest for this aspect of psychopathology include both the left parietal lobe and its connections to the thalamus, which are important for body schema representation[74] and also the emotional limbic network.

Line drawings

Using line drawings of underweight, normal weight, and overweight female bodies, Uher and colleagues[75] found a highly consistent pattern of brain activity related to body shape processing in healthy women and in women with eating disorders. Compared with a control condition (line drawings of houses), the body images activated in all groups the lateral prefrontal cortex, lateral fusiform gyrus, and inferior parietal cortex. However, responses in the occipitotemporal and parietal cortices were less strong in patients with eating disorders. Aversion ratings in the eating disorder group correlated positively with activity in the right apical medial prefrontal cortex and negatively with the activity in the left lateral fusiform gyrus. Thus, parts of the network that are engaged in processing female body shapes appear underactive in women with eating disorders.

Self- versus non–self body images

In accordance with the findings in the Uher and colleagues[75] study, Sachdev and colleagues[76] found that processing of non–self-images generated a response in similar brain areas in eating disorder patients (AN) and control subjects. This consisted of an activation of the inferior and middle frontal gyri (somewhat higher in AN), superior and inferior parietal lobules, posterior lobe of the cerebellum, and the thalamus. However the processing of self-images differed in that people with AN had a lack of activation of the brain regions involved in emotional and perceptual processing whereas controls had greater activation in the middle frontal gyri, insula, precuneus, and occipital regions to images of themselves.[76]

Distorted body images

Distorted self-images presented to people with AN activated the "fear network," namely the right amygdala, the right gyrus fusiformis, and brainstem regions[77] and in the dorsolateral prefrontal cortex and inferior parietal lobule.[78]

Disgust

Brain responses following the viewing of disgusting and highly repulsive pictures did not differ between BN patients and controls and included activation of the left amygdala and the occipitotemporal visual cortex.[79] The hypothesis of elevated global disgust sensitivity in BN patients could not be supported. This is consistent with the finding of Uher and colleagues[68] in both AN and BN.

Reward

People with AN are able to deprive themselves of the reward of food and there has been interest in their response to general reward tasks. Recovered RAN subjects had a stronger caudate response to a simple monetary reward task than comparison women. This change in caudate hemodynamic signal (during either wins or losses) was associated with trait anxiety. Moreover, in the anterior ventral striatum, recovered RAN patients had similar responses to both win and loss conditions whereas comparison women distinguished between positive and negative feedback. This suggests that individuals with AN may have a decreased sensitivity to reward.[80]

NEUROTRANSMISSION/RECEPTOR FUNCTIONING
Anorexia Nervosa

Dopamine

It has been speculated that dopamine-related disturbance of reward mechanisms might contribute to altered hedonics of feeding behavior and the anhedonic temperament in AN. Frank and colleagues[81] demonstrated higher dopamine D2/D3 receptor binding in recovered AN subjects in the anteroventral striatum, suggesting either decreased intrasynaptic dopamine concentration or increased D2/D3 receptor density or affinity to be present in AN. Moreover, in the AN group, dopamine binding potential in the dorsal caudate and dorsal putamen correlated positively with harm avoidance. This observation supports the view that the dopamine abnormalities in AN might contribute to the characteristic harm avoidance or increased physical activity.[81]

Serotonin

There is growing evidence that a disturbance in serotonin function may be involved in the etiology and pathogenesis of eating disorders[82] and may account for the relation with impulse dyscontrol and mood problems.[83]

Several potential physiologic confounding factors limit the interpretation of findings of serotonin function in the acute illness state (such as reduced levels of estrogens, reduced food intake, fatty acids displacing tryptophan from albumin, resulting in an increase in free tryptophan, and 5-hydroxytryptamine [5-HT] serotonin turnover in the brain), and many studies have been done in people who have recovered from their illness.

Serotonin 2A receptors Audenaert and colleagues[84] reported decreased 5-hydroxy-tryptamine 2A (5HT2A) binding in the left frontal cortex and bilaterally in parietal and occipital cortices in people with AN using SPECT.[84] In another SPECT study from the same group, 5HT2A binding was significantly reduced in the parietal cortex in AN-BP in comparison with RAN.[85] A decrease in 5HT2A binding was also found in PET studies in recovered patients.[86,87] One study showed decreased 5HT2A receptor binding in the mesial temporal, parietal, and occipital cortical areas and in subgenual and pregenual cingulated cortex.[87] Similarly, AN-BP patients had reduced 5HT2A binding in the left subgenual cingulated, left parietal cortex, and right occipital cortex.[86] In another study by the same group in acutely ill AN patients, 5HT2A binding was found to be normal.[88] This suggests that there may be state-related changes in 5HT2A function, which can mask trait-related anomalies.

Serotonin 1A receptors In contrast, Serotonin 1A receptor (5HT1A) activity is increased in prefrontal and lateral orbital frontal regions, mesial and lateral temporal areas, the parietal cortex, and the dorsal raphe nucleus.[88] Recovered AN-BP patients also have increased 5HT1A binding in several cortical brain areas (cingulate, mesial and lateral temporal, medial and lateral orbital frontal, parietal and prefrontal cortices) and the dorsal raphe nucleus.[89] Increased 5-HTT binding was found in recovered RAN patients.[90]

The neuroimaging–genetics interface

In a small pilot study, SS homozygous individuals for the functional polymorphism of the promoter region of the 5-HTT gene (5-HTTLPR) had reduced 5-HTT binding in the dorsal caudate when compared with LL subjects.[90] However, the allele distributions of 5-HTTLPR were similar in the eating disorder group and the control group.

Relationship of changes in serotonin receptor function with psychopathology

Harm avoidance is a personality/temperament concept that refers to a general level of trait anxiety. Positive correlations between this anxiety measure and 5HT2A binding have been described in the in the temporal cortex[86] and supragenual cingulate, frontal, and parietal brain regions[88] of recovered AN patients. This is regardless of any abnormality in overall 5HT2A receptor activity.[88] In addition, harm avoidance is associated with the 5HT1A postsynaptic binding in the mesial temporal and cingulate regions in the recovered RAN subgroup but not recovered AN-BP subgroup.[89] In addition, a negative relationship between temporal 5HT2A binding potential and novelty seeking has been reported as has been a negative association between the 5HT2A binding potential in diverse cortical areas and drive for thinness in AN-BP patients.[86]

Overall, these results suggest that there is a persistent disturbance of brain 5-HT neuronal function in AN, which relates to key aspects of the psychopathology. It is uncertain whether this is a trait-related vulnerability factor or whether it represents a scar from the illness. Furthermore, it is uncertain whether these changes result from an alteration in the affinity (such as the proportion of receptors occupied by tonic transmitter levels) or in the number of receptors available.

Bulimia Nervosa

Dopamine

In a study by Tauscher and colleagues,[91] the administered ligand was [^{123}I] β-carbo-methoxy-3-β-(4-iodophenyl)-tropane (B-CIT), which has the ability to assess not only serotonin but also dopamine binding sites. Acutely ill BN subjects have a reduced striatal dopamine transporter availability.

Serotonin

Serotonin 2A receptors In a sample of acutely ill bulimia nervosa, purging-type (BN-P) patients, cortical 5-HT2A receptor activity (SPECT) was not dissimilar to that in controls.[85] Using PET, Kaye and colleagues[83] found that women who had recovered from BN had a reduction of medial orbital frontal cortex 5HT2A binding.

Serotonin 1A receptors 5HT1A binding is higher in BN patients than in control subjects in diverse brain regions, with the most robust differences in the angular gyrus, the medial prefrontal cortex, and the posterior cingulate cortex.[92]

Serotonin transporter Koskela and colleagues[93] studied the 5-HTT availability (SPET) in the midbrain and the thalamus in (purging or non-purging) BN and non-affected female twin pair members and found no HTT binding differences between the groups, but a post hoc subgroup analysis revealed that the BN-P had higher 5-HTT binding than that in the healthy women in the midbrain, but not in the thalamus. Reduced 5-HT transporter availability was found in the hypothalamus and thalamus in BN,[91] especially in the group with a longer duration of illness.[91]

Opioid

The endogeneous opioid system is thought to be implicated in the "liking" aspects of food intake. Opioid system abnormalities that have been demonstrated in BN consist of a lower mu opioid receptor binding in the left insular cortex, the primary gustatory cortex.[94] The authors speculated that cyclic behavioral patterns of food restriction and bingeing could induce a downregulation of the opioid receptors as a result of chronically increased endogeneous opioid release. Receptor binding correlated negatively with recent fasting behavior, which is in line with data on insular activation when food is perceived as rewarding and in a state of hunger, but not in a satiated state.[95,96]

OBESITY

Functional neuroimaging provides an increasingly important tool for investigating how different regions of the brain work in concert to orchestrate normal eating behaviors and how they conspire to produce obesity and other eating disorders.[97,98]

Resting State and Obesity

Compared with lean subjects, brain metabolic activity in obese subjects is significantly higher in the bilateral parietal somatosensory cortex, in the regions where sensation to the mouth, lips, and tongue are located. The enhanced activity in somatosensory regions involved with sensory processing of food in the obese subjects could make them more sensitive to the rewarding properties of food related to palatability and could contribute to overeating.[99] In another study by the same researchers, whole brain metabolism and striatal metabolism were not found to be abnormal in obese subjects.[100]

Obesity and Symptom Provocation

Nuclear functional imaging

Simply looking at a portion of food as compared with looking at a picture of a landscape results in higher right perfusion of the parietal and temporal cortices in obese women, but not in controls (SPECT study). In addition, in the obese women the activation of the right parietal cortex was associated with an enhanced feeling of hunger when looking at food.[101]

The sensory experience of food is a primary reinforcer of eating. Del Parigi and colleagues[102] developed a PET paradigm with rCBF assessment in response to the oral administration of 2 mL of a liquid meal (Ensure Plus, 1.5 kcal/mL) after a 36-hr period of fasting. Lean and obese groups differed in response to the sensory experience of food in several regions. Greater increases in the middle-dorsal insula and midbrain and greater decreases in the posterior cingulate, temporal, and orbitofrontal cortices were found in the obese than those in the lean group. The percentage of body fat, glycemia, and dietary disinhibition independently correlated with the neural response to the sensory experience of the meal in the middle-dorsal insular cortex. This suggests that obesity is associated with an abnormal brain response to the sensory aspects of a liquid meal after a prolonged fast, especially in areas of the primary gustatory cortex.[102]

Leptin exerts its anorexogenic effect through binding to specific hypothalamic receptors. Hypothalamus blood flow (SPECT) was inversely correlated with leptin levels during exposure to food in obese subjects, but not in normal-weight individuals.[103] Although this is an interesting observation, the complexity of the numerous biochemical processes taking place in the hypothalamus, with orexogenic and anorexogenic effects, makes further interpretation difficult.

fMRI

Food and reward

To test the hypothesis that the increased motivational potency of foods in obese individuals is mediated in part by a hyperactive reward system, Stoeckel at al[104] investigated the activation of reward system to pictures of high-calorie and low-calorie foods in obese and normal-weight women. Pictures of high-calorie foods produced significantly greater activation in the obese group than that in controls in the following brain areas: medial and lateral orbitofrontal cortex, amygdala, nucleus accumbens/ventral striatum, medial prefrontal cortex, insula, anterior cingulate cortex, ventral pallidum, caudate, putamen, and hippocampus. In addition, in the high- versus low-calorie contrast, the obese group also exhibited a larger difference than the controls in all of the same regions (except for the putamen). In contrast, in the control group, greater activation by high-calorie foods was seen only in dorsal caudate and by low-calorie food pictures in the lateral orbitofrontal cortex, medial prefrontal cortex, and anterior cingulate cortex.

Obese women selectively activated the dorsal striatum, a region related to reward anticipation and habit learning, while viewing high-caloric foods.[105] Tastants activated the insula more in hungry obese and post-obese subjects than in hungry normal-weight individuals.[106]

In summary, this greater activation in response to pictures of high-calorie foods in obese women might mediate motivational effects of food cues.

Hypothalamus abnormality

A functional abnormality of the hypothalamus, a key player in the regulation of energy intake and feeding behavior, may be related to excess energy intake and obesity. The existence of differential hypothalamic functions in lean and obese humans has been shown.[107] After glucose ingestion, lean subjects demonstrated an inhibition of the fMRI signal in the areas corresponding to the paraventricular and ventromedial nuclei. In obese subjects, this inhibitory response was markedly attenuated and delayed when compared.

Leptin and brain activation

Leptin replacement in 3 adults with a missense mutation in the ob gene normalized body weight and eating behavior. During viewing of food-related stimuli, leptin replacement reduced brain activation in regions linked to hunger (insula, parietal and temporal cortex) whereas it enhanced activation in regions linked to inhibition and satiety (prefrontal cortex). Leptin appears to modulate feeding behavior through these circuits, suggesting therapeutic targets for human obesity.[108]

Obesity and Receptor/NT

Overeating in obese individuals not only shares similarities with drug addiction on a clinical level, with the loss of control and compulsive drug taking behavior, but also the underlying biological mechanisms have commonalities. Reductions in striatal dopamine D2 receptors have been documented in obese subjects (similar findings are present in various forms of addictions).[109] Moreover, D2 receptor levels (PET) were found to have an inverse relationship to the BMI of the obese subjects. One hypothesis to explain this is that decreased levels of D2 receptors predispose subjects to search for reinforcers (in the case of the obese subjects, for food) to activate D2-regulated reward circuits. However, methodologically it cannot be ruled out that these findings were due to augmentation in concentration of extracellular dopamine. Nevertheless, this seemed very unlikely because pharmacologic evidence points toward an association between the enhanced dopamine activity and reduced food intake.[100,109]

Serotonergic mechanisms

The serotonin neurotransmitter system has been studied less intensely in obesity than in eating disorders. Diminished 5-HTT binding was found in the midbrain of binge-eating obese subjects compared with their non-bingeing counterparts.[110] Moreover, successful treatment (combined group psychotherapy and fluoxetine) resulted in a significant increase in 5-HTT binding only in the binge-eating subgroup of obese subjects.[111]

Diffusion Weighed Imaging

Obesity is characterized by an altered distribution of body fluid. Diffusion-weighted imaging (DWI) has enabled researchers to now also demonstrate brain diffusion changes in regions related to satiety and hunger (hypothalamus, hippocampal gyrus, amygdala, insula, cerebellum, and midbrain) in obese as compared with control subjects.[112] This indicates altered fluid distribution (intra/extracellular) and/or vasogenic edema in these brain areas of obese subjects. Morbidly obese subjects differ from other obese individuals with regard to brain diffusion in the orbitofrontal and occipital cortex.

Bingeing

Salient food stimuli

Investigating binge eating as a separate entity is hard, but researchers have attempted to overcome this by comparing obese binge eaters and non-bingeing obese individuals.

Exposure to food generated a greater cerebral blood flow increase (SPECT study) in the left than in the right hemisphere, especially in the frontal and prefrontal regions, in obese binge-eating women. The left (pre)frontal perfusion correlated with the increase in hunger.[113] In line with this are the results from an fMRi study by Geliebter and colleagues,[114] who compared brain activation to visually and auditory presented food stimuli in a group of obese and normal-weight binge eaters and control subjects, 3 hours after eating a meal.[114] The obese binge-eating group had greater activation in the frontal cortex (premotor area and inferior frontal gyrus), and in the occipital and temporal lobe (fusiform gyrus). These studies suggest that food stimuli are more salient in the obese binge-eating group.

SUMMARY

The body of literature on neuroimaging studies in eating disorders has grown exponentially over the last 2 decades and has contributed a better insight into the clinical eating disorders. In summary, global and regional reduced resting state perfusion and metabolism have been found in eating disorders, associated with the nutritional state of patients. Furthermore, eating disorder patients have been shown to respond differently from control subjects when presented with disease-related cues such as food images and tastants and body images. In addition, neurotransmitter system abnormalities have been reported, with evidence being the strongest for the serotonin system. Furthermore, it was demonstrated that dopamine and related reward systems function differently from healthy controls. Dopamine-mediated reward systems may contribute to obesity and serotonin system anomalies to binge eating.

Several factors might help explain apparently incongruent data. Firstly, methodological issues play an important role. Subject selection, sample size (and the related issues of lack of power), nutritional state, and other sample characteristics might influence the results. In addition, the imaging technique and the procedures used have a strong impact on the outcome of an experiment. Data analysis techniques have significantly improved, and these allow us for more accurate group comparisons (eg, by allowing a correction for partial volume loss).

An important aspect that needs to be taken into consideration when looking at neuroimaging data is the study sample characteristics. It is a clinical reality that eating disorders have a high comorbidity with other psychiatric disorders, especially mood and anxiety disorders. More than half (56.2%) of the patients with AN, 94.5% with BN, 78.9% with binge-eating disorder, 63.6% with subthreshold binge-eating disorder, and 76.5% with any binge eating met criteria for at least 1 of the core disorders listed in the fourth edition of the Diagnostic and Statistical Manual of Mental Disorders (DSM-IV).[115] Furthermore, from a dimensional perspective there is subsyndromal overlap with other disorders, for example, obsessive-compulsive traits are found to be a risk factor for AN. This illustrates that it is difficult to recruit a homogeneous study sample with high conformity in their associated clinical characteristics, and this further complicates the interpretation. Brain perfusion and activation abnormalities have been reported in these comorbid psychiatric disorders and neurotransmitter system abnormalities. Thus, it is essential for investigators to assess comorbidity and report not on only on categorical diagnoses but assess at least mood and anxiety levels. This information could be included in the imaging data analysis, or results should be at least interpreted against this background.

Functional imaging findings with disease-specific cues in patient groups should be interpreted with caution. These may be merely correlates of the disorder rather than biomarkers that may relate etiology.

In eating disorder research, investigators have focused on either structural or functional brain imaging techniques, but the interpretation of functional data has always suffered from the sometimes insufficient knowledge about structural anomalies. With regard to the data analysis, most good recent studies use partial volume corrections to correct for brain volume changes and thus allow a more accurate reading of the results of functional imaging studies. Nevertheless, future research would benefit from the application of structural (including MRS) and functional techniques in the same sample to facilitate linking findings in both approaches.

As in other domains of science and medicine, there is a need for replication studies and novel paradigms that take into account the limitations of previous studies. Moreover, several interesting and promising paradigms have been applied in healthy controls, with potential implications for those with disturbed eating patterns.

REFERENCES

1. Peters JC, Wyatt HR, Donahoo WT, et al. From instinct to intellect: the challenge of maintaining healthy weight in the modern world. Obes Rev 2002;3(2):69–74.
2. Treasure JL. Getting beneath the phenotype of anorexia nervosa: the search for viable endophenotypes and genotypes. Can J Psychiatry 2007;52(4):212–9.
3. Finlayson G, King N, Blundell JE. Is it possible to dissociate 'liking' and 'wanting' for foods in humans? A novel experimental procedure. Physiol Behav 2007; 90(1):36–42.
4. Finlayson G, King N, Blundell J. The role of implicit wanting in relation to explicit liking and wanting for food: implications for appetite control. Appetite 2008; 50(1):120–7.

5. Macmillian M. Restoring Phineas Gage: a 150th retrospective. J Hist Neurosci 2000;9:46–66.
6. Uher R, Treasure J. Brain lesions and eating disorders. J Neurol Neurosurg Psychiatry 2005;76(6):852–7.
7. Gagel O. Magersucht. vol. 5. Berlin: Springer; 1953.
8. Martin F. Pathologie des aspects neurologiques et psychiatriques des quelques manifestations carentielles avec troubles digestifs et neuro-endocriniens etude des alterations du systeme nerveux central dans deux cas d' anorexie survenue chez la jeune fille (dite anorexie mentale). Acta Neurol Belg 2008;52(1958): 816–30 [French].
9. Dolan RJ, Mitchell J, Wakeling A. Structural brain changes in patients with anorexia nervosa. Psychol Med 1988;18(2):349–53.
10. Krieg JC, Lauer C, Leinsinger G, et al. Brain morphology and regional cerebral blood flow in anorexia nervosa. Biol Psychiatry 1989;25(8):1041–8.
11. Palazidou E, Robinson P, Lishman WA. Neuroradiological and neuropsychological assessment in anorexia nervosa. Psychol Med 1990;20(3):521–7.
12. Golden NH, Ashtari M, Kohn MR, et al. Reversibility of cerebral ventricular enlargement in anorexia nervosa, demonstrated by quantitative magnetic resonance imaging. J Pediatr 1996;128(2):296–301.
13. Swayze VW, Andersen A, Arndt S, et al. Reversibility of brain tissue loss in anorexia nervosa assessed with a computerized Talairach 3-D proportional grid. Psychol Med 1996;26(2):381–90.
14. Katzman DK, Lambe EK, Mikulis DJ, et al. Cerebral gray matter and white matter volume deficits in adolescent girls with anorexia nervosa. J Pediatr 1996;129(6): 794–803.
15. Swayze VW, Andersen AE, Andreasen NC, et al. Brain tissue volume segmentation in patients with anorexia nervosa before and after weight normalization. Int J Eat Disord 2003;33(1):33–44.
16. Katzman DK, Zipursky RB, Lambe EK, et al. A longitudinal magnetic resonance imaging study of brain changes in adolescents with anorexia nervosa. Arch Pediatr Adolesc Med 1997;151(8):793–7.
17. Castro-Fornieles J, Bargallo N, Lazaro L, et al. A cross-sectional and follow-up voxel-based morphometric MRI study in adolescent anorexia nervosa. J Psychiatr Res 2008, in press.
18. Krieg JC, Lauer C, Pirke KM. Structural brain abnormalities in patients with bulimia nervosa. Psychiatry Res 1989;27(1):39–48.
19. Hoffman GW, Ellinwood EH Jr, Rockwell WJ, et al. Cerebral atrophy in bulimia. Biol Psychiatry 1989;25(7):894–902.
20. Husain MM, Black KJ, Doraiswamy PM, et al. Subcortical brain anatomy in anorexia and bulimia. Biol Psychiatry 1992;31(7):735–8.
21. Laessle RG, Krieg JC, Fichter MM, et al. Cerebral atrophy and vigilance performance in patients with anorexia nervosa and bulimia nervosa. Neuropsychobiology 1989;21(4):187–91.
22. McCormick LM, Keel PK, Brumm MC, et al. Implications of starvation-induced change in right dorsal anterior cingulate volume in anorexia nervosa. Int J Eat Disord 2008, in press.
23. Giordano GD, Renzetti P, Parodi RC, et al. Volume measurement with magnetic resonance imaging of hippocampus-amygdala formation in patients with anorexia nervosa. J Endocrinol Invest 2001;24(7):510–4.
24. Connan F, Murphy F, Connor SE, et al. Hippocampal volume and cognitive function in anorexia nervosa. Psychiatry Res 2006;146(2):117–25.

25. Neumarker KJ, Bzufka WM, Dudeck U, et al. Are there specific disabilities of number processing in adolescent patients with Anorexia nervosa? Evidence from clinical and neuropsychological data when compared to morphometric measures from magnetic resonance imaging. Eur Child Adolesc Psychiatry 2000;9(Suppl 2):II111–21.

26. Lambe EK, Katzman DK, Mikulis DJ, et al. Cerebral gray matter volume deficits after weight recovery from anorexia nervosa. Arch Gen Psychiatry 1997;54(6): 537–42.

27. Wagner A, Greer P, Bailer UF, et al. Normal brain tissue volumes after long-term recovery in anorexia and bulimia nervosa. Biol Psychiatry 2006;59(3):291–3.

28. Muhlau M, Gaser C, Ilg R, et al. Gray matter decrease of the anterior cingulate cortex in anorexia nervosa. Am J Psychiatry 2007;164(12):1850–7.

29. Peters A, Schweiger U, Pellerin L, et al. The selfish brain: competition for energy resources. Neurosci Biobehav Rev 2004;28(2):143–80.

30. Schlemmer HP, Mockel R, Marcus A, et al. Proton magnetic resonance spectroscopy in acute, juvenile anorexia nervosa. Psychiatry Res 1998;82(3):171–9.

31. Roser W, Bubl R, Buergin D, et al. Metabolic changes in the brain of patients with anorexia and bulimia nervosa as detected by proton magnetic resonance spectroscopy. Int J Eat Disord 1999;26(2):119–36.

32. Kato T, Shioiri T, Murashita J, et al. Phosphorus-31 magnetic resonance spectroscopic observations in 4 cases with anorexia nervosa. Prog Neuropsychopharmacol Biol Psychiatry 1997;21(4):719–24.

33. Ohrmann P, Kersting A, Suslow T, et al. Proton magnetic resonance spectroscopy in anorexia nervosa: correlations with cognition. Neuroreport 2004;15(3): 549–53.

34. Castro-Fornieles J, Bargallo N, Lazaro L, et al. Adolescent anorexia nervosa: cross-sectional and follow-up frontal gray matter disturbances detected with proton magnetic resonance spectroscopy. J Psychiatr Res 2007;41(11):952–8.

35. Pannacciulli N, Del PA, Chen K, et al. Brain abnormalities in human obesity: a voxel-based morphometric study. Neuroimage 2006;31(4):1419–25.

36. Haltia LT, Viljanen A, Parkkola R, et al. Brain white matter expansion in human obesity and the recovering effect of dieting. J Clin Endocrinol Metab 2007; 92(8):3278–84.

37. Matochik JA, London ED, Yildiz BO, et al. Effect of leptin replacement on brain structure in genetically leptin-deficient adults. J Clin Endocrinol Metab 2005; 90(5):2851–4.

38. Glahn DC, Thompson PM, Blangero J. Neuroimaging endophenotypes: strategies for finding genes influencing brain structure and function. Hum Brain Mapp 2007;28(6):488–501.

39. Malhi GS, Lagopoulos J. Making sense of neuroimaging in psychiatry. Acta Psychiatr Scand 2008;117(2):100–17.

40. Chuang KH, van GP, Merkle H, et al. Mapping resting-state functional connectivity using perfusion MRI. Neuroimage 2008;40(4):1595–605.

41. Herholz K, Krieg JC, Emrich HM, et al. Regional cerebral glucose metabolism in anorexia nervosa measured by positron emission tomography. Biol Psychiatry 1987;22(1):43–51.

42. Delvenne V, Goldman S, Biver F, et al. Brain hypometabolism of glucose in low-weight depressed patients and in anorectic patients: a consequence of starvation? J Affect Disord 1997;44(1):69–77.

43. Delvenne V, Goldman S, De MV, et al. Brain glucose metabolism in anorexia nervosa and affective disorders: influence of weight loss or depressive symptomatology. Psychiatry Res 1997;74(2):83–92.
44. Delvenne V, Goldman S, De MV, et al. Brain glucose metabolism in eating disorders assessed by positron emission tomography. Int J Eat Disord 1999; 25(1):29–37.
45. Delvenne V, Lotstra F, Goldman S, et al. Brain hypometabolism of glucose in anorexia nervosa: a PET scan study. Biol Psychiatry 1995;37(3):161–9.
46. Delvenne V, Goldman S, De MV, et al. Brain hypometabolism of glucose in anorexia nervosa: normalization after weight gain. Biol Psychiatry 1996;40(8):761–8.
47. Kojima S, Nagai N, Nakabeppu Y, et al. Comparison of regional cerebral blood flow in patients with anorexia nervosa before and after weight gain. Psychiatry Res 2005;140(3):251–8.
48. Takano A, Shiga T, Kitagawa N, et al. Abnormal neuronal network in anorexia nervosa studied with I-123-IMP SPECT. Psychiatry Res 2001;107(1):45–50.
49. Naruo T, Nakabeppu Y, Deguchi D, et al. Decreases in blood perfusion of the anterior cingulate gyri in anorexia nervosa restrictors assessed by SPECT image analysis. BMC Psychiatry 2001;1:2.
50. Nozoe S, Naruo T, Yonekura R, et al. Comparison of regional cerebral blood flow in patients with eating disorders. Brain Res Bull 1995;36(3):251–5.
51. Key A, O'Brien A, Gordon I, et al. Assessment of neurobiology in adults with anorexia nervosa. Eur Eat Disorders Rev 2006;14:308–14.
52. Yonezawa H, Otagaki Y, Miyake Y, et al. No differences are seen in the regional cerebral blood flow in the restricting type of anorexia nervosa compared with the binge eating/purging type. Psychiatry Clin Neurosci 2008;62(1):26–33.
53. Gordon I, Lask B, Bryant-Waugh R, et al. Childhood-onset anorexia nervosa: towards identifying a biological substrate. Int J Eat Disord 1997;22(2):159–65.
54. Chowdhury U, Gordon I, Lask B, et al. Early-onset anorexia nervosa: is there evidence of limbic system imbalance? Int J Eat Disord 2003;33(4):388–96.
55. Gordon CM, Dougherty DD, Fischman AJ, et al. Neural substrates of anorexia nervosa: a behavioral challenge study with positron emission tomography. J Pediatr 2001;139(1):51–7.
56. Krieg JC, Holthoff V, Schreiber W, et al. Glucose metabolism in the caudate nuclei of patients with eating disorders, measured by PET. Eur Arch Psychiatry Clin Neurosci 1991;240(6):331–3.
57. Frank GK, Bailer UF, Meltzer CC, et al. Regional cerebral blood flow after recovery from anorexia or bulimia nervosa. Int J Eat Disord 2007;40(6):488–92.
58. Miller KK, Deckersbach T, Rauch SL, et al. Testosterone administration attenuates regional brain hypometabolism in women with anorexia nervosa. Psychiatry Res 2004;132(3):197–207.
59. Goethals I, Vervaet M, Audenaert K, et al. Does regional brain perfusion correlate with eating disorder symptoms in anorexia and bulimia nervosa patients? J Psychiatr Res 2007;41(12):1005–11.
60. Delvenne V, Goldman S, Simon Y, et al. Brain hypometabolism of glucose in bulimia nervosa. Int J Eat Disord 1997;21(4):313–20.
61. Andreason PJ, Altemus M, Zametkin AJ, et al. Regional cerebral glucose metabolism in bulimia nervosa. Am J Psychiatry 1992;149(11):1506–13.
62. Wu JC, Hagman J, Buchsbaum MS, et al. Greater left cerebral hemispheric metabolism in bulimia assessed by positron emission tomography. Am J Psychiatry 1990;147(3):309–12.

63. Hagman JO, Buchsbaum MS, Wu JC, et al. Comparison of regional brain metabolism in bulimia nervosa and affective disorder assessed with positron emission tomography. J Affect Disord 1990;19(3):153–62.

64. Frank GK, Kaye WH, Greer P, et al. Regional cerebral blood flow after recovery from bulimia nervosa. Psychiatry Res 2000;100(1):31–9.

65. Naruo T, Nakabeppu Y, Sagiyama K, et al. Characteristic regional cerebral blood flow patterns in anorexia nervosa patients with binge/purge behavior. Am J Psychiatry 2000;157(9):1520–2.

66. Nozoe S, Naruo T, Nakabeppu Y, et al. Changes in regional cerebral blood flow in patients with anorexia nervosa detected through single photon emission tomography imaging. Biol Psychiatry 1993;34(8):578–80.

67. Ellison Z, Foong J, Howard R, et al. Functional anatomy of calorie fear in anorexia nervosa. Lancet 1998;352(9135):1192.

68. Uher R, Murphy T, Brammer MJ, et al. Medial prefrontal cortex activity associated with symptom provocation in eating disorders. Am J Psychiatry 2004;161(7):1238–46.

69. Uher R, Brammer MJ, Murphy T, et al. Recovery and chronicity in anorexia nervosa: brain activity associated with differential outcomes. Biol Psychiatry 2003;54(9):934–42.

70. Santel S, Baving L, Krauel K, et al. Hunger and satiety in anorexia nervosa: fMRI during cognitive processing of food pictures. Brain Res 2006;1114(1):138–48.

71. Wagner A, Aizenstein H, Mazurkewicz L, et al. Altered insula response to taste stimuli in individuals recovered from restricting-type anorexia nervosa. Neuropsychopharmacology 2008;33(3):513–23.

72. Aron AR, Fletcher PC, Bullmore ET, et al. Stop-signal inhibition disrupted by damage to right inferior frontal gyrus in humans. Nat Neurosci 2003;6(2):115–6.

73. Frank GK, Wagner A, Achenbach S, et al. Altered brain activity in women recovered from bulimic-type eating disorders after a glucose challenge: a pilot study. Int J Eat Disord 2006;39(1):76–9.

74. McGlynn SM, Schacter DL. Unawareness of deficits in neuropsychological syndromes. J Clin Exp Neuropsychol 1989;11(2):143–205.

75. Uher R, Murphy T, Friederich HC, et al. Functional neuroanatomy of body shape perception in healthy and eating-disordered women. Biol Psychiatry 2005;58(12):990–7.

76. Sachdev P, Mondraty N, Wen W, et al. Brains of anorexia nervosa patients process self-images differently from non-self-images: an fMRI study. Neuropsychologia 2008;46(8):2161–8.

77. Seeger G, Braus DF, Ruf M, et al. Body image distortion reveals amygdala activation in patients with anorexia nervosa—a functional magnetic resonance imaging study. Neurosci Lett 2002;326(1):25–8.

78. Wagner A, Ruf M, Braus DF, et al. Neuronal activity changes and body image distortion in anorexia nervosa. Neuroreport 2003;14(17):2193–7.

79. Schienle A, Stark R, Shafer A, et al. Disgust and disgust sensitivity in bulimia nervosa: an fMRI study. Eur Eat Disorders Rev 2004;12:42–50.

80. Wagner A, Aizenstein H, Venkatraman VK, et al. Altered reward processing in women recovered from anorexia nervosa. Am J Psychiatry 2007;164(12):1842–9.

81. Frank GK, Bailer UF, Henry SE, et al. Increased dopamine D2/D3 receptor binding after recovery from anorexia nervosa measured by positron emission tomography and [11c]raclopride. Biol Psychiatry 2005;58(11):908–12.

82. Kaye W. Neurobiology of anorexia and bulimia nervosa. Physiol Behav 2008; 94(1):121–35.
83. Kaye WH, Frank GK, Meltzer CC, et al. Altered serotonin 2A receptor activity in women who have recovered from bulimia nervosa. Am J Psychiatry 2001;158(7): 1152–5.
84. Audenaert K, Van Laere K, Dumont F, et al. Decreased 5-HT2a receptor binding in patients with anorexia nervosa. J Nucl Med 2003;44(2):163–9.
85. Goethals I, Vervaet M, Audenaert K, et al. Comparison of cortical 5-HT2A receptor binding in bulimia nervosa patients and healthy volunteers. Am J Psychiatry 2004;161(10):1916–8.
86. Bailer UF, Price JC, Meltzer CC, et al. Altered 5-HT(2A) receptor binding after recovery from bulimia-type anorexia nervosa: relationships to harm avoidance and drive for thinness. Neuropsychopharmacology 2004;29(6):1143–55.
87. Frank GK, Kaye WH, Meltzer CC, et al. Reduced 5-HT2A receptor binding after recovery from anorexia nervosa. Biol Psychiatry 2002;52(9):896–906.
88. Bailer UF, Frank GK, Henry SE, et al. Exaggerated 5-HT1A but normal 5-HT2A receptor activity in individuals ill with anorexia nervosa. Biol Psychiatry 2007; 61(9):1090–9.
89. Bailer UF, Frank GK, Henry SE, et al. Altered brain serotonin 5-HT1A receptor binding after recovery from anorexia nervosa measured by positron emission tomography and [carbonyl11C]WAY-100635. Arch Gen Psychiatry 2005;62(9): 1032–41.
90. Bailer UF, Frank GK, Henry SE, et al. Serotonin transporter binding after recovery from eating disorders. Psychopharmacology (Berl) 2007;195(3):315–24.
91. Tauscher J, Pirker W, Willeit M, et al. [123I] beta-CIT and single photon emission computed tomography reveal reduced brain serotonin transporter availability in bulimia nervosa. Biol Psychiatry 2001;49(4):326–32.
92. Tiihonen J, Keski-Rahkonen A, Lopponen M, et al. Brain serotonin 1A receptor binding in bulimia nervosa. Biol Psychiatry 2004;55:871–3.
93. Koskela AK, Keski-Rahkonen A, Sihvola E, et al. Serotonin transporter binding of [123I]ADAM in bulimic women, their healthy twin sisters, and healthy women: a SPET study. BMC Psychiatry 2007;7:19.
94. Bencherif B, Guarda AS, Colantuoni C, et al. Regional mu-opioid receptor binding in insular cortex is decreased in bulimia nervosa and correlates inversely with fasting behavior. J Nucl Med 2005;46(8):1349–51.
95. Tataranni PA, Gautier JF, Chen K, et al. Neuroanatomical correlates of hunger and satiation in humans using positron emission tomography. Proc Natl Acad Sci U S A 1999;96(8):4569–74.
96. Small DM, Zatorre RJ, Dagher A, et al. Changes in brain activity related to eating chocolate: from pleasure to aversion. Brain 2001;124(Pt 9):1720–33.
97. DelParigi A, Pannacciulli N, Le DN, et al. In pursuit of neural risk factors for weight gain in humans. Neurobiol Aging 2005;26(Suppl 1):50–5.
98. Tataranni PA, DelParigi A. Functional neuroimaging: a new generation of human brain studies in obesity research. Obes Rev 2003;4(4):229–38.
99. Wang GJ, Volkow ND, Felder C, et al. Enhanced resting activity of the oral somatosensory cortex in obese subjects. Neuroreport 2002;13(9):1151–5.
100. Wang GJ, Volkow ND, Logan J, et al. Brain dopamine and obesity. Lancet 2001; 357(9253):354–7.
101. Karhunen LJ, Lappalainen RI, Tammela L, et al. Subjective and physiological cephalic phase responses to food in obese binge-eating women. Int J Eat Disord 1997;21(4):321–8.

102. DelParigi A, Chen K, Salbe AD, et al. Sensory experience of food and obesity: a positron emission tomography study of the brain regions affected by tasting a liquid meal after a prolonged fast. Neuroimage 2005;24(2):436–43.
103. Karhunen LJ, Lappalainen RI, Vanninen EJ, et al. Serum leptin and regional cerebral blood flow during exposure to food in obese and normal-weight women. Neuroendocrinology 1999;69(3):154–9.
104. Stoeckel LE, Weller RE, Cook EW III, et al. Widespread reward-system activation in obese women in response to pictures of high-calorie foods. Neuroimage 2008;41(2):636–47.
105. Rothemund Y, Preuschhof C, Bohner G, et al. Differential activation of the dorsal striatum by high-calorie visual food stimuli in obese individuals. Neuroimage 2007;37(2):410–21.
106. DelParigi A, Chen K, Salbe AD, et al. Persistence of abnormal neural responses to a meal in postobese individuals. Int J Obes Relat Metab Disord 2004;28(3): 370–7.
107. Matsuda M, Liu Y, Mahankali S, et al. Altered hypothalamic function in response to glucose ingestion in obese humans. Diabetes 1999;48(9):1801–6.
108. Baicy K, London ED, Monterosso J, et al. Leptin replacement alters brain response to food cues in genetically leptin-deficient adults. Proc Natl Acad Sci U S A 2007;104(46):18276–9.
109. Wang GJ, Volkow ND, Thanos PK, et al. Similarity between obesity and drug addiction as assessed by neurofunctional imaging: a concept review. J Addict Dis 2004;23(3):39–53.
110. Kuikka JT, Tammela L, Karhunen L, et al. Reduced serotonin transporter binding in binge eating women. Psychopharmacology (Berl) 2001;155(3):310–4.
111. Tammela LI, Rissanen A, Kuikka JT, et al. Treatment improves serotonin transporter binding and reduces binge eating. Psychopharmacology (Berl) 2003; 170(1):89–93.
112. Alkan A, Sahin I, Keskin L, et al. Diffusion-weighted imaging features of brain in obesity. Magn Reson Imaging 2008;26(4):446–50.
113. Karhunen LJ, Vanninen EJ, Kuikka JT, et al. Regional cerebral blood flow during exposure to food in obese binge eating women. Psychiatry Res 2000;99(1): 29–42.
114. Geliebter A, Ladell T, Logan M, et al. Responsivity to food stimuli in obese and lean binge eaters using functional MRI. Appetite 2006;46(1):31–5.
115. Hudson JI, Hiripi E, Pope HG Jr, et al. The prevalence and correlates of eating disorders in the National Comorbidity Survey Replication. Biol Psychiatry 2007; 61(3):348–58.

Leptin-Mediated Neuroendocrine Alterations in Anorexia Nervosa: Somatic and Behavioral Implications

Timo D. Müller[a], Manuel Föcker, MD[a], Kristian Holtkamp, MD[b], Beate Herpertz-Dahlmann, MD[b], Johannes Hebebrand, MD[a],*

KEYWORDS

- Hyperactivity • Semi-starvation • Osteoporosis • Amenorrhea
- Hypoleptinemia • Hyperleptinema • Weight loss

In 1953, Kennedy[1] postulated that circulating signals from the periphery that change in relation to body fat stores inform the brain about changes in body fat mass and that the brain in response to these signals adjusts food intake and energy balance to achieve body weight maintenance. The first peripheral hormone implicated in the regulation of food intake was the pancreatic hormone insulin.[2] Positional cloning of the mouse *obese (ob)* gene in 1994 led to the discovery of leptin, a 16-kDa protein that is mainly secreted by white adipocytes and that, in relation to body fat mass, enters the brain through the bloodstream to activate central neuronal circuits to reduce food intake and to increase energy expenditure.[3]

Leptin is secreted into the bloodstream in a pulsatile manner and shows a diurnal variation in normal and overweight individuals, with an increase of about 50% during the night.[4] In anorectic individuals, however, this diurnal variation of leptin secretion is strikingly reduced.[5,6] Plasma levels of leptin further correlate with the amount of body fat.[7] Individuals with a low body fat mass (eg, patients with anorexia nervosa [AN]) have consistently been reported to show low to undetectable plasma levels of leptin.[8] Additionally, even after correction for body mass index (BMI) or body fat mass, plasma levels of leptin have repeatedly been shown to be higher in females than in males.[7,9,10]

This work was supported by grants from the Federal Ministry of Education and Research (NGFN2; 01GS0482, 01GS0483) and (01GV0602 360372), the European Union (FP6 LSHMCT-2003-503041), and the Deutsche Forschungsgemeinschaft (DFG; HE 1446/4-1).

[a] Department of Child and Adolescent Psychiatry and Psychotherapy, University of Duisburg-Essen, Virchowstrasse 174, 45147 Essen, Germany

[b] Department of Child and Adolescent Psychiatry and Psychotherapy, University Clinics, RWTH Aachen, Neuenhofer Weg 21, 52074 Aachen, Germany

* Corresponding author.

E-mail address: johannes.hebebrand@uni-duisburg-essen.de (J. Hebebrand).

Child Adolesc Psychiatric Clin N Am 18 (2008) 117–129
doi:10.1016/j.chc.2008.07.002
1056-4993/08/$ – see front matter

A multiple regression analysis with BMI and percent body fat as fixed variables further revealed that testosterone is negatively correlated with plasma levels of leptin in boys, but not in girls, thus indicating that higher androgen concentrations are at least partly responsible for the observed lower leptin concentrations in boys.[10] Plasma levels of leptin, however, decline on food deprivation and become similar in both sexes after a 36-hour fast.[11]

Since its discovery in 1994, a tremendous amount of research has focused on leptin-mediated signaling pathways, revealing that leptin is not only a key hormone implicated in the regulation of energy balance but it is also a pleiotropic hormone involved in various neuroendocrine and behavioral alterations associated with profound changes in energy stores. The observation that obese leptin-deficient *ob/ob* mice show endocrine abnormalities similar to those observed in semi-starved *wild-type* mice, together with the observation that prevention of the starvation-induced fall in leptin by exogenous leptin supplementation substantially blunts the changes in the hypothalamic–pituitary–adrenal (HPA), –gonadal (HPG), and –thyroid (HPT) axes, has led to the hypothesis that leptin is a key hormone mediating the neuroendocrine response to semi-starvation.[12] Indeed, hypoleptinemia induced by profound weight loss turned out to mediate various physiologic and endocrinologic alterations associated with reduced body weight, such as modulation of bone formation,[13–15] inflammation,[16,17] reproduction,[18–21] and the regulation of the HPA[12,22,23] and HPA–thyroidT axis.[24]

As leptin plays an important role in the adaptation of an organism to semi-starvation, AN can be considered as a model disorder to elucidate the relationship between hypoleptinemia induced by profound weight loss and the somatic, behavioral, and neuroendocrine alterations associated with semi-starvation. Moreover, patients with AN share many physiologic, endocrinologic, and behavioral features with healthy subjects who voluntarily or involuntarily lost a substantial amount of body weight, such as osteopenia/osteoporosis, amenorrhea, hyperactivity, hypothermia, bradycardia, reduced basal metabolic rate, and activation of the HPA axis.[8] However, even though AN shares many neuroendocrine and behavioral similarities with healthy subjects undergoing semi-starvation, the diagnostically relevant psychopathological features clearly distinguishing AN from weight reduced healthy subjects are the intense fear of gaining weight and the undue influence of body weight on self-evaluation.

In light of the postulated critical role of leptin in the adaptation of an organism to semi-starvation, the focus of this review is to summarize the pivotal role of leptin in the neuroendocrine response to profound weight loss, with special emphasis on AN. In particular, we focus on the effects of semi-starvation–induced hypoleptinemia on the HPA and HPG axis, bone formation, and the hyperactivity in patients with AN. Additionally, we highlight the consolidated findings obtained in the "activity-based anorexia" rat model, which serves as an animal model for AN.

LEPTIN LEVELS IN PATIENTS WITH AN

Hypoleptinemia is a cardinal feature of acute AN, and in most studies mean leptin levels only rarely exceed 2 µg/L^{-1} on referral;[8] the low leptin levels are typically below those of healthy gender- and age-matched controls and reflect the low fat mass. The highest plasma leptin levels in patients with AN were reported by Grinspoon and colleagues[25] with 5.6 ± 3.7 µg/L^{-1}; the variation in mean leptin concentration might at least partly be explained by the time point of blood sampling, because weight regain leads to an increase in leptin secretion. This time point varies among the different studies from "at a baseline visit"[26,27] or "within the first days upon referral"[18,19,28–34] to "at the end of a 3-week nutritional stabilization phase" or "after a minimum weight gain of

10%."[35] Other studies do not specify when during the course of treatment blood was sampled.[8] Leptin levels, however, can only be compared between studies when blood is collected at the same point in time, optimally within the first 1 to 3 days on referral, as leptin levels expeditiously increase on initiation of a refeeding therapy;[20,29,34,36,37] accordingly, leptin levels have increased from those observed on admission after 30 days of refeeding[36] or after a body weight gain of 5%.[37] However, several lines of evidence further indicate that the increase in leptin levels on refeeding is also dependent on the severity of hypoleptinemia; patients with exceedingly low plasma levels of leptin on admission show only slight linear increases in the initial phase of weight regain, which is typically followed by a subsequently more rapid increase.[20,29] Several studies have further shown that hyperleptinemia can ensue from the therapeutically induced weight gain in both female[20,29] and male[19] patients with AN, thus indicating that hyperleptinemia in these patients might contribute to difficulties in long-term weight restoration and body weight maintenance. However, not all studies have been able to confirm this finding,[34] possibly because of different rates of therapeutically induced weight gain or differences in the second time point at which patients' blood was sampled.

In most studies plasma levels of leptin were highly correlated with percent body fat[5,20,25,27,34,38] and, to a lesser extent, with BMI on referral;[5,20,25,27,29] only few studies failed to detect a clear correlation[39,40] including the first study to analyze leptin levels in AN patients using an ELISA.[39]

HYPOTHALAMIC–PITUITARY–ADRENAL AXIS

Generally, activation of the HPA axis in response to acute stress conditions is mediated through an increased secretion of hypothalamic corticotropin-releasing hormone (CRH), which is transported through the portal system to the pituitary where CRH stimulates the production of adrenocorticotropic hormone (ACTH); increased secretion of glucocorticoids from the adrenal gland ensues.[41]

Hypercortisolism has consistently been reported in patients with acute AN.[5,14,31,41–47] This is partly provoked by an increased secretion of CRH in the hypothalamus and partly by an increased half-life of cortisol due to a decreased cortisol metabolism.[5,41] Serum levels of cortisol, however, decline on weight regain[48,49] and become similar to those observed in controls after weight reconstitution.[48]

In accordance with the findings in AN patients, activation of the HPA axis is increased in voluntarily fasted healthy subjects[50–52] as well as in rats[53] and mice[12,22] undergoing semi-starvation; corticosterone levels are increased. In 1996, Ahima and colleagues[12] first postulated that semi-starvation–induced hypoleptinemia mediates the activation of the HPA axis under severe conditions of reduced energy availability. The hypothesis was based on the observation that leptin supplementation blunts hypercorticosteronemia in semi-starved *wild-type* mice[12] and in obese leptin deficient *ob/ob* mice.[22,54] Additionally, the stress-induced increase in hypothalamic CRH release was inhibited by leptin supplementation in a dose-dependent manner.[22]

AMENORRHEA AND REPRODUCTIVE FUNCTION

Secondary amenorrhea defined as the absence of at least 3 consecutive menstrual cycles in postmenarchal females represents the fourth edition of Diagnostic and statistical manual of mental disorders diagnostic criterion for AN.[55] However, secondary amenorrhea is not confined to patients with AN; also healthy females with relatively low body fat mass, for example, underweight women,[30] women with anorexia athletica,[38] and elite women athletes[56] show an elevated incidence of amenorrhea and disturbances in menstrual function. The observation that delayed puberty and menstrual irregularities are frequently observed in relatively thin girls has, long before the discovery of leptin, led to the hypothesis that a critical amount of body weight or body fat mass is required for the onset and maintenance of cyclical ovulation.[57]

In the state of semi-starvation the occurrence of amenorrhea reflects the physiologic neuroendocrine adaptation; adequate energy stores to sustain a pregnancy and to provide adequate nutrition to both the fetus and the mother are not available. Based on the observation that both rodents[58,59] and humans[60,61] with mutations in the leptin receptor gene or with leptin deficiency due to mutations in the leptin gene are amenorrheic and that infertility of obese leptin-deficient ob/ob mice can be restored by exogenous leptin supplementation,[58,59] it was postulated that initiation and maintenance of the human menstrual cycle requires endogenous plasma levels of leptin above a specific threshold value; accordingly amenorrhea ensues on attainment of subthreshold leptin levels. We have determined that this threshold value is around 2 μg/L.[30] Accordingly, plasma levels of leptin turned out to be a better predictor of amenorrhea than BMI, fat mass, or percent body fat,[30] thus indicating that the drop in leptin levels mediated by profound weight loss represents the first step of a neuroendocrine cascade that shuts off the HPG axis. Further studies confirmed that a drop in leptin levels below a critical threshold lowers the production of central gonadotropin-releasing hormone (GnRH), leading to decreased levels of the gonadotropins follicle-stimulating hormone (FSH) and luteinizing hormone (LH), which in turn entails a curtailment of ovarian estrogen production.[18,30,62,63] Several studies further indicate that cocaine- and amphetamine-regulated transcript (CART) might be an important mediator of leptin's action on GnRH secretion[64,65] and that the drop in leptin levels below a critical threshold suppresses GnRH secretion through an upregulation of CART in the hypothalamus.[8,65]

In patients with AN the increase in leptin levels due to a refeeding therapy leads to increments of FSH and LH secretion when leptin levels exceed 1.2 μg/L (FSH)[20] and 1.85 μg/L (LH),[18] respectively. Accordingly, treatment of amenorrheic women with recombinant leptin increased mean LH levels and LH pulse frequency after 2 weeks and increased maximal follicular diameter, the number of dominant follicles, ovarian volume, and estradiol levels over a period of 3 months;[66] these females did not fulfill criteria for AN at the time of the study. However, in patients with acute AN, increments of leptin levels and subsequently of the gonadotropins are not able to rapidly restore regular menstruation; 85% of adolescents with AN resumed menses within 6 months after restoration of 90% of standard weight.[67] Obviously, it takes time for the reproduction axis to normalize, including the renewed growth of the ovaries.

BONE FORMATION

A persisting decrease in bone mineral density (BMD) is one of the most profound long-term consequences of prolonged AN,[8,68,69] and the association of BMD deficiency with AN has consistently been shown in both female[68–72] and male patients with AN.[73] The peak physiologic calcium accretion and bone mass accrual is between age 11 and 16 years[74–76] and this time coincides with the highest incidence for the development of AN.[77] Sufficient energy availability is crucial for bone mass development during this period, and prolonged semi-starvation at this age is an important risk factor for the development and persistence of osteopenia and osteoporosis later in life.[8] Indeed, the decrease in BMD is not immediately restored on weight regain[69,70,78–80] and 1 study even reported persisting BMD deficiency more than 10 years after the diagnosis of AN.[78] Accordingly, osteopenia and osteoporosis have consistently been described in 50% to 92% and 13% to 38% of patients with AN, respectively.[25,81] In light of these long-term complications, it is not surprising that anorectic patients show a 7-fold increased incidence of spontaneous fractures[82] and 1 study even reported a 57% cumulative incidence of fractures at the hip, radius, and spine 40 years after the diagnosis of AN.[83]

Semi-starvation–induced hypercortisolism is implicated in the development of BMD deficiency, and thus osteopenia and osteoporosis, as high serum levels of cortisol inhibit bone formation, increase bone resorption, impair calcium absorption from the gut, and affect the secretion of several hormones implicated in bone metabolism.[13,14,84,85] Leptin, however, is indirectly involved in the frequently observed BMD deficiency in AN, because semi-starvation–induced hypoleptinemia entails hypercortisolism due to activation of the HPA axis. Several lines of evidence further indicate that leptin also directly influences bone metabolism; leptin is known to stimulate the expression and secretion of central CART,[86] which inhibits bone loss through inhibition of bone resorption.[87] Thus, semi-starvation–induced hypoleptinemia in combination with an autonomic dysfunction might at least partly explain the consistently observed impairment of bone metabolism in patients with AN.[8]

HYPERACTIVITY IN PATIENTS WITH AN AND SEMI-STARVED RATS

Elevated levels of physical activity are commonly observed in patients with AN[8,28,33,88–93] and some investigators view this phenomenon as a core clinical symptom of AN.[8,88,91,94] In light of the lack of a consistent operational definition of "hyperactivity," excessive exercise is described in 31% to 80% of patients with AN.[91] In some studies, patients with AN were reported to have an addictive, obsessive-compulsive drive to exercise.[90,91,95] The hypothesis that physiologic mechanisms due to semi-starvation underlie this phenomenon was supported by the observation that rats increase their running wheel activity up to 300% to 500% within a few days, when food is either supplied for only a limited period per day (eg, 1–2 h/d)[96–99] or when food is restricted to 60% of the ad libitum food intake.[32] In the most extreme cases, in which food was only supplied for 1 h/d, rats even ran themselves to death within approximately 21 days.[100] This phenomenon called "activity based anorexia" (ABA)[101] or "semi-starvation–induced hyperactivity" (SIH) is considered as an animal model of AN,[8,32,91,98] which shows several symptoms of AN, such as weight loss, low adiposity, hypothermia, low leptin levels, high levels of physical activity, and, in females amenorrhea.[91]

In 2000, Exner and colleagues[32] first postulated that semi-starvation–induced hypoleptinemia triggers SIH. The hypothesis was confirmed experimentally by way of subcutaneous implantation of mini-pumps containing leptin or vehicle in rats undergoing semi-starvation; vehicle treated rats increased their activity up to 300% within 7 days, whereas the activity of the leptin treated rats remained at baseline.[32] A second experiment showed that leptin normalized activity levels even after SIH had set in.[32] The suppression of SIH by exogenous application of leptin was subsequently confirmed by an independent group.[98]

The SIH triggered by hypoleptinemia in rats suggests that the same mechanism might underlie the hyperactivity in patients with AN. Indeed, Exner and colleagues[32] reported the highest levels of restlessness (assessed by self-ratings) in patients with AN when leptin levels and body weight were at their lowest. Additionally, activity levels decreased when leptin levels and body mass increased owing to inpatient treatment.[32] Consistently, serum leptin levels were negatively correlated with motor restlessness (assessed by expert ratings using visual analog scales) in 61 females with

AN.[33] The result was independently confirmed in 27 adolescents with AN, in whom motor restlessness was assessed by expert ratings using the Structured Inventory for Anorectic and Bulimic Syndromes (SIAB).[33] To corroborate these findings, various qualities of physical activity (excessive exercise, motor and inner restlessness) were assessed by accelerometry and self- and expert ratings in an independent sample of 26 inpatients with AN; leptin levels were significantly associated with all qualities of activity and restlessness.[28]

Semi-starvation–induced hyperactivity is seemingly not confined to patients with AN. Thus, survivors of captivity after World War II reported an increase in activity, productivity, and creativity in the initial phase of reduced food availability.[91,102,103] Additionally, voluntary periods of severe food restriction ("fasting cures") are practiced frequently in the European population as part of a traditional self-care health-promoting activity, and these voluntary fasting cures have been shown to be associated with mood enhancement, leptin depletion, and activation of the HPA axis.[50,51]

The increase in activity levels in times of reduced energy availability has been interpreted as increased foraging behavior. Thus, in evolutionary terms, starvation-induced increase in activity levels might be a phylogenetically old pathway to increase the odds for survival.[91] The decrease in activity due to application of leptin as a satiety signal supports this hypothesis.

The molecular mechanisms underlying the induction of SIH by hypoleptinemia remain unclear. Several leptin-mediated first- and second-order systems in the brain and the periphery might be associated with the effect of leptin on SIH. These could act in concert; alternatively, a single system underlies SIH. The hypothalamic melanocortinergic (MC) system[86] might be involved in the leptin-mediated effect on SIH, because MC receptor expression is increased in the ventromedial hypothalamus of SIH rats, suggesting that a hyperactive MC system underlies the SIH phenotype.[104] However, central infusion of alpha-melanocyte—stimulating hormone[105] or agouti-related protein[99] had no effect on total daily running activity. Other possible pathways downstream of the leptin receptor that might be implicated in SIH are the serotonergic/dopaminergic system or the HPA axis. The increase in glucocorticoids mediated by semi-starvation–induced activation of the HPA axis might play an important role in the development of SIH, because SIH was completely suppressed in adrenalectomized rats and restored after corticosterone treatment.[106,107] Additionally, application of corticosterone increases locomotor activity in ad libitum-fed rats[108] and mice.[109] In accordance with the animal models, urinary free cortisol has recently been shown to correlate with activity levels (measured by accelerometry) in 36 women with acute AN.[110]

NEURONAL FUNCTIONS

Recently, several studies have demonstrated that the actions of leptin are not restricted to the hypothalamus and the hypothalamus–pituitary axis. Instead, many other brain areas including brain stem, cerebellum, amygdala, substantia nigra, and especially the hippocampus are highly enriched with leptin receptors. New findings indicate an enhancement of N-methyl-D-aspartic acid receptor function and hippocampal long-term potentiation by leptin and thus underline the importance of this hormone in hippocampal learning and memory function.[111] Accordingly, memory impairments are observed in leptin-insensitive rodents, whereas leptin administration improves memory processes. Interestingly, severely underweight anorectic patients also display memory deficits, especially concerning working memory, which often alleviate with weight gain.[112]

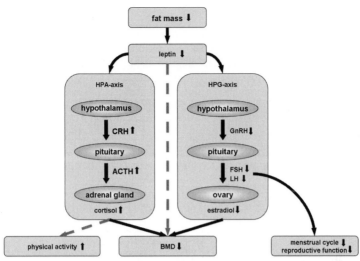

Fig. 1. Semi-starvation–induced alterations of the hypothalamus–pituitary–adrenal (HPA) and –gonadal (HPG) axis in patients with anorexia nervosa. ACTH, adrenocorticotropic hormone; GnRH, gonadotropin-releasing hormone; FSH, follicle-stimulating hormone; LH, luteinizing hormone; BMD, bone mineral density; ↑, increased; ↓, decreased; dashed line, indirect influence; continuous line, direct influence.

SUMMARY

The crucial role of leptin in the neuroendocrine alterations associated with AN is indisputable (**Fig. 1**). Plasma levels of leptin are strikingly reduced during the acute phase of the disorder and increase on weight regain. Whereas hypercortisolism rapidly normalizes on weight restoration, disturbances of ovarian function and decreased BMD can persist for several months up to years after body weight has been restored to normal values. The degree of hypoleptinemia in the acute phase of AN can be considered as an indicator of the severity of the disorder; the lower the leptin level, the more semi-starvation has progressed, and the less adipose tissue exerts its pleiotropic function on other tissues. Accordingly, secretion of gonadotropins (FSH, LH) decreases when leptin levels drop below specific thresholds, thus entailing the development of amenorrhea. Hypoleptinemia-induced hyperactivity reminds us of the difficulty to distinguish between primary and secondary (semi-starvation induced) psychopathological symptoms in AN.

In light of the pivotal role of leptin in mediating the neuroendocrine alterations associated with semi-starvation, the determination of leptin levels should become part of the routine clinical evaluation at referral.[8] It was previously also discussed to include hypoleptinemia as a diagnostic criterion of AN.[94] A prerequisite of that recommendation would be the definition of both the normal reference range and the range of leptin levels observed in patients with AN. As leptin levels potentially differ from those on admission after initiation of weight restoration, the time point of blood sampling needs to be considered when comparing different studies. Measurement of leptin levels may potentially help to detect AN early on during childhood and to assess the severity of the disorder.

REFERENCES

1. Kennedy GC. The role of depot fat in the hypothalamic control of food intake in the rat. Proc R Soc Lond B Biol Sci 1953;140:578–96.
2. Woods SC, Lotter EC, McKay LD, et al. Chronic intracerebroventricular infusion of insulin reduces food intake and body weight of baboons. Nature 1979;282:503–5.
3. Zhang Y, Proenca R, Maffei M, et al. Positional cloning of the mouse obese gene and its human homologue. Nature 1994;372:425–32.
4. Licinio J, Mantzoros C, Negrao AB, et al. Human leptin levels are pulsatile and inversely related to pituitary-adrenal function. Nat Med 1997;3:575–9.
5. Stoving RK, Vinten J, Handberg A, et al. Diurnal variation of the serum leptin concentration in patients with anorexia nervosa. Clin Endocrinol (Oxf) 1998;48: 761–8.
6. Balligand JL, Brichard SM, Brichard V, et al. Hypoleptinemia in patients with anorexia nervosa: loss of circadian rhythm and unresponsiveness to short-term refeeding. Eur J Endocrinol 1998;138:415–20.
7. Maffei M, Halaas J, Ravussin E, et al. Leptin levels in human and rodent: measurement of plasma leptin and ob RNA in obese and weight-reduced subjects. Nat Med 1995;1:1155–61.
8. Hebebrand J, Muller TD, Holtkamp K, et al. The role of leptin in anorexia nervosa: clinical implications. Mol Psychiatry 2007;12:23–35.
9. Havel PJ, Kasim-Karakas S, Dubuc GR, et al. Gender differences in plasma leptin concentrations. Nat Med 1996;2:949–50.
10. Wabitsch M, Blum WF, Muche R, et al. Contribution of androgens to the gender difference in leptin production in obese children and adolescents. J Clin Invest 1997;100:808–13.
11. Maccario M, Aimaretti G, Corneli G, et al. Short-term fasting abolishes the sex-related difference in GH and leptin secretion in humans. Am J Physiol Endocrinol Metab 2000;279:E411–6.
12. Ahima RS, Prabakaran D, Mantzoros C, et al. Role of leptin in the neuroendocrine response to fasting. Nature 1996;382:250–2.
13. Heer M, Mika C, Grzella I, et al. Changes in bone turnover in patients with anorexia nervosa during eleven weeks of inpatient dietary treatment. Clin Chem 2002;48:754–60.
14. Heer M, Mika C, Grzella I, et al. Bone turnover during inpatient nutritional therapy and outpatient follow-up in patients with anorexia nervosa compared with that in healthy control subjects. Am J Clin Nutr 2004;80:774–81.
15. Elefteriou F. Neuronal signaling and the regulation of bone remodeling. Cell Mol Life Sci 2005;62:2339–49.
16. Loffreda S, Yang SQ, Lin HZ, et al. Leptin regulates proinflammatory immune responses. FASEB J 1998;12:57–65.
17. Gualillo O, Eiras S, Lago F, et al. Elevated serum leptin concentrations induced by experimental acute inflammation. Life Sci 2000;67:2433–41.
18. Ballauff A, Ziegler A, Emons G, et al. Serum leptin and gonadotropin levels in patients with anorexia nervosa during weight gain. Mol Psychiatry 1999;4:71–5.
19. Wabitsch M, Ballauff A, Holl R, et al. Serum leptin, gonadotropin, and testosterone concentrations in male patients with anorexia nervosa during weight gain. J Clin Endocrinol Metab 2001;86:2982–8.
20. Holtkamp K, Mika C, Grzella I, et al. Reproductive function during weight gain in anorexia nervosa. Leptin represents a metabolic gate to gonadotropin secretion. J Neural Transm 2003;110:427–35.

21. Bluher S, Mantzoros CS. Leptin in reproduction. Curr Opin Endocrinol Diabetes Obes 2007;14:458–64.
22. Heiman ML, Ahima RS, Craft LS, et al. Leptin inhibition of the hypothalamic-pituitary-adrenal axis in response to stress. Endocrinology 1997;138:3859–63.
23. Malendowicz LK, Rucinski M, Belloni AS, et al. Leptin and the regulation of the hypothalamic-pituitary-adrenal axis. Int Rev Cytol 2007;263:63–102.
24. Martin NM, Smith KL, Bloom SR, et al. Interactions between the melanocortin system and the hypothalamo-pituitary-thyroid axis. Peptides 2006;27:333–9.
25. Grinspoon S, Gulick T, Askari H, et al. Serum leptin levels in women with anorexia nervosa. J Clin Endocrinol Metab 1996;81:3861–3.
26. Misra M, Soyka LA, Miller KK, et al. Serum osteoprotegerin in adolescent girls with anorexia nervosa. J Clin Endocrinol Metab 2003;88:3816–22.
27. Misra M, Miller KK, Almazan C, et al. Hormonal and body composition predictors of soluble leptin receptor, leptin, and free leptin index in adolescent girls with anorexia nervosa and controls and relation to insulin sensitivity. J Clin Endocrinol Metab 2004;89:3486–95.
28. Holtkamp K, Herpertz-Dahlmann B, Hebebrand K, et al. Physical activity and restlessness correlate with leptin levels in patients with adolescent anorexia nervosa. Biol Psychiatry 2006;60:311–3.
29. Hebebrand J, Blum WF, Barth N, et al. Leptin levels in patients with anorexia nervosa are reduced in the acute stage and elevated upon short-term weight restoration. Mol Psychiatry 1997;2:330–4.
30. Kopp W, Blum WF, von Prittwitz S, et al. Low leptin levels predict amenorrhea in underweight and eating disordered females. Mol Psychiatry 1997;2:335–40.
31. Eckert ED, Pomeroy C, Raymond N, et al. Leptin in anorexia nervosa. J Clin Endocrinol Metab 1998;83:791–5.
32. Exner C, Hebebrand J, Remschmidt H, et al. Leptin suppresses semi-starvation induced hyperactivity in rats: implications for anorexia nervosa. Mol Psychiatry 2000;5:476–81.
33. Holtkamp K, Herpertz-Dahlmann B, Mika C, et al. Elevated physical activity and low leptin levels co-occur in patients with anorexia nervosa. J Clin Endocrinol Metab 2003;88:5169–74.
34. Haas V, Onur S, Paul T, et al. Leptin and body weight regulation in patients with anorexia nervosa before and during weight recovery. Am J Clin Nutr 2005;81:889–96.
35. Tolle V, Kadem M, Bluet-Pajot MT, et al. Balance in ghrelin and leptin plasma levels in anorexia nervosa patients and constitutionally thin women. J Clin Endocrinol Metab 2003;88:109–16.
36. Haluzik M, Papezova M, Nedvidkova J, et al. Serum leptin levels in patients with anorexia nervosa before and after partial refeeding, relationships to serum lipids and biochemical nutritional parameters. Physiol Res 1999;48:197–202.
37. Vaisman N, Hahn T, Karov Y, et al. Changes in cytokine production and impaired hematopoiesis in patients with anorexia nervosa: the effect of refeeding. Cytokine 2004;26:255–61.
38. Matejek N, Weimann E, Witzel C, et al. Hypoleptinaemia in patients with anorexia nervosa and in elite gymnasts with anorexia athletica. Int J Sports Med 1999;20:451–6.
39. Hebebrand J, van der Heyden J, Devos R, et al. Plasma concentrations of obese protein in anorexia nervosa. Lancet 1995;346(8990):1624–5.
40. Mantzoros C, Flier JS, Lesem MD, et al. Cerebrospinal fluid leptin in anorexia nervosa: correlation with nutritional status and potential role in resistance to weight gain. J Clin Endocrinol Metab 1997;82:1845–51.

41. Licinio J, Wong ML, Gold PW. The hypothalamic-pituitary-adrenal axis in anorexia nervosa. Psychiatry Res 1996;62:75–83.
42. Kennedy SH, Brown GM, McVey G, et al. Pineal and adrenal function before and after refeeding in anorexia nervosa. Biol Psychiatry 1991;30:216–24.
43. Monteleone P, Martiadis V, Colurcio B, et al. Leptin secretion is related to chronicity and severity of the illness in bulimia nervosa. Psychosom Med 2002;64:874–9.
44. Weinbrenner T, Zittermann A, Gouni-Berthold I, et al. Body mass index and disease duration are predictors of disturbed bone turnover in anorexia nervosa. A case-control study. Eur J Clin Nutr 2003;57:1262–7.
45. Weinbrenner T, Zuger M, Jacoby GE, et al. Lipoprotein metabolism in patients with anorexia nervosa: a case-control study investigating the mechanisms leading to hypercholesterolaemia. Br J Nutr 2004;91:959–69.
46. Misra M, Miller KK, Bjornson J, et al. Alterations in growth hormone secretory dynamics in adolescent girls with anorexia nervosa and effects on bone metabolism. J Clin Endocrinol Metab 2003;88:5615–23.
47. Misra M, Miller KK, Cord J, et al. Relationships between serum adipokines, insulin levels, and bone density in girls with anorexia nervosa. J Clin Endocrinol Metab 2007;92:2046–52.
48. Gold PW, Gwirtsman H, Avgerinos PC, et al. Abnormal hypothalamic-pituitary-adrenal function in anorexia nervosa. Pathophysiologic mechanisms in underweight and weight-corrected patients. N Engl J Med 1986;314:1335–42.
49. Gwirtsman HE, Kaye WH, George DT, et al. Central and peripheral ACTH and cortisol levels in anorexia nervosa and bulimia. Arch Gen Psychiatry 1989;46:61–9.
50. Michalsen A, Kuhlmann MK, Ludtke R, et al. Prolonged fasting in patients with chronic pain syndromes leads to late mood-enhancement not related to weight loss and fasting-induced leptin depletion. Nutr Neurosci 2006;9:195–200.
51. Michalsen A, Schneider S, Rodenbeck A, et al. The short-term effects of fasting on the neuroendocrine system in patients with chronic pain syndromes. Nutr Neurosci 2003;6:11–8.
52. Fichter MM, Pirke KM. Effect of experimental and pathological weight loss upon the hypothalamo-pituitary-adrenal axis. Psychoneuroendocrinology 1986;11:295–305.
53. Djordjevic J, Cvijic G, Davidovic V. Different activation of ACTH and corticosterone release in response to various stressors in rats. Physiol Res 2003;52:67–72.
54. Stephens TW, Basinski M, Bristow PK, et al. The role of neuropeptide Y in the antiobesity action of the obese gene product. Nature 1995;377:530–2.
55. American Psychiatric Association. In: Diagnostic and statistical manual of mental disorders DSM-IV. 4th edition. (text revision). Washington, DC: American Psychiatric Publishing; 2000RH, LD, MD, et al. 2007;56:569–79.
56. De Souza MJ, Metzger DA. Reproductive dysfunction in amenorrheic athletes and anorexic patients: a review. Med Sci Sports Exerc 1991;23:995–1007.
57. Frisch RE, McArthur JW. Menstrual cycles: fatness as a determinant of minimum weight for height necessary for their maintenance or onset. Science 1974;185:949–51.
58. Chehab FF, Lim ME, Lu R. Correction of the sterility defect in homozygous obese female mice by treatment with the human recombinant leptin. Nat Genet 1996;12:318–20.
59. Mounzih K, Lu R, Chehab FF. Leptin treatment rescues the sterility of genetically obese ob/ob males. Endocrinology 1997;138:1190–3.

60. Strobel A, Issad T, Camoin L, et al. A leptin missense mutation associated with hypogonadism and morbid obesity. Nat Genet 1998;18:213–5.
61. Clement K, Vaisse C, Lahlou N, et al. A mutation in the human leptin receptor gene causes obesity and pituitary dysfunction. Nature 1998;392:398–401.
62. Audi L, Mantzoros CS, Vidal-Puig A, et al. Leptin in relation to resumption of menses in women with anorexia nervosa. Mol Psychiatry 1998;3:544–7.
63. Chan JL, Mantzoros CS. Role of leptin in energy-deprivation states: normal human physiology and clinical implications for hypothalamic amenorrhoea and anorexia nervosa. Lancet 2005;366:74–85.
64. Parent AS, Lebrethon MC, Gerard A, et al. Leptin effects on pulsatile gonadotropin releasing hormone secretion from the adult rat hypothalamus and interaction with cocaine and amphetamine regulated transcript peptide and neuropeptide Y. Regul Pept 2000;92:17–24.
65. Chan JL, Mantzoros CS. Leptin and the hypothalamic-pituitary regulation of the gonadotropin-gonadal axis. Pituitary 2001;4:87–92.
66. Welt CK, Chan JL, Bullen J, et al. Recombinant human leptin in women with hypothalamic amenorrhea. N Engl J Med 2004;351:987–97.
67. Golden NH, Jacobson MS, Schebendach J, et al. Resumption of menses in anorexia nervosa. Arch Pediatr Adolesc Med 1997;151:16–21.
68. Bachrach LK, Guido D, Katzman D, et al. Decreased bone density in adolescent girls with anorexia nervosa. Pediatrics 1990;86:440–7.
69. Soyka LA, Misra M, Frenchman A, et al. Abnormal bone mineral accrual in adolescent girls with anorexia nervosa. J Clin Endocrinol Metab 2002;87:4177–85.
70. Bachrach LK, Katzman DK, Litt IF, et al. Recovery from osteopenia in adolescent girls with anorexia nervosa. J Clin Endocrinol Metab 1991;72:602–6.
71. Misra M, Miller KK, Almazan C, et al. Alterations in cortisol secretory dynamics in adolescent girls with anorexia nervosa and effects on bone metabolism. J Clin Endocrinol Metab 2004;89:4972–80.
72. Soyka LA, Grinspoon S, Levitsky LL, et al. The effects of anorexia nervosa on bone metabolism in female adolescents. J Clin Endocrinol Metab 1999;84:4489–96.
73. Castro J, Toro J, Lazaro L, et al. Bone mineral density in male adolescents with anorexia nervosa. J Am Acad Child Adolesc Psychiatry 2002;41:613–8.
74. Bonjour JP, Theintz G, Buchs B, et al. Critical years and stages of puberty for spinal and femoral bone mass accumulation during adolescence. J Clin Endocrinol Metab 1991;73:555–63.
75. Theintz G, Buchs B, Rizzoli R, et al. Longitudinal monitoring of bone mass accumulation in healthy adolescents: evidence for a marked reduction after 16 years of age at the levels of lumbar spine and femoral neck in female subjects. J Clin Endocrinol Metab 1992;75:1060–5.
76. Bailey DA, Martin AD, McKay HA, et al. Calcium accretion in girls and boys during puberty: a longitudinal analysis. J Bone Miner Res 2000;15:2245–50.
77. Katzman DK. Medical complications in adolescents with anorexia nervosa: a review of the literature. Int J Eat Disord 2005;37(Suppl):S52–9 [discussion: S87–9].
78. Brooks ER, Ogden BW, Cavalier DS. Compromised bone density 11.4 years after diagnosis of anorexia nervosa. J Womens Health 1998;7:567–74.
79. Golden NH. Osteopenia and osteoporosis in anorexia nervosa. Adolesc Med 2003;14:97–108.

80. Mika C, Holtkamp K, Heer M, et al. A 2-year prospective study of bone metabolism and bone mineral density in adolescents with anorexia nervosa. J Neural Transm 2007;114:1611–8.
81. Misra M, Klibanski A. Anorexia nervosa and osteoporosis. Rev Endocr Metab Disord 2006;7:91–9.
82. Rigotti NA, Neer RM, Skates SJ, et al. The clinical course of osteoporosis in anorexia nervosa. A longitudinal study of cortical bone mass. JAMA 1991;265: 1133–8.
83. Lucas AR, Beard CM, O'Fallon WM, et al. 50-year trends in the incidence of anorexia nervosa in Rochester, Minn.: a population-based study. Am J Psychiatry 1991;148:917–22.
84. Misra M, Prabhakaran R, Miller KK, et al. Prognostic indicators of changes in bone density measures in adolescent girls with anorexia nervosa-II. J Clin Endocrinol Metab 2008;93:1292–7.
85. Chiodini I, Torlontano M, Carnevale V, et al. Skeletal involvement in adult patients with endogenous hypercortisolism. J Endocrinol Invest 2008;31:267–76.
86. Schwartz MW, Woods SC, Porte D Jr, et al. Central nervous system control of food intake. Nature 2000;404:661–71.
87. Elefteriou F, Ahn JD, Takeda S, et al. Leptin regulation of bone resorption by the sympathetic nervous system and CART. Nature 2005;434:514–20.
88. Casper RC. Behavioral activation and lack of concern, core symptoms of anorexia nervosa? Int J Eat Disord 1998;24:381–93.
89. Casper RC. The 'drive for activity' and "restlessness" in anorexia nervosa: potential pathways. J Affect Disord 2006;92:99–107.
90. Holtkamp K, Hebebrand J, Herpertz-Dahlmann B. The contribution of anxiety and food restriction on physical activity levels in acute anorexia nervosa. Int J Eat Disord 2004;36:163–71.
91. Hebebrand J, Exner C, Hebebrand K, et al. Hyperactivity in patients with anorexia nervosa and in semistarved rats: evidence for a pivotal role of hypoleptinemia. Physiol Behav 2003;79:25–37.
92. van Elburg AA, Hoek HW, Kas MJ, et al. Nurse evaluation of hyperactivity in anorexia nervosa: a comparative study. Eur Eat Disord Rev 2007;15:425–9.
93. van Elburg AA, Kas MJ, Hillebrand JJ, et al. The impact of hyperactivity and leptin on recovery from anorexia nervosa. J Neural Transm 2007;114:1233–7.
94. Hebebrand J, Casper R, Treasure J, et al. The need to revise the diagnostic criteria for anorexia nervosa. J Neural Transm 2004;111:827–40.
95. Davis C, Katzman DK, Kirsh C. Compulsive physical activity in adolescents with anorexia nervosa: a psychobehavioral spiral of pathology. J Nerv Ment Dis 1999; 187:336–42.
96. Dwyer DM, Boakes RA. Activity-based anorexia in rats as failure to adapt to a feeding schedule. Behav Neurosci 1997;111:195–205.
97. Morse AD, Russell JC, Hunt TW, et al. Diurnal variation of intensive running in food-deprived rats. Can J Physiol Pharmacol 1995;73:1519–23.
98. Hillebrand JJ, Koeners MP, de Rijke CE, et al. Leptin treatment in activity-based anorexia. Biol Psychiatry 2005;58:165–71.
99. Hillebrand JJ, Kas MJ, Scheurink AJ, et al. AgRP(83-132) and SHU9119 differently affect activity-based anorexia. Eur Neuropsychopharmacol 2006;16: 403–12.
100. Hall JF, Hanford PV. Activity as a function of a restricted feeding schedule. J Comp Physiol Psychol 1954;47:362–3.

101. Epling WF, Pierce WD, Stefan L. A theory of activity-based anorexia. Int J Eat Disord 1981;3:27–47.
102. Schilling F. Selbstbeobachtungen im Hungerzustand. Beiträge aus der Allgemeinen Medizin 1948;6:41–67.
103. Seemann W. Über Hungerreaktionen von Kriegsgefangenen. Psyche 1950;4: 107–19.
104. Kas MJ, van Dijk G, Scheurink AJ, et al. Agouti-related protein prevents self-starvation. Mol Psychiatry 2003;8:235–40.
105. Hillebrand JJ, Kas MJ, Adan RA. Alpha-MSH enhances activity-based anorexia. Peptides 2005;26:1690–6.
106. Challet E, le Maho Y, Robin JP, et al. Involvement of corticosterone in the fasting-induced rise in protein utilization and locomotor activity. Pharmacol Biochem Behav 1995;50:405–12.
107. Lin WJ, Singer G, Papasava M. The role of adrenal corticosterone in schedule-induced wheel running. Pharmacol Biochem Behav 1988;30:101–6.
108. Wolkowitz OM. Prospective controlled studies of the behavioral and biological effects of exogenous corticosteroids. Psychoneuroendocrinology 1994;19: 233–55.
109. Pechnik RN, Kariagina A, Hartvig E, et al. Developmental exposure to corticosterone: behavioral changes and differential effects on leukemia inhibitory factor (LIF) and corticotropin-releasing hormone (CRH) gene expression in the mouse. Psychopharmacology (Berl) 2006;185:76–83.
110. Klein DA, Mayer LE, Schebendach JE, et al. Physical activity and cortisol in anorexia nervosa. Psychoneuroendocrinology 2007;32:539–47.
111. Harvey J. Leptin regulation of neuronal excitability and cognitive function. Curr Opin Pharmacol 2007;7:643–7.
112. Kemps E, Tiggemann M, Wade T. Selective working memory deficits in anorexia nervosa. Eur Eat Disord Rev 2006;14:97–103.

Overview of Treatment Modalities in Adolescent Anorexia Nervosa

Beate Herpertz-Dahlmann, MD[a],*, Harriet Salbach-Andrae, PhD[b]

KEYWORDS
- Anorexia nervosa • Adolescence • Inpatient treatment
- Day care management • Review

The aim of this article is to scrutinize and compare the benefits of distinct treatment settings for anorexia nervosa (AN) and to review the different treatment modalities that have proven helpful in the management of young patients with AN. Unfortunately, with the exception of outpatient family therapy, there is a dearth of controlled studies on the treatment of adolescent AN, which results in most of the recommendations being made based on mainstream clinical opinion with little empiric standing. To date, there are no multisite comparison trials of different treatment methods with large sample sizes in inpatient, day patient, or outpatient settings.

TREATMENT SETTINGS

This section deals primarily with inpatient and day care management, because different types of outpatient treatment are described in more detail in articles by Le Grange and Eisler and Schmidt elsewhere in this issue.

Inpatient Treatment

Inpatient treatment is considered the treatment of choice for severely undernourished young AN patients, especially in Europe. However, this point of view has been challenged recently. Results of a randomized effectiveness study have demonstrated

This research was supported by the German Ministry for Education and Research (01GV0602 360372).

[a] Departments of Child and Adolescent Psychiatry and Psychotherapy, RWTH Aachen University, Neuenhofer Weg 21, 52074 Aachen, Germany

[b] Department of Child and Adolescent Psychiatry, Psychosomatic and Psychotherapy Charité - Universitätsmedizin Berlin, Campus Virchow Klinikum, Augustenburger Platz 1, DE - 13353 Berlin, Germany

* Corresponding author.

E-mail address: bherpertz-dahlmann@ukaachen.de (B. Herpertz-Dahlmann).

Child Adolesc Psychiatric Clin N Am 18 (2008) 131–145
doi:10.1016/j.chc.2008.07.010
1056-4993/08/$ – see front matter
childpsych.theclinics.com

that inpatient treatment may not provide advantages over outpatient treatment in adolescent AN.[1]

In the United States, about half of patients seeking treatment for AN are admitted to inpatient treatment.[2] The mean duration of inpatient treatment for 15- to 24-year-old young people in Germany was 49.8 days, with overall costs of €12.800 € /patient in 1998.[3] In the United States, the average length of stay for each inpatient decreased from 149.5 days in 1984 to 23.7 days in 1998.[4] Instead, residential treatment options for individuals with AN or bulimia nervosa (BN) are becoming increasingly common. The average length of residential treatment was 83 days for patients with eating disorders, with an average cost per day of $956.00.[5]

Admission to the hospital is a clinical decision based on multiple factors that should always include the patient and her family, even when it is involuntarily. Criteria for considering admission to hospital are summarized in **Table 1**.

Most clinicians believe that multidisciplinary inpatient units experienced in the treatment of adolescent AN are the most effective settings for restoration of healthy body weight and for a fundamental change in overvaluation of weight and shape. However, there are no controlled studies to compare the outcomes of inpatient treatment on a general pediatric or adolescent psychiatric ward to a specialized inpatient program for eating disorders (see also Ref.[6]).

Involuntary Treatment and Coercive Pressure

Involuntary treatment of eating disorders has always been a controversial issue. It is used rarely in adolescent patients and only in life-threatening situations. Some early research argued that patients legally admitted for involuntary treatment have negative memories of their hospitalization and might not experience any benefit. However, recent studies from the United States and United Kingdom report that short-term responses of the legally committed patients were just as good as the responses of the patients who had voluntarily agreed to treatment.[7,8] Detained patients gained as much weight during the hospital stay as those who were voluntarily admitted, but took longer to meet their weight goals. Most of the involuntarily treated patients later affirmed the necessity of their treatment and complied with the treatment process. In the British study,[7] involuntarily admitted patients had more aversive childhoods, displayed more self-harm behaviors, had more previous admissions to hospital, and had a higher mortality rate at long-term follow-up. Note that both studies included adolescent patients. Russell[9] maintains that involuntarily treated patients often realize some time later that the professional staff, their family members, and legal authorities

Table 1	
Criteria for inpatient care in adolescent AN	
Medical Criteria	**Psychosocial Criteria**
BMI less than the third percentile	Severe social isolation
Rapid weight loss, low energy intake, refusal to drink	High parental criticism, dysfunctional family interactions
Medical complications (eg, hypokalemia, alkalosis, severe bradycardia, pancreas or liver affection)	Lack of outpatient facilities or insufficient response to outpatient treatment trials
Severe psychiatric comorbidity such as depression or OCD	

take their illness seriously. Moreover, the patients and their parents may even feel relieved to hand over the responsibility for their health to a professional team.

Even voluntarily admitted patients often perceive subtle or direct pressure by their parents, friends, or teachers. In a recent study by Guarda and colleagues[10] patients' perceptions about their need for hospitalization and the coerciveness of the admission process were evaluated. Patients younger than 18 years reported more perceived coercion and tended to disagree with hospitalization than did adult patients. After 2 weeks of treatment, nearly half of the patients who denied needing admission had changed their minds to believing that they did indeed need to be admitted. However, the large majority of those who had changed their minds were adults, whereas the adolescents still did not endorse the need for hospitalization. Thus, it might be more difficult to persuade anorectic adolescents than adults of the seriousness of their illness, which points to the necessity of involving caretakers of eating disordered adolescents in treatment procedures.

This is also true for treatment adherence. One-third to one-half of anorectic inpatients drop out of treatment prematurely,[11–13] which is substantially higher than the rates reported in general psychiatry. Predictors of dropout in adults were a higher number of previous hospitalizations, especially in those who dropped out in the earliest phase of treatment and the binge–purge subtype of AN.[11,14]

Relapse rates of 25% to 40% have been reported during the first year after admission.[15–18] In a multisite follow-up study of adolescent AN in Western and Eastern Europe, significant predictors of readmission were paternal alcoholism, eating disorder in infancy, physical hyperactivity, lower weight increase at first admission, and lower BMI at first discharge.[18] Other studies have identified high mean scores on the Eating Attitudes Test, lower mean age, previous treatments for eating disorders, severity of obsessive compulsive disorder (OCD) symptoms, and excessive exercise immediately after discharge.

However, up to now it has not been clarified whether there is a paucity in the quality of inpatient treatment in adolescent AN or whether AN per se takes a protracted and distressful course.

Full-Time Inpatient Hospital Treatment Versus Outpatient Treatment in Adolescent Anorexia Nervosa

In a very early, randomized controlled trial that compared inpatient and outpatient treatment, the investigators found limited evidence that outpatient treatment was as effective as inpatient treatment in adolescents not ill enough to warrant emergency medical treatment.[19] In this study, inpatient treatment was characterized by a multimodal approach, including dietary counseling and individual and family therapy. In the second arm of the trial, patients received twelve outpatient sessions with varying amounts of individual and family therapy. In the third option, patients and parents were treated separately with 10 group meetings for the anorectic patient and the parents, respectively. Both outpatient options also received dietary counseling. After 1 year, weight gains in all 3 treatment groups were significant, with the largest gains in the outpatient groups.[19] This comparative study was biased by the fact that many patients randomized to inpatient treatment did not accept it. There was a 2-year follow-up investigation for the outpatient group treated with a package of individual and family therapy. Of the original 20 patients, 12 were rated as well or nearly well according to Morgan and Russell criteria.[20]

There is some inconclusive evidence that hospital inpatient care may adversely affect outcome in young patients. In a British study, 21 of 75 patients who had received inpatient treatment had a significantly worse outcome than the 51 patients never admitted to the hospital.[21] This study, too, was biased by several factors, including the problem that the time of follow-up varied between 2 and 7 years, although it is well known that a longer time of follow-up is associated with a better outcome. In addition, treatment modalities differed significantly between settings. Only those treated on an outpatient basis received family therapy, which is the only treatment method that has proven to be relatively successful in adolescent AN.

In another controlled trial, 167 young people with AN were randomized to inpatient treatment, to a specialized eating disorder outpatient service with a manualized treatment program, or to treatment as usual at a child and adolescent mental health service.[1] According to the results of this study, there was no advantage of inpatient over outpatient management. Indeed, inpatient treatment predicted a poor prognosis, and specialist outpatient management did not result in a better outcome than general child and adolescent mental health service. However, these findings are difficult to interpret. First, the duration of treatment differed significantly among the 3 arms of the trial, with inpatient treatment lasting a mean of 15 weeks and the 2 outpatient arms lasting 6 months. Inpatient treatment was not followed by any kind of outpatient care. Second, adherence to treatment regimens varied substantially. Unsurprisingly, inpatient treatment had the highest dropout rate. All participants were evaluated on an intention-to-treat-based analysis, although several of the outpatients subsequently engaged in more intensive forms of treatment. Third, with the exception of the specialist outpatient management, treatment components were not manualized. The investigators argue that despite the caveats, the study provides insight into a more naturalistic use of services in the United Kingdom.

In sum, basic questions about inpatient treatment have not been adequately addressed or answered. There is some evidence that inpatient treatment is helpful for severely malnourished or medically at-risk patients. However, there are no evidence-based criteria for admission to inpatient treatment, and the specific goals of inpatient treatment are not agreed on. Accordingly, there is no established consensus about the most effective length of inpatient care or about the comparative role of different treatment modalities. In addition, it is still unclear whether different age groups (eg, adults versus adolescents) may profit from different treatment settings.[22]

Day Care Management

In addition to financial benefit, day-patient treatment may have some advantages over inpatient care. Day-patient care allows the patient to have extensive contact with her family, school, and peers. New skills learned at the day-patient program may be transferred home immediately, and alternate social roles or coping strategies will be more easily generalized from the therapeutic milieu to everyday situations. Nevertheless, there is only 1 survey in the literature based on a systematic database search of eating disorder day-hospital-treatment programs.[23] This study mainly focused on 3 institutions, 1 in the United States 1 in Canada, and 1 in Germany. Findings from these treatment locations suggest that the day-treatment programs led to significant weight gain and an improvement in specific and general psychopathology in AN patients. The outcome did not depend significantly on the number of days spent in day care. Older adolescents were included in these partial day programs; however, there was no information on the influence of age on outcome.

Significant differences between day care units exist in terms of criteria for admission (eg, minimal body weight, repeated outpatient failure), time spent in treatment, and posttreatment care. Some institutions operate 7 days/week, whereas others are open only 4 days/week.

To our knowledge, there is only 1 study that has compared day-patient and inpatient treatment.[24] In this study, 13 consecutively admitted day patients were matched with corresponding inpatients. After inpatient treatment, patients had gained a greater amount of weight and reached a more favorable overall outcome. However, this study was biased by an extremely small sample size and nonrandomization. Therefore, randomized controlled trials between day care management and inpatient treatment are urgently needed. In the United States, the pressure to reduce the length of stay for hospitalized patients and reduced insurance coverage for management of eating disorders has led to a hurried transmission into less intensive settings. In contrast, the high costs for the treatment of adolescent AN in Germany reflects the fact that most of the patients are admitted to inpatient treatment. However, both situations depend more on health care policies than on empiric standing. Adolescent anorectic patients may experience the care of the professional staff in a hospital setting as supportive, whereas life outside the hospital is seen as tough and the resumption of responsibilities too stressful. A return to hospitalization related to relapse of the eating disorder is probably seen as an escape and not as a failure.[21] Instead, the time spent outside the unit after day treatment might provide a better opportunity to gain mastery in everyday life (concerning eating and non-eating behavior) and thus might contribute to a better relapse prevention. At present, the authors are conducting a 5-site controlled study supported by the German Ministry for Education and Research. In this investigation, children and adolescents between 11 and 17 years of age are randomized to either day-patient or inpatient service after a 3-week admission to an inpatient unit. Treatment approaches are manualized, and apart from the setting, modalities are exactly the same. Up to now, more than 60 patients fulfilling fourth edition of the Diagnostic and Statistical Manual of Mental Disorders (DSM-IV) criteria for AN have been enrolled in this study.

MULTIMODAL TREATMENT APPROACH

Although it has not yet been systematically assessed in controlled trials, there is some clinical evidence that a multidisciplinary behavioral treatment program in an inpatient or day-care setting is effective to restore a healthy body weight and better psychological and social functioning. This can be achieved by a multimodal treatment approach based on the following main components:

(1) Nutritional rehabilitation and treatment of medical complications
(2) Nutritional counseling to restore healthy eating behavior
(3) Individual therapy to help the patient to correct dysfunctional thoughts and improve self-esteem
(4) Group therapy
(5) Family (or parent) counseling or therapy.

In addition, comorbid disorders, especially depressive, anxious, or obsessive-compulsive symptoms should be alleviated.

To prevent more adolescents from dropping out of treatment, it may be helpful to introduce some sort of "motivational enhancement intervention" to engage them in therapy and reduce ambivalence and resistance to change. In adolescent inpatients, low motivation to change was a reliable predictor of readmission to hospital.[25] Recent studies suggest that motivational interviewing, which has been used in the treatment of addiction, may be helpful in short-term treatment outcomes in adolescent AN[26,27] (for a description see the article by Schmidt, elsewhere in this issue). In an Australian study group, motivational enhancement therapy was used in the beginning of inpatient treatment to foster longer-term motivation and promote treatment continuation.[28]

Nutritional Rehabilitation

Nutritional rehabilitation and nutritional counseling are described here in more detail, because in our opinion it is an important component of inpatient and day care treatment in adolescent AN.

The goal of nutritional rehabilitation in emaciated AN patients is the restoration of normal body weight. In general, a healthy body weight may be considered the weight at which menstruation reoccurs. However, by clinical experience, we know that many anorectic patients do not resume menstruation in the first months of treatment despite reaching a reasonable weight. Some researchers have recommended assessing ovarian maturity as a reliable measure of adequate target weight.[29] In the German guidelines for the treatment of adolescent eating disorders, the 25th age-adjusted BMI percentile is defined as target weight for girls younger than 18 years, including premenstrual patients. Accordingly, goals for weight have to be adapted continuously to account for increases in age and height. Several clinicians prefer a target weight range to a definite weight target.[30] Discussing a target weight range or weight target is recommended toward the end of the initial phase of treatment, when the patient may be less distressed at the prospect of further weight gain.

Given the severe caloric restraint characteristic of adolescent AN patients, renutrition should be started at a low caloric level of 900 to 1000 kcal/d; in severe cases, intake should be even less. Too high a caloric replacement may lead to the so-called "refeeding syndrome," with cardiac, renal, and neurologic complications. In addition, patients may complain of "feeling extremely full" because of delayed gastric emptying. The number of calories should be increased stepwise over a period of 1 or 2 weeks until the patient arrives at 2200 to 2500 kcal/d depending on her height and age. With the help of a behavioral program, an average weight gain of 500 to 1000 g/wk (1–2 lb/wk) in inpatient settings and 300 to 500 g/wk in day care management should be achieved.[31] In some patients, calorie levels should be adjusted several times owing to changes in resting energy expenditure and activity levels. Because of dehydration or edema, it may be necessary to weigh the patient daily at the beginning of refeeding; afterward weighing twice a week is sufficient to ensure the expected weight gain.

During the early stages of inpatient treatment, it is necessary to advise the patient about the potential adverse physical consequences of starvation and to support her compliance with the refeeding program. A normalization of body weight is needed to reverse the physical and mental consequences of malnutrition, such as starvation-associated depression and obsessive behavior. In the United States, clinicians are under increasing pressure to transfer AN patients from inpatient treatment to less expensive settings. However, several studies on adolescent patients suggest that restoration to full weight, in contrast to partial weight, confers a more favorable prognosis.[32,33] On the other hand, a too rapid and large weight gain may be followed by hyperleptinemia in previously starved patients, which likely promotes reduction of food intake and increase in energy expenditure, resulting in a premature relapse. A modest but regular weight gain is probably associated with a more favorable short-term outcome.[34]

Nutritional Counseling

Eating disordered patients are well informed about caloric intent and the amount of fat in different food items, although they have insufficient knowledge of adequate nutritional requirements. To reestablish a normal eating behavior, an individualized meal plan is developed for each patient, consisting of 3 main meals and 3 snacks. It is always designed with the patient, and takes her personal likes or dislikes into account. The meal plan is built on caloric needs and recommended food components, including a sufficient amount of protein, carbohydrates, and fat. Patients should be encouraged to expand their meal choices to previously "forbidden foods" to enrich a severely restricted diet. At the beginning of treatment it is often helpful for the adolescent patient to get the size of her meal portioned or to get detailed information on portion size by seeing pictures or food models. If the adolescent has great difficulty restoring normal eating habits, it is often helpful to provide a "human model" for the patient to imitate. In the authors' department, a nurse demonstrates how to take a normal bite, finish a meal in a reasonable time, and incorporate all food groups, such as fats and desserts, in a setting separate from the other patients.

In addition to individual nutritional advice, nutritional group programs are helpful. In weekly psychoeducational sessions, patients are informed about things like standard nutritional recommendations, necessity of fat intake for absorption of fat-soluble vitamins, and consequences of starvation for bone metabolism and growth of height. Anorectic patients often avoid or feel ashamed of eating with others or in unknown places or situations, which might contribute to their social isolation. For this reason, cooking sessions and staff-supported visits to restaurants, school cafeterias, and food courts are also part of the group program to help patients to gain necessary skills for eating in public or with their peers. Finally, it is important to involve the family in the reestablishment of normal eating patterns. Parents often do not know what to say to help patients with their meal plans or their meal sizes. In addition, during the meal, there is often a high level of parental criticism focused on the patient. For that reason, it is often helpful to arrange staff-supported family meals with the parents, siblings, and the patient attending.

There is scant research on the importance of nutritional counseling on the outcome of adolescent AN treatment. In a post-hospitalization study in adult AN by Pike and colleagues[35] nutritional counseling was compared with cognitive-behavioral therapy (CBT). CBT was found to lead to lower dropout rates, a higher percentage of favorable outcomes, and a longer time to relapse. However, in most multidisciplinary treatment approaches, nutritional counseling is complementary to, not a substitute for, individual psychotherapy.

Individual Psychotherapy

There are virtually no controlled studies on individual psychotherapy in adolescent AN. In adults, therapeutic approaches comprise CBT, interpersonal therapy (IPT), cognitive analytic therapy (CAT), focal psychoanalytic therapy and specialist supportive clinical management (SSCM) (for a review see Ref.[36]). Several of these studies focused on CBT, which has proven effective in the treatment of BN (a more thorough survey of this treatment modality is given in the article by Schmidt, elsewhere in this issue). However, in AN, individual CBT has probably no advantage over other forms of individual treatment.

In a recent study on underweight outpatients with AN or subthreshold AN (age range, 17–40 years), CBT was compared with IPT and nonspecific supportive clinical management,[37] which was later described as SSCM.[38] Intriguingly, the results favored SSCM, which led to better outcomes than IPT when global outcome ratings were compared. Therapeutic response to CBT fell between IPT and SSCM. SSCM combines the principles of supportive psychotherapy and clinical management, which was delivered by a clinician experienced in the treatment of eating disorders. Besides a regular monitoring of body weight, clinical management comprised several components of psychoeducation, including explanations about the etiology, symptoms, course, and outcome of the eating disorder. The patient received nutritional education and advice, and a target weight range was set during treatment. These strategies, which aimed at improving the core symptoms of AN, were embedded in a reliable and supportive relationship between clinician and patient, which fostered working together in an environment of empathy and acceptance.[38]

Although the results of this study are interesting, they cannot be generalized to most of the patients with AN. Mean BMI at baseline was high (17.3 + 1.1) and because there was no follow-up investigation, the number of relapses after the end of treatment is unknown.

Body Image Therapy

Bruch[39] is credited as being the first to define a "perceptual and conceptual disturbance or disorder of body image" in patients with AN. In the DSM-IV,[40] distorted body image is defined as a "disturbance in the way in which one's body weight or shape is experienced, with undue influence of body weight or shape on self evaluation." Many studies have shown the association between eating pathology and disturbed body image (eg,[41]). Beyond that, a negative body image seems to have an essential role in the development and maintenance of AN.[42,43] The large number of studies concerning the assessment of negative body image in AN stands in contrast to the few attempts to influence the way these patients actually experience their bodies. Although treatment programs specifically targeting body image concerns have been developed,[44–46] no randomized controlled trials for adolescent and adult eating disorders exist. Cognitive-behavioral body image therapy includes body exposure, desensitization through specific "do it yourself" exercises, and full-length "mirror confrontation." Moreover, cognitive techniques are used to identify and modify negative body-related thoughts.[47] In nonclinical samples, evidence for the effectiveness of cognitive-behavioral body image therapy has been found.[48,49] A pilot study by Key and colleagues[50] assessed the role of mirror confrontation in the desensitization of a body image treatment within an inpatient program for AN. They found that body image treatment involving sustained mirror confrontation was more effective than body image treatment without mirror confrontation. Unfortunately, the sample size was small and no information about the effect on weight gain was given. Another study, which was executed with women suffering from AN, BN, EDNOS (eating disorder not otherwise specified), and healthy controls, demonstrated that the extent of negative cognitions and emotions evoked by looking in a mirror can be reduced by cognitive-behavioral body image therapy aiming at an improvement of body image.[51] This study, too, was biased by a small sample size and the lack of an eating disordered control group. Because body image therapy is often applied in inpatient and day care management of adolescent AN, evidence-based studies on the effect of body image therapy should be conducted.

Group Psychotherapy

Group psychotherapy is generally recognized as an important form of psychotherapy for AN patients and is usually implemented in inpatient and outpatient settings. Although it is difficult to specifically address individual (eg, comorbid) problems and issues, group therapy is cost-effective compared with individual therapy and provides support and motivation. Despite the listed advantages, only 1 randomized controlled study has examined the efficacy of outpatient group psychotherapy for the treatment of AN in adolescence to date[19] (as aforementioned). No controlled trial has yet compared the effectiveness of individual versus group psychotherapy in AN. Comparison of group CBT and individual CBT for adult patients with BN showed no significant differences between both groups at follow-up.[52] Additional studies should examine whether group psychotherapy is as effective as individual psychotherapy in AN. Program descriptions of multifamily therapy have been published. A more detailed description of this form of family-based therapy is given by Le Grange and Eisler, elsewhere in this issue.

Dialectical behavior therapy (DBT) is an empirically supported treatment that comprises (a) a skills training group to enhance skill capabilities, (b) individual psychotherapy sessions to conduct behavioral and solution analyses on target behaviors and to improve client motivation, and (c) intersession telephone availability to enhance skills generalization and therapeutic relationship issues. It targets emotion regulation and was originally developed for female adult multiproblem outpatients diagnosed with borderline personality disorder (BPD).[53] Interest in DBT has grown recently and researchers have begun to apply DBT to other clinical populations in inpatient and outpatient settings (eg, Ref.[54]). Wisniewski and Kelly[55] presented a case for applying DBT to the treatment of AN and BN patients. Telch and colleagues[56] and Safer and colleagues[57] adapted DBT for patients with binge eating disorder and BN. These results revealed preliminary evidence suggesting that DBT may be an effective treatment for these eating disorders in adults. To date, only 2 studies exist on the effectiveness of DBT for adolescent patients suffering from AN and BN.[58,59] The results of these pilot studies suggest that DBT seems to be a promising treatment for inpatient and outpatient settings for these adolescents; however, further evaluation is required before any firm conclusions can be drawn.

Family-based Interventions

Family-based therapy (FBT) has gradually been established over the last decade as an important therapeutic strategy for adolescents with AN. In this context, families seem to be an important resource for the recovery of young anorectic patients. Built on Minuchin's work, the first controlled FBT study with adolescents and young adults was initiated by Russell at the Maudley's hospital in London. In their study, FBT with younger and non-chronic anorectic patients was more effective than individual supportive therapy. Since then, the Maudsley research group has conducted several studies. Their results are described in another article by Le Grange and Eisler in this issue.

Most of these family-based interventions were performed on an outpatient basis, although some of the participating patients required admission to inpatient treatment because of insufficient weight gain or starvation-associated medical risks.[60] In some of the investigations, patients had to have a minimal body weight more than 75% ideal body weight (IBW) or were even in the low range of normal weight. Therefore, findings of outpatient family therapy in adolescent AN may not be transferred to severely emaciated patients. In another well-known study by Robin and colleagues in Detroit,[61] about half of the sample was hospitalized at the beginning of therapy and stayed on the ward until their weight had increased to more than 80% of ideal body weight.

Besides the "state of the art" FBT, only a few models of family-based interventions exist. Geist and colleagues[62] compared the effect of family therapy with family group psychoeducation. Most of the treatment sessions took place in an inpatient setting. The investigators concluded that group psychoeducation involving parents and anorectic adolescents was as effective as family therapy with regard to eating disorder or general psychopathology. Finally, Uehara and colleagues[63] reported that 52-hour sessions of family psychoeducation led to a significant reduction in the emotional involvement of relatives of adult female patients with eating disorders. Since then, some research groups have developed psychoeducation programs to involve parents or whole families in the therapeutic process instead of or complementary to "typical" FBT. In a project by Zucker and colleagues[64] 16 families whose children were receiving outpatient treatment participated in a 16-session group treatment. Only parents attended the group, and group sizes ranged from 7 to 12 participants. The program adapted elements of DBT, learning theory and social cognitive. Topics of the sessions included etiology of eating disorders, parenting style, behavior modification, role modeling (parents as models of healthy behavior), family mealtimes, emotion regulation, and communication. The parental response to the intervention was positive in the sense that parents acknowledged the program to be an essential part of the management of their child's eating disorder and as a result decreased the burden they experienced.

The eating disorder research group at the authors' department also designed a program of group psychoeducation for parents to increase the understanding of the disorder and to promote high transparency with regard to our treatment strategy (**Table 2**). In accordance with the program by Zucker and colleagues,[64] it was aimed

Table 2 Psychoeducation program for parents of eating disordered patients	
Topic	**Contents**
Session 1	
Etiology, symptoms, medical complications of AN, importance of weight gain in adolescence	Physiologic and psychologic consequences of semi-starvation, short-term and long-term consequences of malnourishment (eg, osteoporosis), compulsive need for exercise, significance of target weight
Session 2	
Concept and goals of inpatient treatment program	Criteria for admission to inpatient treatment, components and aims of treatment program, (eg, individual and group psychotherapy, family-based interventions)
Session 3	
Nutritional counseling	Caloric needs for weight restoration and weight maintenance, overall and specific nutritional needs in adolescence, food components, reintroduction of "forbidden food"
Session 4	
Relapse prevention and outpatient treatment	Necessity of long-term "aftercare," how to identify first signs of relapse, criteria for readmission, what to tell teachers and neighbors
Session 5	
Role of the family in eating disorders, feelings of shame and guilt	Active role of the parents to help the adolescent recover, negative effects of parental criticism on outcome, improvement of parenting skills

only at the parents of the authors' eating disordered inpatients and outpatients. They received detailed information about the group psychoeducation at the first contact to the eating disorder service. The program was limited to 5 dates of 90 minutes, which took place 1 day every week in the late afternoon. The group was guided by a child and adolescent psychiatrist, a nutritional scientist, and an occupational therapist specialized in work with eating disordered patients. In a preliminary evaluation, parents of 142 patients were invited to anonymously fill out a satisfaction questionnaire, which was returned by 115 (81%) of the parents. Most (77%) of those who had returned the evaluation sheet rated the group psychoeducation as a helpful way to cope with their child's disorder and 85% would recommend other parents to take part in the program.[65]

Relatives of patients with eating disorders show high levels of emotional distress, which may contribute to dysfunctional coping.[66] Through group psychoeducation programs, parents are provided with relevant information on the illness and intervention strategies. This seems to reduce conflicts between patients, parents, and therapists, which are usually common in the treatment of eating disorders. In learning about the biological mechanisms, etiology, and symptomatology of eating disorders, parents are relieved of guilt and shame for being the agent of the child's disorder.

In conclusion, group psychoeducation for parents of adolescents with eating disorders may represent a useful and economic method in the multimodal treatment of eating disorders.

SUMMARY AND RECOMMENDATIONS FOR FURTHER RESEARCH

Evidence-based findings on the effect of different treatment methods for adolescent AN are limited. Family therapy is considered to be an effective treatment for adolescent patients. However, few data show that FBT is more helpful than other forms of treatment. In addition, it is not clear whether FBT is of any benefit to severely underweight patients or whether psychoeducational interventions prove to be effective help for the parents or the patient. We do not know which kind of individual psychotherapy should be recommended for adolescent AN.

There is no consensus on whether and how target weight should be set. An investigation in the United Kingdom and Europe has demonstrated considerable variation. Although most of the institutions relied on age-related norms in the treatment of adolescent AN, weight targets ranged from the 10th to the 75th percentile for those who used BMI percentiles and between 17.5 and 21 kg/m² for those using absolute values.[30] Recent studies have demonstrated that nonspecific treatment forms were as effective for AN as specific and intensive psychotherapeutic methods.[1,37] The contribution of nonspecific factors to the establishment and maintenance of a strong relationship between the clinician and the adolescent AN patient may be most important for adherence to the treatment process and relapse prevention.

The most urgent questions that have to be resolved by additional research are (1) How can we prevent young patients from dropping out of treatment? (2) What kinds of treatments are effective in severely underweight patients? (3) Which intensity of treatment (inpatient, day patient, or outpatient) is necessary at different stages of the illness? (4) Which treatment modality (medication, different forms of psychotherapy) is most effective for relapse prevention? (5) What is the cost/benefit relationship?

Anorectic adolescents have a much better outcome than their adult counterparts. Many recent follow-up studies point to a recovery rate of about 70% in adolescent AN, and mortality rate is close to zero. This should encourage us to intensify our search for effective treatment interventions in adolescent AN.

REFERENCES

1. Gowers SG, Clark A, Roberts C, et al. Clinical effectiveness of treatments for anorexia nervosa in adolescents. Br J Psychiatry 2007;91:427–35.
2. Agras WS, Brandt HA, Bulic CM, et al. Report of the National institutes of health workshop on overcoming barriers to treatment research in anorexia nervosa. Int J Eat Disord 2004;35(4):509–21.
3. Krauth C, Buser K, Vogel H. How high are the costs of eating disorders—anorexia nervosa and bulimia nervosa—for German society. Eur J Health Econ 2002;3: 244–50.
4. Wiseman CV, Sunday SR, Klapper F, et al. Changing patterns of hospitalization in eating disorder patients. Int J Eat Disord 2001;30(1):69–74.
5. Frisch MJ, Herzog DB, Franko DL. Residential treatment for eating disorders. Int J Eat Disord 2006;39(5):434–42.
6. Guarda AS. Treatment of anorexia nervosa: insights and obstacles. Physiol Behav 2008;94(1):113–20.
7. Ramsay R, Ward A, Treasure J, et al. Compulsory treatment in anorexia nervosa. Short-term benefits and long-term mortality. Br J Psychiatry 1999;175:147–53.
8. Watson TL, Bowers WA, Andersen AE. Involuntary treatment of eating disorders. Am J Psychiatry 2000;157:1806–10.
9. Russell GF. Involuntary treatment in anorexia nervosa. Psychiatr Clin North Am 2001;24(2):337–49.
10. Guarda AS, Pinto AM, Coughlin JW, et al. Perceived coercion and change in perceived need for admission in patients hospitalized for eating disorders. Am J Psychiatry 2007;164:108–14.
11. Kahn C, Pike KM. In search of predictors of dropout from inpatient treatment for anorexia nervosa. Int J Eat Disord 2001;30:237–44.
12. Zeeck A, Hartmann A, Buchholz C, et al. Drop outs from in-patient treatment in anorexia nervosa. Acta Psychiatr Scand 2005;111(1):29–37.
13. Vandereycken W, Pierloot R. Drop-out during in-patient treatment of anorexia nervosa: a clinical study of 133 patients. Br J Med psychol 1983;56(2):145–56.
14. Woodside DB, Carter JC, Blackmore E. Predictors of premature termination of inpatient treatment for anorexia nervosa. Am J Psychiatry 2004;161(12):2277–81.
15. Herpertz-Dahlmann B, Müller B, Herpertz S, et al. Prospective ten-year follow-up in adolescent anorexia nervosa—course, outcome and psychiatric comorbidity. J Child Psychol Psychiatry 2001;42:603–12.
16. Carter JC, Blackmore E, Sutandar-Pinnock K, et al. Relapse in anorexia nervosa: a survival analysis. Psychol Med 2004;34(4):671–9.
17. Castro J, Gila A, Puig J, et al. Predictors of rehospitalization after total weight recovery in adolescents with anorexia nervosa. Int J Eat Disord 2004;36:22–30.
18. Steinhausen H, Grigoroiu-Serbanescu M, Boyadjieva S, et al. Course and predictors of rehospitalization in adolescent anorexia nervosa in a multisite study. Int J Eat Disord 2008;41(1):29–36.
19. Crisp AH, Norton KR, Gowers S, et al. A controlled study of the effect of therapies aimed at adolescent and family psychopathology in anorexia nervosa. Br J Psychiatry 1991;159:325–33.
20. Gowers SG, Norton KR, Halek C, et al. Outcome of outpatient psychotherapy in a random allocation treatment study of anorexia nervosa. Int J Eat Disord 1994; 15:165–77.
21. Gowers SG, Weetman J, Shore A, et al. Impact of hospitalisation on the outcome of adolescent anorexia nervosa. Br J Psychiatry 2000;176:138–41.

22. Fairburn CG. Evidence-based treatment of anorexia nervosa. Int J Eat Disord 2005;37:S26–30.
23. Zipfel S, Reas DL, Thornton C, et al. Day hospitalization programs for eating disorders: a systematic review of the literature. Int J Eat Disord 2002;31: 105–17.
24. Zeeck A, Hartmann A, Wetzler-Burmeister E, et al. Comparison of inpatient and day clinic treatment of anorexia nervosa. Z Psychosom Med Psychother 2006; 52(2):190–203.
25. Ametller L, Castro J, Serrano E, et al. Readiness to recover in adolescent anorexia nervosa: prediction of hospital admission. J Child Psychol Psychiatry 2005;46(4):394–400.
26. Gowers S, Smyth B. The impact of a motivational assessment interview on initial response to treatment in adolescent anorexia nervosa. Eur Eat Disord Rev 2004; 12:87–93.
27. Schmidt U. Engagement and motivational interviewing. In: Graham P, editor. Cognitive behaviour therapy for children and families. Cambridge, UK: Cambridge University Press; 2005. p. 67–83.
28. Dean HY, Touyz SW, Rieger E, et al. Group motivational enhancement therapy as an adjunct to inpatient treatment for eating disorders: a preliminary study. Eur Eat Disord Rev 2007;16:265–7.
29. Key A, Mason H, Allan R, et al. Restoration of ovarian and uterine maturity in adolescents with anorexia nervosa. Int J Eat Disord 2002;32:319–25.
30. Roots P, Hawker J, Gowers SG. The use of target weights in the inpatient treatment of adolescent anorexia nervosa. Eur Eat Disorders Rev 2006;14:323–8.
31. Wilson GT, Shafran R. Eating disorders guidelines from NICE. Lancet 2005;365: 79–81.
32. Lock J, Litt I. What predicts maintenance of weight for adolescents medically hospitalized for anorexia nervosa. Eat Disord 2003;11(1):1–7.
33. Howard WT, Evans KK, Quintero-Howard CV, et al. Predictors of success or failure of transition to day hospital treatment for inpatients with anorexia nervosa. Am J Psychiatry 1999;156:1697–702.
34. Holtkamp K, Herpertz-Dahlmann B, Mika C, et al. Elevated physical activity and low leptin levels co-occur in patients with anorexia nervosa. J Clin Endocrinol Metab 2003;88:5169–74.
35. Pike KM, Walsh BT, Vitousek K, et al. Cognitive behaviour therapy in the posthospitalization treatment of anorexia nervosa. Am J Psychiatry 2003;160:2046–9.
36. Bulik CM, Berkman ND, Brownley KA, et al. Anorexia nervosa treatment: a systematic review of randomized controlled trials. Int J Eat Disord 2007;40(4):310–20.
37. McIntosh VW, Jordan J, Luty SE, et al. Three Psychotherapies for anorexia nervosa: a randomized, controlled trial. Am J Psychiatry 2005;162:741–7.
38. McIntosh VW, Jordan J, Luty SE, et al. Specialist supportive clinical management for anorexia nervosa. Int J Eat Disord 2006;39:625–32.
39. Bruch H. Perceptual and conceptual disturbances in anorexia nervosa. Psychosom Med 1962;24:187–94.
40. American Psychiatric Association. Diagnostic and statistical manual of mental disorders. 4th edition. Washington, DC: American Psychiatric Association; 1994. p. 545.
41. Gardner RM, Bokenkamp ED. The role of sensory and nonsensory factors in body size estimations of eating disorder subjects. J Clin Psychol 1996;52:3–15.
42. Killen JD, Taylor CB, Hayward C, Haydel KF, et al. Weight concerns influence the development of eating disorders: a 4-year prospective study. J Consult Clin Psychol 1996;64:936–40.

43. Stice E. Risk and maintenance factors for eating pathology: a meta-analytic review. Psychol Bull 2002;128:825–48.
44. Cash TF, Grant JR. Cognitive-behavioural treatment of body image disturbances. In: Van Hasselt VB, Hersen M, editors. Sourcebook of psychological treatment manuals for adult disorders. New York: Plenum Press; 1996. p. 567–614.
45. Rosen JC. Cognitive-behavioural body-image therapy. In: Garner DM, Garfinkel PE, editors. Handbook of treatment for eating disorders. New York: Guilford; 1998. p. 188–201.
46. Vocks S, Legenbauer T. Körperbildtherapie bei Anorexia und Bulimia nervosa. Ein kognitiv-verhaltenstherapeutisches Behandlungsprogramm. Göttingen: Hogrefe; 2005 [in German].
47. Cash TF, Hrabosky JI. Treatment of body image disturbances. In: Thompson JK, editor. Handbook of eating disorders and obesity. New Jersey: John Wiley & Sons; 2004. p. 515–41.
48. Delinsky SS, Wilson GT. Mirror exposure for the treatment of body image disturbance. Int J Eat Disord 2006;39:108–16.
49. Grant JR, Cash TF. Cognitive-behavioral body image therapy: comparative efficacy of group and modest-contact treatments. Behav Ther 1995;26:68–84.
50. Key A, George CL, Beattie D, et al. Body image treatment within an inpatient program for anorexia nervosa: the role of mirror exposure in the desensitization process. Int J Eat Disord 2002;31:185–90.
51. Vocks S, Wächter A, Wucherer M, et al. Look at yourself: can body image therapy affect the cognitive and emotional response to seeing oneself in the mirror in eating disorders? Eur Eat Disord Rev 2008;16:147–54.
52. Chen E, Touyz SW, Beumont PJ, et al. Comparison of group and individual cognitive-behavioral therapy for patients with bulimia nervosa. Int J Eat Disord 2002; 33:241–54.
53. Linehan MM, Armstrong HE, Suarez A, et al. Cognitive-behavioral treatment of chronically parasuicidal borderline patients. Arch Gen Psychiatry 1991;48: 1060–4.
54. Rathus JH, Miller AL. Dialectical behavior therapy adapted for suicidal adolescents. Suicide Life Threat Behav 2002;32:146–57.
55. Wisniewski L, Kelly E. The application of dialectical behavior therapy to the treatment of eating disorders. Cogn Behav Pract 2003;10:131–8.
56. Telch CF, Agras WS, Linehan MM. Dialectical behavior therapy for binge eating disorder. J Consult Clin Psychol 2001;69:1061–5.
57. Safer DL, Lock J, Couturier JL. Dialectical behavior therapy modified for adolescent binge eating disorder: a case report. Cogn Behav Pract 2007;14: 157–67.
58. Salbach H, Klinkowski N, Pfeiffer E, et al. Dialectical behavior therapy for adolescents with anorexia and bulimia nervosa (DBT-AN/ BN)–a pilot study. [[Dialektisch Behaviorale Therapie für jugendliche Patientinnen mit Anorexia und Bulimia nervosa (DBT-AN/BN)–eine Pilotstudie]]. Prax Kinderpsychol Kinderpsychiatr 2007; 56:91–108 [in German].
59. Salbach-Andrae H, Bohnekamp I, Pfeiffer E, Lehmkuhl U, et-al. Dialectical behavior therapy of anorexia and bulimia nervosa among adolescents: a case series. Cogn Behav Pract, in press.
60. Eisler I, Dare C, Hodes M, et al. Family therapy for adolescent anorexia nervosa: the results of a controlled comparison of two family interventions. J Child Psychol Psychiatry 2000;41:727–36.

61. Robin AL, Siegel PT, Moye A, et al. A controlled comparison of family versus individual therapy for adolescents with anorexia nervoxa. J Am Acad Child Adolesc Psychiatry 1999;38:1482–9.
62. Geist R, Heinmaa M, Stephens D, et al. Comparison of family therapy and family group psychoeducation in adolescents with anorexia nervosa. Can J Psychiatry 2000;45:173–8.
63. Uehara T, Kawashima Y, Goto M, et al. Psychoeducation for the families of patients with eating disorders and changes in expressed emotion: a preliminary study. Compr Psychiatry 2001;42:132–8.
64. Zucker NL, Marcus M, Bulik C. A group parent-training program: a novel approach for eating disorder management. Eat Weight Disord 2006;11(2):78–82.
65. Holtkamp K, Herpertz-Dahlmann B, Vloet T, et al. Group psychoeducation for parents of adolescents with eating disorders: the Aachen program. Eating Disorders 2005;13:381–90.
66. Treasure J, Murphy T, Szmukler G, et al. The experience of caregiving for severe mental illnesses: a comparison between anorexia nervosa and psychosis. Soc Psychiatry Psychiatr Epidemiol 2001;36(7):343–7.

Cognitive Behavioral Approaches in Adolescent Anorexia and Bulimia Nervosa

U. Schmidt, PhD, MRCPsych

KEYWORDS

- Anorexia nervosa • Bulimia nervosa • Eating disorders
- Adolescents • Children • Cognitive–behavioral therapy

The vast majority of eating disorder (ED) cases have their onset in adolescence.[1] Given the dramatic and highly visible nature of anorexia nervosa (AN), the time to diagnosis is usually short (months), with parents typically being the first to identify the problem. In contrast, bulimia nervosa (BN) may remain a shameful secret for a significant period of time,[2] although adolescents now form most of the BN patients presenting to primary care for help.[1] Thus it is surprising that few studies exist that have assessed the efficacy of psychotherapeutic interventions in adolescents with ED.[3,4] Most of the existing treatment literature on adolescent EDs focuses on family therapy and a broader range of family-based interventions, mainly in AN, but increasingly also in BN.[5–7] Much less is known about the efficacy of cognitive–behavioral treatment (CBT) in adolescents with EDs. This article uses what is known about CBT in adults with ED as a starting point and, after some developmental considerations about CBT in children and adolescents, reviews how CBT might be adapted for adolescents with ED and what the current knowledge base on CBT in adolescents is. The article is concluded with some thoughts on future developments in this area.

COGNITIVE–BEHAVIORAL THERAPY IN EATING DISORDERS: WHAT DO WE KNOW FROM RESEARCH IN ADULTS?

A specific form of CBT for BN (CBT-BN) was developed by Fairburn and colleagues[8] and focuses on addressing bulimic behaviors and cognitions, such as overvalued beliefs about weight, shape, or appearance. This treatment is recommended by the NICE [National Institute for Health and Clinical Excellence] guidelines[4] as the treatment of choice for BN and binge eating disorder (BED) in adults. It is underpinned by a solid evidence base that suggests that CBT-BN is at least as effective as other treatments

Section of Eating Disorders, Institute of Psychiatry, PO Box 59, De Crespigny Park, London SE5 8AF, UK
E-mail address: u.schmidt@iop.kcl.ac.uk

Child Adolesc Psychiatric Clin N Am 18 (2008) 147–158
doi:10.1016/j.chc.2008.07.011
1056-4993/08/$ – see front matter © 2008 Elsevier Inc. All rights reserved.

if not superior in producing recovery from BN.[9] Thirty percent to 40% of people are symptom-free at the end of treatment, with gains maintained at longer-term follow-up. In recent years attempts have been made to increase the efficacy of CBT for bulimic disorders. For example, Fairburn and colleagues[10] have developed a new model of treatment for all EDs, the so-called "transdiagnostic model." In addition to focusing on ED symptoms, this model tackles areas in which these patients commonly experience problems (such as perfectionism, low self-esteem, affective instability, and interpersonal problems). Cooper and coworkers[11] and Waller and colleagues[12] have also developed promising adaptations to CBT-BN, although to date there has been no comparison of CBT-BN with these more sophisticated approaches.[13]

In contrast to the situation in BN, there is no leading therapy for adults with AN.[14] Only 3 randomized controlled trials (RCTs) have examined the role of CBT in the treatment of adults with AN. In 1 of these, CBT was found to be superior at preventing relapse after inpatient treatment than nutritional counseling.[15] In a second trial, CBT, interpersonal therapy, and specialist supportive clinical management (SSCM) were compared in outpatients with AN, with SSCM producing the best outcomes.[16] Finally, in a third study comparing CBT with fluoxetine in AN, alone or in combination, dropout rates from both treatments were too high to estimate treatment effects.[17] Reasons for the poor CBT treatment adherence and poor outcomes in adults with AN are complex. It seems that CBT for AN has largely been adapted from that for other disorders (eg, BN) without a clear underlying model of the core disease-maintaining factors for AN.

COGNITIVE–BEHAVIORAL THERAPY FOR CHILDREN AND ADOLESCENTS WITH EATING DISORDER
Developmental Considerations

What is cognitive–behavioral therapy all about?
Bolton,[18] in a thoughtful overview of theoretic and developmental issues in cognitive behavior therapy for children and adolescents, suggests

> A common characterization of the theory behind CBT, consistent with its background in cognitive psychology, is that behaviour is regulated by appraisals of stimuli, rather than by the stimuli themselves. 'Stimuli' mean events in the world but also events within the body, and mental states of others, and of the self. Appraisals may be verbal, but they may also be in sensori or sensori-motor code (eg, threat perception is an appraisal that does not require verbal coding). 'Behaviour' involves motor behaviour, but also affective responses. A way of expressing the core working assumption of CBT is thus that appraisals – the meaning assigned to stimuli, or the way they are represented – are critical in the regulation of affect and behaviour.

From this definition it follows that to be able to use CBT, young persons have to be able to build theories and reflect on their own thinking. This activity involves the ability to understand connections between beliefs, the ability to evaluate thoughts as bad, clever, stupid, useless, and so forth, the recognition that mental states may be more or less under the person's control, and the possession of insight into other people's mental states (ie, theory of mind).[18]

Cognitive development and cognitive–behavioral therapy
Brain development, in particular development of the prefrontal cortex (an area involved in decision-making, forward planning, and emotional control), undergoes significant modification starting at puberty, continuing throughout adolescence, and is complete only around the age of 20 to 22 years (for review see).[19] Nonetheless, there

is widespread agreement among experts that adolescents can and do benefit from CBT.[20] Although cognitive abilities and sophistication in adolescents are highly variable, adolescents "...are both information processors and theorists. They are continually observing their experience, storing it in memory, retrieving it for reflection, and attributing meaning to it."[20]

What about pre-pubertal children? CBT can and has been used in this group, too.[18] However, a meta-analysis of CBT outcome studies in children and adolescents found markedly larger effect sizes in studies on adolescents than those in younger children,[21] supporting the notion that the level of cognitive development does determine the ability to use CBT successfully. Having said that, Bolton[18] reminds us that metacognition, that is, the ability to reflect on your thinking, "comes in various shapes and sizes and many kinds if not all begin to have made their appearance already in young childhood." Given that the majority of young people with EDs develop their problem post-pubertally, we can be fairly sure that they usually will have the cognitive ability to use a cognitive–behavioral approach to treatment.

Finally, it is also important to note that although children and adolescents may have limitations in the area of cognitive development, "the child and adolescent have views of themselves and the world that are less fixed and so far more open to new possibilities." In contrast, "by the time of adulthood, people have had the time, capacity and need to build up styles and systems of belief around problematic behaviour, including entrenched secondary appraisals that unfortunately exacerbate and maintain the problem."[18] Thus adolescents' greater cognitive malleability affords them an advantage in terms of being able to change more readily. This is borne out by the treatment outcome literature in EDs, which suggests that early treatment (ie, in adolescence) has much better outcomes than later treatment (ie, in adulthood).[2]

Social development and cognitive–behavioral therapy

Adolescence is a time of increasing autonomy from the family of origin, with conflict rising and closeness and time spent together decreasing in early to mid adolescence, and a reversal of this pattern as adulthood approaches. Yet practically and emotionally adolescents continue to depend on and need their parents. Adolescents do best with authoritative parenting, that is, where clear boundaries are combined with warmth and autonomy granting.[20] Of significance in the context of EDs, parents typically buy and prepare food and determine the family rules, beliefs, and culture around eating.

Adolescence is also a time of the growing importance of peer relationships, including sexual relationships. This brings challenges, risks, and opportunities for the young person. Of specific relevance to EDs, Wilson and Sysko[22] (quoting Striegel-Moore)[23] point out that teenage girls are socialized to evaluate themselves in terms of appearance and derive their self-esteem and sense of personal identity through others' approval of their physical attractiveness.

Thus, all in all, the young person's problems need to be understood in the context of family and peer relationships, and the clinical case conceptualization needs to reflect this.[24]

The evidence on whether and how parents should be involved in psychological treatment of adolescents is mixed, and it depends on multiple factors, including the nature of the young person's difficulties and the parents' style, their own difficulties, and availability.[20,24] Given the medical risks of AN and the often limited treatment motivation of young people with this condition, in most cases it is imperative that parents are involved intensively in the treatment, whereas in BN the situation is much less clear cut.

Treatment motivation

CBT typically assumes a motivated patient who wants to change. However, treatment motivation of many adolescents with an ED (especially those with AN) is low, because they are often brought to the clinic by their parents, and may not see the need for changing themselves or may only see the benefits of the disorder (eg, weight loss increasing peer approval).[25] Surpirsingly, a study that compared treatment-seeking adolescents with BN and adults with BN in terms of their treatment motivation found no difference between the 2 groups.[26] Motivation to change was high in both age groups, but confidence in the ability to change or self-efficacy was low in both groups.

How can developmental knowledge help the therapist?

Weisz and Hawley[20] note that "developmental findings are essentially group trends." Therefore, developmental research will *not* tell a therapist what specific issues to address in a given case. Nonetheless, developmental knowledge can help therapy in several ways by alerting therapists to issues for which they should be vigilant, such as having a developmentally informed awareness of risk factors. This is important because the therapist can then ask the right sort of questions, and this can help to prioritize the focus for interventions and select appropriate candidate interventions.

How Should Cognitive–Behavioral Therapy be Adapted for Adolescents with Eating Disorders?

The general principles of how psychological therapies need to be adapted for adolescents have been identified by Weisz and Hawley,[20] who suggest that interventions for adolescents need to (1) focus on motivation and engagement of the young person, and (2) be flexible in treatment structure and contents to accommodate the developmental variability of adolescents. These investigators also suggest that modularized treatments, using a toolbox approach, might be particularly useful to adolescents. Finally, they emphasize the need to involve parents flexibly. These points are underscored by 2 thoughtful articles of how CBT can be adapted for adolescents with bulimic disorders.[22,27] In the following sections, some of the adaptations of CBT for adolescents with ED that have emerged within the work from the author's group and the evidence that supports it are outlined.

Motivation and engagement

The author and her group have adapted the principles and techniques of motivational interviewing (MI) and of motivational enhancement therapy (MET)[28] for use with young people with EDs[29] and integrated this into a cognitive-behavioral framework.[25,30,31] The empathic, respectful, accepting style of MI fits well with teenagers' wish to be taken seriously and their need for autonomy. Adaptations to the classical MI approach include the use of a more structured way of eliciting concerns from young persons,[25] the use of writing tasks,[32,33] and the use of externalization, that is, getting young people to think of the ED as separate from themselves. The practice of giving feedback on clinical symptoms and risks is an essential part of MET, and the author and her group have shown that this improves outcome in patients with BN.[34] More recently, this has included giving feedback on the particular neuropsychological information processing style typically found in EDs (such as cognitive rigidity, set-shifting impairments, and attention to detail at the expense of the bigger picture) and how this might affect the person.[35] Feedback is given verbally and in a letter from the therapist to the patient. Research has shown that these letters are highly valued by patients and make them feel more involved in their treatment.[36] Together, these techniques help to engage young people in treatment in a way that sets the therapist apart from other authority figures and presents new and interesting information.[37]

The standard MI techniques for building motivation for change can all be used with adolescents, such as exploring readiness and confidence to change, pros and cons of change, looking forward and backward, and exploring values and value–behavior congruence. Especially in AN, a key feature is an exploration of the valued function of the anorexia in the person's life together with the identification of relevant pro-anorexia beliefs, which are usually closely linked to the reasons the person has for not wanting to change[38,39] and which are believed to maintain the disorder.[30] A conversation about the things that young people value about AN sheds light on underlying beliefs they may have about themselves, others, and the world at large, their values and personal rules. For example, a young person who believes that the anorexia makes her special and makes others notice and admire her may have core beliefs about being boring and unlovable.

Case formulation and treatment planning
In our practice a collaboratively developed longitudinal cognitive-behavioral case formulation is shared with the patient as a diagram and a letter.[31] The practice of writing formulation letters is derived from cognitive analytic therapy.[40] A treatment plan is developed, based on the formulation.

Working toward change
Many of the standard CBT techniques underpinning symptomatic change, such as self-monitoring, goal setting, problem solving, cognitive restructuring, and carefully planned behavioral experiments, can be readily used in adolescents with ED. In addition, we have found specifically constructed therapeutic writing tasks to be a useful therapeutic tool that fits well with adolescents' wish for privacy and control.

Using writing in cognitive–behavioral treatment
There is a large and sound body of research supporting the use of writing about traumatic or negative life events as a tool for processing these.[41,42] Young people with EDs, especially those with AN, are often much more able to express their thoughts and feelings on paper than face-to-face. Thus, the author and her group use written tasks throughout treatment. For example, early on the author and her group use "letters to AN as a friend or as an enemy" to explore the positive and negative aspects of AN in the person's life. Moreover, these letters serve to externalize the disorder. The author and her group use the term "anorexic voice" or more personalized epithets to refer to AN symptoms. Writing tasks set in the future, either with an ED or without the ED, allow individuals to take a broader perspective on their illness and think about other goals, values, and life directions that they would like to take. Later on in the therapy, writing tasks focused on the role of the ED in the person's life or on key events or relationships are used to reduce emotional avoidance and foster the processing of emotionally salient material while giving young people control over what and how much they feel able to divulge. Writing about difficult events from different people's perspectives aids cognitive restructuring and decentering. It can also help patients get away from an excessive focus on detail and instead to see the bigger picture "in life." Writing also allows young people to come to terms with upsetting things, finding new solutions to difficulties and new meanings. These tasks are presented to patients as homework assignments, but always offered as something that they may wish to "try out." Further details about the use of these writing tasks can be found elsewhere.[32,33]

Involvement of parents of people with eating disorders

In the author and his group's model of ED treatment, involvement of the family is integral. The younger the patient and the higher the medical risk, the more intensively the parents will need to be involved in treatment. Separate and joint sessions are helpful. Parents of young people with ED have deficits in skills and knowledge about managing ED symptoms.[43] Moreover, they benefit from an introduction to what CBT is all about and how this might help their child. Among a range of interventions for carers, the author and her group have recently developed a Web-based CBT-based intervention for parents/carers of young people with AN.[44] The program is formulation-based and includes parallel CBT formulations of the young person's difficulties and the parents' response to this, to illustrate how parental and child behaviors interact with each other. Key components include teaching parents relevant skills to communicate motivationally with the young person about their ED, while remaining firm about "non-negotiables." The program also teaches parents how to give mealtime support to the young person with AN and how to deal with other difficult behaviors that the young person displays (eg, binge–purge behaviors or self-harm). Finally, it teaches parents how to look after their own needs. In an "offline" pilot evaluation of this program, parents' anxiety and depression decreased significantly, and negative experience of caregiving and expressed emotion reduced.[45] A randomized controlled trial of this approach is underway. This program can be used to support the young person's CBT by giving the parents separate but complementary information and skills training, building on the same model.

Evidence Base for CBT in Adolescents with Different Eating Disorders

The evidence base for CBT in adolescents with EDs is small and of variable quality.

Anorexia nervosa

A small randomized, controlled study compared manual-based CBT with behavioral family therapy in 25 adolescents and young adults with AN.[46] Participants in both treatment groups received 21 to 25 sessions of therapy over 1 year. No significant outcome differences between treatment groups were found in nutritional status, eating behaviors, mood, self-esteem, and family communication. Fifteen patients (60% of the total sample) had a "good" outcome (defined as maintaining weight within 10% of average body weight and regular menstrual cycles) at posttreatment and at 6 months' follow-up. Most of the patients did not reach symptomatic recovery. The study almost certainly was underpowered, and conclusions that can be drawn are limited.

One large RCT (n = 167)[47] evaluated the effectiveness of 3 treatments for adolescents (aged 12–18 years) with AN, comparing inpatient, specialist outpatient, and general child and adolescent mental health service (CAMHS) treatment within a UK National Health Service context. The specialist outpatient treatment was a manualized treatment and consisted of an initial MI, individual CBT plus parental feedback (12 sessions), parental counseling with the patient (between 4 to 8 sessions depending on patients' age), dietetic therapy (4 sessions with parental involvement as required), multimodal feedback, and monitoring (weight, self-report, and clinician-rated questionnaire) (4 sessions). The treatment was designed to last 6 months. The CBT, parental counseling, and feedback components of the treatment were provided by the same therapist and the dietetic component of the treatment was provided by an experienced dietitian. It is not clear what CBT model was used, whether the study therapists were trained CBT therapists, and how treatment fidelity was assessed. All 3 groups made considerable progress at 1 year, with further improvement by 2 years, but full recovery rates were low (33% at 2 years). Adherence to inpatient treatment was poor (50%). On an intention-to-treat analysis, neither inpatient nor specialist outpatient therapy demonstrated advantages over general CAMHS treatment. Some CAMHS outpatients were subsequently admitted on clinical grounds. A cost-effectiveness analysis suggested that the specialist outpatient group was less costly over the 2-year follow-up (mean total cost, £26,738 GBP) than the inpatient (£34,531 GBP) and general outpatient treatment (£40,794 GBP) groups, but this result was not statistically significant.[48]

Bulimia nervosa
A small case series (n = 7) of adolescents with binge eating syndromes (BN, EDNOS, BED) was treated with a version of CBT-BN adapted for an adolescent population with promising outcomes.[49]

Guided CBT self-care treatment
One randomized controlled study[7] compared family therapy with cognitive-behavioral guided self-care in adolescents with BN or related disorders. The guided self-care condition used a manual[50] previously tested in adults with BN.[51] The Flesh-Kincade reading age suggests that eighth graders (age, 13–14 years) can read this manual. There are accompanying workbooks for the patient and "close others" and a clinician's guide.[52] Patients had 10 weekly sessions, 3 follow-up sessions (monthly), and 2 optional sessions with a "close other," usually a parent. The therapist's role was to motivate the patients and guide them through the workbook to fit their needs.

Treatment was adapted for adolescents as follows: Initially treatment focused on the function of bulimia in the person's life and built motivation to change. Information about how bulimic symptoms are maintained was introduced, using self-monitoring of thoughts, feelings, and behaviors. Problem solving with behavioral experiments and goal setting were used to help patients alter vicious cycles of behavior. A case formulation was developed collaboratively. After 10 sessions the therapist wrote a good-bye letter. The follow-up sessions focused on relapse prevention. Regular homework accompanied the treatment. The sessions with a "close other" addressed how they could help the patient.

The individual guided self-care treatment showed earlier improvement on bingeing, but otherwise no differences in clinical outcomes compared with family therapy. However, individual treatment appeared to be more acceptable because a significant proportion of the young people eligible for participation (28%) cited not wanting to involve their families as their main reason for nonparticipation. This may not reflect clinical practice, where initial reluctance to involve the family can be resolved over time. The design allowed adolescents to involve "close others" other than parents in treatment, and a quarter of randomized patients did so.[53] These patients were older, less likely to live at home, and had more chronic symptoms, more comorbidity, and poorer relationships with their parents. This suggests the need to offer at least some individual therapy to these young people.

Internet-based cognitive–behavioral therapy for adolescents with bulemia nervosa
There is evidence that adolescents may prefer self-help to more traditional routes of care.[54] Because they are computer literate and socialize well through electronic means, one way of delivering treatment to them in a way that is appealing, accessible, and disseminable is to deliver CBT using the Internet. With this in mind we conducted a cohort study ("the BYTE study") involving 101 adolescents with BN or EDNOS assessing the feasibility, acceptability, and clinical outcomes of a Web-based CBT package (Overcoming bulimia online).[55,56] Participants were recruited from UK ED clinics or from *beat*, a UK-wide charity specializing in EDs. The program consisted

of 8 interactive online CBT sessions, peer support through message boards for participants and parents, and contact with an e-mail support clinician. Patients' bulimic symptomatology was assessed by interview with the eating disorders examination (EDE)[57] at baseline and posttreatment at 3 and 6 months. Qualitative questionnaires were also administered to determine patients' attitudes to and experience of the treatment package. There were significant reductions in objective bingeing, vomiting, global EDE score, and service contacts from baseline to 3 months, and this reduction was maintained at 6 months. Participants' views of the intervention were positive. The Web-based intervention was feasible, acceptable to participants, and effective in producing and maintaining reductions in bulimic symptomatology. The intervention has the potential to be used as a first step in the treatment of adolescents with BN.[56]

Eating Disorder not Otherwise Specified

There has recently been considerable interest in those EDs that do not fulfill precise diagnostic criteria, that is, those currently classified as EDNOS.[58] The RCT mentioned here[7] included EDNOS patients. Compared with BN patients, these patients binged, vomited, and purged significantly less and were less preoccupied with food. They had more depression and had more current and childhood obsessive-compulsive disorder. About 66.6% of EDNOS versus 27.8% of BN patients abstained from bingeing and vomiting after 1 year. However, diagnosis did not moderate the treatment outcome. Costs did not differ between groups. The study concludes that EDNOS in adolescents is not trivial. It has milder ED symptoms but more comorbidity than BN. Implications for clinical practice arise from this because it needs to be carefully assessed whether comorbid symptoms need treatment in their own right. Psychological case formulations may need to be adapted to accommodate comorbidity either as potential vulnerability or maintaining factors for the ED.[59]

No evidence is available on CBT treatment of binge EDBED in adolescents.

DISCUSSION

In contrast to other psychological disorders in adolescents where CBT has widely been used,[60] CBT for adolescents with EDs is as yet in its infancy. This is particularly surprising in the area of bulimic disorders where CBT is the treatment of choice for the adult form of the disorder. It is perhaps less surprising in AN, where the evidence base on use of CBT in adults is limited, and the efficacy of this approach is as yet uncertain.

Despite the limited existing evidence, in BN there is some suggestion that individual CBT-based approaches in adolescents may at least be as effective as family therapy and perhaps more acceptable.[7] Useful suggestions have been made as to how to adapt CBT treatment procedures for BN for adolescents.[22,27]

In AN the problem is more complex, in that it is not clear whether existing CBT models developed for adults "hit the spot." For example, most CBT models of AN focus on weight and shape concerns, and this may not be appropriate for many cases of AN, where weight loss is driven by some other valued function of the anorexia. The author and her group's model of treatment of AN is a culture-free cognitive-interpersonal model[30] and can account for and accommodate different valued functions of AN. This is currently being tested in adults, but the treatment approach based on this would seem to fit well with the needs of adolescents, given its motivational and modularized nature and involvement of parents.

An interesting approach to CBT with children and adolescents is that of Dummett,[61] who has emphasized the importance of incorporating developmental, attachment, familial, systemic, and other perspectives into therapy and has developed a generic template for a systemic CBT formulation that includes these different perspectives. This formulation can be developed collaboratively and shared between young people and their families. CBT for EDs could usefully adapt this approach.

Much more work is required to increase the evidence base on the efficacy of CBT in adolescents with ED. In addition, future studies should address whether there are particular subgroups of adolescents with ED for whom CBT works more or less well. Finally, understanding mediators, moderators, and the therapy process is another promising and much needed area for future research.[62]

SUMMARY

Despite the demonstrated efficacy of CBT in the treatment of a wide range of child and adolescent disorders and in adults with bulimic disorders, CBT for adolescents with EDs remains poorly studied. Adaptations of CBT for adolescents with BN exist but need further study. CBT models appropriate for use in adolescents with AN have also been developed but as yet need to be tested.

ACKNOWLEDGMENT

This work was supported by the ARIADNE program (Applied Research into Anorexia Nervosa and Not Otherwise Specified Eating Disorders), funded by a Department of Health NIHR Program Grant for Applied Research (Reference number RP-PG-0606-1043) to U. Schmidt, J. Treasure, K. Tchanturia, H. Startup, S. Ringwood, S. Landau, M. Grover, I. Eisler, I. Campbell, J. Beecham, M. Allen, and G. Wolff. The views expressed herein are not necessarily those of DH/NIHR.

REFERENCES

1. Currin L, Schmidt U, Treasure J, et al. Time trends in eating disorder incidence. Br J Psychiatry 2005;186:132–5.
2. Currin L, Schmidt U. A critical analysis of the utility of an early intervention approach in the eating disorders. J Ment Health 2005;14:1–14.
3. Berkman ND, Bulik CM, Brownley KA, et al. Management of eating disorders. Evid Rep Technol Assess (Full Rep) 2006;135:1–166.
4. National Collaborating Centre for Mental Health. Eating disorders: core interventions in the treatment and management of anorexia nervosa, bulimia nervosa and related eating disorders. Leicester (UK): British Psychological Society and Gaskell; 2004.
5. Eisler I. The empirical and theoretical base of family therapy and multiple family day therapy for adolescent anorexia nervosa. J Fam Ther 2005;27:104–31.
6. le Grange D, Crosby RD, Rathouz PJ, et al. A randomized controlled comparison of family-based treatment and supportive psychotherapy for adolescent bulimia nervosa. Arch Gen Psychiatry 2007;64:1049–56.
7. Schmidt U, Lee S, Perkins S, et al. A randomized controlled trial of family therapy and cognitive-behavioral guided self-care for adolescents with bulimia nervosa or related disorders. Am J Psych 2007;164:591–8.
8. Fairburn CG, Marcus M, Wilson G. Cognitive-behavioral therapy for binge eating and bulimia nervosa: a comprehensive treatment manual. In: Fairburn CG, Wilson GT, editors. Binge eating: nature, assessment and treatment. New York: Guilford Press; 1993. p. 361–404.
9. Wilson GT, Grilo CM, Vitousek KM. Psychological treatment of eating disorders. Am Psychol 2007;62:199–216.

10. Fairburn CG, Cooper Z, Shafran R. Cognitive behaviour therapy for eating disorders: a "transdiagnostic" theory and treatment. Behav Res Ther 2003;41: 509–28.
11. Cooper MJ, Wells A, Todd G. A cognitive model of bulimia nervosa. Br J Clin Psychol 2004;43(Pt 1):1–16.
12. Waller G, Cordery H, Corstorphine E, et al. Cognitive behavioral therapy for eating disorders. Cambridge, UK: Cambridge University Press; 2007.
13. Van den Eynde F, Schmidt U. Treatment of bulimia nervosa and binge eating disorder. Psychiatry 2007;7:161–6.
14. Fairburn CG. Evidence-based treatment of anorexia nervosa. Int J Eat Disord 2005;37(Suppl):S26–30 [discussion S41–2].
15. Pike KM, Walsh BT, Vitousek K, et al. Cognitive behavior therapy in the posthospitalization treatment of anorexia nervosa. Am J Psychiatry 2003;160:2046–9.
16. McIntosh VV, Jordan J, Carter FA, et al. Three psychotherapies for anorexia nervosa: a randomized, controlled trial. Am J Psychiatry 2005;162:741–7.
17. Halmi KA, Agras WS, Crow S, et al. Predictors of treatment acceptance and completion in anorexia nervosa: implications for future study designs. Arch Gen Psychiatry 2005;62:776–81.
18. Bolton D. Cognitive behaviour therapy for children and adolescents: some theoretical and developmental issues. In: Graham P, editor. Cognitive behaviour therapy for children and families. Cambridge, UK: Cambridge University Press; 2005. p. 9–24.
19. Keverne EB. Understanding well-being in the evolutionary context of brain development. Philos Trans R Soc Lond, B, Biol Sci 2004;359:1349–58.
20. Weisz JR, Hawley KM. Developmental factors in the treatment of adolescents. J Consult Clin Psychol 2002;70:21–43.
21. Durlak JA, Fuhrman T, Lampman C. Effectiveness of cognitive-behavior therapy for maladapting children: a meta-analysis. Psychol Bull 1991;110:204–14.
22. Wilson GT, Sysko R. Cognitive-behavioural therapy for adolescents with bulimia nervosa. Eur Eat Dis Rev 2006;14:8–16.
23. Striegel-Moore RH. Etiology of binge eating: a developmental perspective. In: Fairubrn CG, Wilson GT, editors. Binge eating: nature, assessment and treatment. New York: Guilford Press; 1993. p. 144–72.
24. Drinkwater J. Cognitive case formulation. In: Graham P, editor. Cognitive behaviour therapy for children and families. Cambridge, UK: Cambridge University Press; 2005. p. 9–24.
25. Treasure J, Schmidt U. Eating disorders. In: Arkowitz H, Westra H, Miller W, et al, editors. Motivational interviewing in psychotherapy and mental health. New York: Guilford Publications; 2007.
26. Perkins S, Schmidt U, Eisler I, et al. Motivation to change in recent onset and long-standing bulimia nervosa: are there differences? Eat Weight Disord 2007; 12:61–9.
27. Lock J. Adjusting cognitive behavior therapy for adolescents with bulimia nervosa: results of case series. Am J Psychother 2005;59:267–81.
28. Miller WR, Rollnick S. Motivational interviewing. Preparing people for change. 2nd edition. New York: The Guilford Press; 2002.
29. Schmidt U. Engagement and motivational interviewing. In: Graham P, editor. Cognitive behaviour therapy for children and families. Cambridge University Press; 2005. p. 67–83.
30. Schmidt U, Treasure J. Anorexia nervosa: valued and visible. A cognitive-interpersonal maintenance model and its implications for research and practice. Br J Clin Psychol 2006;45:343–66.

31. Lavender A, Schmidt U. Case formulation of complex eating disorders. In: Tarrier N, editor. Complex case formulation in CBT. Hove (UK): Brunner-Routledge; 2006.

32. Schmidt U, Bone G, Hems S, et al. Structured therapeutic writing tasks as an adjunct to treatment in eating disorders. European Eat Dis Review 2002;10:1–17.

33. Wade T, Schmidt U. Writing therapies for eating disorders treatment. In: Paxton S, Hay P, editors. Treatment approaches for body dissatisfaction and eating disorders: evidence and practice. Melbourne, Australia: IP Communications.

34. Schmidt U, Landau S, Pombo-Carril MG, et al. Does feedback improve the outcome of guided self-care in bulimia nervosa? A preliminary randomised controlled trial. Br J Clin Psychol 2006;45:111–21.

35. Lopez C, Roberts ME, Tchanturia K, et al. Using neuropsychological feedback therapeutically in treatment for anorexia nervosa: two illustrative case reports. Eur Eat Disord Rev 2008 Feb 21 [Epub ahead of publication].

36. Humfress H, Igel V, Lamont A, et al. The effect of a brief motivational intervention on community psychiatric patients' attitudes to their care, motivation to change, compliance and outcome: a case control study. J Ment Health 2002;11:155–66.

37. Ingersoll KS, Wagner CC, Gharib S. Motivational groups for community substance abuse. Programs. Richmond (VA): Mid-Atlantic Addiction Technology Transfer Center/Center for Substance Abuse Treatment; 2000.

38. Serpell L, Neiderman M, Haworth E, et al. The use of the Pros and Cons of Anorexia Nervosa (P-CAN) scale with children and adolescents. J Psychosom Res 2003;54:567–71.

39. Serpell L, Teasdale JD, Troop NA, et al. The development of the P-CAN, a measure to operationalize the pros and cons of anorexia nervosa. Int J Eat Dis 2004; 36:416–33.

40. Ryle A. Cognitive analytic therapy: developments in theory and practice. Chichester (UK): Wiley; 1995.

41. Pennebaker JW. Opening up: the healing power of expressing emotions. New York: Guilford Press; 1997.

42. Pennebaker JW. Writing to heal: a journal for recovering from trauma & emotional upheaval. Oakland (CA): New Harbinger Publications; 2004.

43. Whitney J, Murray J, Gavan K, et al. Experience of caring for someone with anorexia nervosa: qualitative study. Br J Psychiatry 2005;187:444–9.

44. Schmidt U, Williams C, Eisler I, et al. Overcoming anorexia online. Effective caring. A web-based programme for carers of people with AN. Media Innovations Ltd; 2008.

45. Grover M. Paper given at the Academy of Eating Disorders' International Conference. Seattle, Washington; May, 16, 2008.

46. Ball J, Mitchell P. A randomized controlled study of cognitive behavior therapy and behavioral family therapy for anorexia nervosa patients. Eating Disorders 2004;12:303–14.

47. Gowers SG, Clark A, Roberts C, et al. Clinical effectiveness of treatments for anorexia nervosa in adolescents: randomised controlled trial. Br J Psychiatry 2007;191:427–35.

48. Byford S, Barrett B, Roberts C, et al. Economic evaluation of a randomised controlled trial for anorexia nervosa in adolescents. Br J Psychiatry 2007;191: 436–40.

49. Schapman-Williams AM, Lock J, Couturier J. Cognitive-behavioral therapy for adolescents with binge eating syndromes: a case series. Int J Eat Dis 2006;39: 252–5.

50. Schmidt U, Treasure J. Getting better bit(e) by bit(e). A treatment manual for sufferers of bulimia nervosa. Hove (UK): Psychology Press; 1997.
51. Perkins SJ, Murphy R, Schmidt U, et al. Self-help and guided self-help for eating disorders. Cochrane Database Syst Rev 2006;3:CD004191.
52. Treasure J, Schmidt U. The clinicians guide to getting better bit(e) by bit(e). Hove (UK): Psychology Press; 1997.
53. Perkins S, Schmidt U, Eisler I, et al. Why do adolescents with BN choose not to involve their parents in treatment? Eur Child Adolesc Psychiatry 2005;14:376–85.
54. Oliver MI, Pearson N, Coe N, et al. Help-seeking behaviour in men and women with common mental health problems: cross-sectional study. Br J Psychiatry 2005;186:297–301.
55. Williams CJ, Aubin SD, Cottrell D, et al. Overcoming bulimia: a self-help package. Leeds (UK): University of Leeds Press; 1998. Available at: www.calipso.co.uk. Accessed September 14, 2008.
56. Pretorius N, Arcelus J, Beecham J, et al. The feasibility, acceptability, and efficacy of a web-based CBT intervention for adolescents with bulimia nervosa, submitted for publication.
57. Fairburn CG, Cooper Z. The eating disorders examination. In: Fairburn CG, Wilson GT, editors. Binge eating: nature, assessment and treatment. 12th edition. New York: Guilford Press; 1993. p. 317–60.
58. Norring C, Palmer B. EDNOS, eating disorders not otherwise specified. Hove (UK): Routledge; 2005.
59. Schmidt U, Lee S, Perkins S, et al. Do adolescents with eating disorder not otherwise specified or full-syndrome bulimia nervosa differ in clinical severity, comorbidity, risk factors, treatment outcome or cost? Int J Eat Disord 2008 Apr 23 [Epub ahead of print].
60. Graham P, editor. Cognitive behaviour therapy for children and families. Cambridge, UK: Cambridge University Press; 2005.
61. Dummett N. Processes for systemic cognitive-behavioural therapy with children, young people and families. Behav Cognit Psychother 2006;34:179–89.
62. Weersing VR, Brent DA. Psychological therapies: a family of interventions. In: Graham P, editor. Cognitive behaviour therapy for children and families. Cambridge, UK: Cambridge University Press; 2005. p. 48–66.

Family Interventions in Adolescent Anorexia Nervosa

Daniel le Grange, PhD[a,b,]*, Ivan Eisler, PhD[c,d]

KEYWORDS

- Children and adolescents • Anorexia nervosa
- Eating disorders • Family therapy

HISTORY OF THE FAMILY'S ROLE IN EATING DISORDERS

The view that the family has a central role in eating disorders can be traced at least as far back as the late 19th century. The views about the role of parents in anorexia nervosa (AN) varied from Lasegue's[1] neutral stance in taking into account the "preoccupations of relatives," to Gull,[2] considering parents as "generally the worst attendants," and Charcot[3] thinking that their influence is "particularly pernicious." These early descriptions did not see parents as playing a helpful role in their daughter's illness, and indeed one of the earliest debates in the literature on AN was about whether it was at all possible to treat the patient without isolating her from her family.[4,5]

During the first half of the 20th century the family continued to be seen primarily as a hindrance to treatment,[6,7] which together with a general notion that the family environment had at least a contributory role in the development of the illness[7,8] generally led to the exclusion of parents from treatment, sometimes referred to pejoratively as a "parentectomy."[9] It is not until the 1960s that the authors find a major shift in thinking about the role of the family in eating disorders in the work of Bruch,[10,11] Palazzoli,[12] and in particular Minuchin and colleagues[13,14] at the Child Guidance Center in Philadelphia. The theoretic models suggested by these investigators, posited specific family mechanisms underpinning the development of AN, which could be targeted by

This work was supported by an International Visiting Fellowship from the University of Sydney, Australia (Dr le Grange).

[a] Section of Child and Adolescent Psychiatry, Department of Psychiatry, The University of Chicago, 5841 South Maryland Avenue, MC3077, Chicago, IL 60637, USA

[b] Eating Disorders Program, The University of Chicago Medical Center, 5841 South Maryland Avenue, MC3077, Chicago, IL 60637, USA

[c] Section of Family Psychology and Family Therapy, Kings College, University of London, Institute of Psychiatry, PO73, de Crespigny Park, London SE5 8AF, UK

[d] Child and Adolescent Eating Disorders Service, South London and Maudsley NHS Foundation Trust, Michael Rutter Centre for Children and Adolescents, Maudsley Hospital, Denmark Hill, SE5 8AZ London, UK

* Corresponding author.

E-mail address: legrange@uchicago.edu (D. le Grange).

Child Adolesc Psychiatric Clin N Am 18 (2008) 159–173
doi:10.1016/j.chc.2008.07.004
1056-4993/08/$ – see front matter © 2008 Elsevier Inc. All rights reserved.

treatment. Thus the psychosomatic family model, developed by Minuchin and colleagues,[14] hypothesizes that the prerequisite for the development of AN was a family process characterized by rigidity, enmeshment, overinvolvement, and conflict avoidance, which occur alongside a physiologic vulnerability in the child, and the child's role as a go-between in cross-generational alliances.[13,14] Minuchin did not place blame on the parents, highlighting the evolving, interactive nature of this process and emphasizing that the psychosomatic model was more than an account of a familial origin for AN. Nonetheless, Minuchin and colleagues still maintained that the psychosomatic family process is a necessary *context* for the development of AN and that the aim of treatment is to *change* the way the family functions.

This conceptual shift of explaining AN as being part of an evolving interactional family context had a profound impact on the development of treatments even though, as described later, the empiric foundation of the "psychosomatic family" model has been shown to be weak. The principal change arose from seeing the family as needing to take an active part in treatment to facilitate the change of some of the patterns of family interaction that had evolved around and had become intertwined with the eating problems. An important aim of the treatment model was to strengthen the parental subsystem to challenge what were seen as problematic cross-generational alliances and over-close, enmeshed relationships that were making it difficult for the parents to respond to their concerns for their daughter's health in an active and united way.[15]

Since the early work of Minuchin and colleagues and some of the other pioneer figures of the family therapy field, such as Palazzoli,[12] Stierlin and Weber,[16] and White,[17] family therapy has gradually established itself as an important treatment approach for adolescent AN supported by growing empiric evidence of its efficacy. This development has undoubtedly been one of the important factors in the major changes in the treatment of eating disorders that the field has witnessed in the past 10 to 15 years.[18]

Paradoxically, alongside the data for the efficacy of family therapy, there has also been growing evidence that the theoretic models, from which the family treatment of eating disorder was derived, are flawed.[19,20] There has been considerable research endeavoring to uncover characteristics that are specific to families in which an offspring has an eating disorder and to test the specific predictions of the psychosomatic family model with generally disappointing and inconsistent findings.[21,22] There is a growing indication that families in which someone has an eating disorder are a heterogeneous group not only with respect to sociodemographic characteristics but also in terms of the nature of the relationships within the family, the emotional climate, and the patterns of family interaction.[20] Although there is some evidence that family therapy is accompanied by changes in family functioning,[23,24] these changes are not necessarily in keeping with the psychosomatic family model and the changes may not apply consistently across all families. This fact inevitably brings to the fore the question of what the targets of effective family interventions should be and what processes underlie any resultant change. This has necessitated a second conceptual shift, away from an emphasis on family etiology of the eating disorder toward an understanding of the evolution of the family dynamics in the context of the development of an eating disorder, which may function as maintenance mechanisms.[19,25] This has gone hand-in-hand with the development of a much more explicitly nonblaming approach to family treatment of adolescent AN in which the family is seen not as the cause of the problem but as a resource to help the young person in the process of recovery.[19,26–28] Before describing the current approaches to family intervention in eating disorders the authors review the existing evidence for their efficacy.

UNCONTROLLED OPEN STUDIES OF FAMILY THERAPY FOR ADOLESCENT ANOREXIA NERVOSA

Over the past 30 years evidence for the usefulness of using family interventions for eating disorders has been steadily accumulating.[29] In their seminal work, Minuchin and his colleagues[14] describe the use of structural family therapy to provide treatment of adolescent AN. In their case series, the Philadelphia team reported a remarkably high recovery rate of 86% with their treatment approach. This result was in stark contrast to most of the earlier accounts of treatment outcome with children and adolescents suffering from AN.[30–32] The patient population was mainly adolescent with a short duration of illness (mean, ~8 months), and was treated largely on an outpatient basis although a proportion also required a brief admission to a pediatric unit. These positive results, combined with the persuasive theoretic model that underpinned their approach, have made the work of the Philadelphia team highly influential despite the methodological weaknesses for which the study has been criticized.[33]

Two similar studies of adolescent AN, 1 in Toronto[34] and 1 in Buenos Aires,[35] have been reported. Family therapy was the primary treatment, but a combination of individual and inpatient treatment was also used. The study reported by Martin[34] was of a 5-year follow-up of 25 adolescent AN patients (mean age, 14.9 years) with a short duration of illness (mean: 8.1 months). Posttreatment data revealed significant improvements. A modest 23% of patients would have met the Morgan and Russell[36] criteria for good outcome, 45% intermediate outcome, and 32% poor outcome. Outcome at follow-up, however, was comparable to Minuchin's results, with 80% of patients having a good outcome, 4% intermediate outcome, and the remaining still in treatment (12%), or relapsed (4%). Herscovici and Bay[35] report the outcome of a series of 30 patients followed up 4 to 8.6 years after their first presentation (mean age, 14.7 years; mean duration of illness, 10.3 months). Whereas 40% of patients were admitted to hospital during the study, 60% had a good outcome, 30% an intermediate outcome, and 10% a poor outcome.

A few other studies have used family therapy as the only treatment. A small number of adolescent patients were seen in outpatient family therapy at the Maudsley Hospital in London (n = 12)[37] and at a general practice-based family therapy clinic in North London (n = 11).[38] Treatment was brief (<6 months) and 90% of patients were reported to have made significant improvements or were recovered at follow-up. Stierlin and Weber[16,39] conducted a larger study and reported on families seen at the Heidelberg Center over a period of 10 years. Forty-two female patients with AN and their families were included in the follow-up. This study differed from the first two in that patients were older (mean age when first seen, 18.2 years), had been ill for longer (on average >3 years), and the majority had previous treatment (56% as inpatients). Therapy lasted on average less than 9 months and used few sessions (mean, 6 months). At a mean follow-up of 4.5 years, less than two thirds were within a normal weight range and were menstruating. No distinctions were made between adolescents and young adults in the report, and the findings are therefore not directly comparable to the other studies described here. Several more recent and larger dissemination studies of manualized family therapy for adolescent AN in the form of uncontrolled studies have been reported,[40–44] which have produced comparable findings. In the only case series of family therapy for children with AN, Lock and colleagues[45] demonstrated that this treatment is just as effective for these younger patients as it is for adolescents with AN. These studies all add to the evidence that children and adolescents do well in treatment when a family intervention is the main form of treatment.

RANDOMIZED CONTROLLED TRIALS OF FAMILY THERAPY FOR ADOLESCENT ANOREXIA NERVOSA

There have been a limited number of randomized controlled trials of family therapy for AN and all have been small. In the first of these, Russell and colleagues[46] at the Maudsley Hospital compared family therapy with individual supportive therapy following in-patient treatment in 80 patients of all ages. Twenty-six of these were adolescents with AN, 21 had an age at onset on or before 18 years, and a duration of illness of less than 3 years. All patients were initially admitted to the hospital for an average of 10 weeks for weight restoration before being randomized to outpatient follow-up treatment. Adolescents with a short duration of illness fared significantly better with family therapy than the control treatment. Although the findings were inconclusive for those whose illness had lasted more than 3 years, these patients generally had a poor outcome. At 5-year follow-up[47] adolescents with a short history of illness and who received family therapy continued to do well, with 90% having a good outcome. Patients who had received individual therapy also continued to improve; however, nearly half still had significant eating disorder symptoms at follow-up.

Three subsequent studies compared different forms of family intervention. In the first 2, Le Grange and colleagues[48] and Eisler and colleagues[23] compared conjoint family therapy (CFT) and separated family therapy (SFT) among a total of 58 patients. In SFT, the adolescent was seen on her own and the parents were seen in a separate session by the same therapist. Both treatments were provided on an outpatient basis. Overall results were similar in these 2 studies with patients showing significant improvements in both CFT and SFT (>60% were classified as having a good or intermediate outcome post-treatment) and small differences between treatments in terms of symptom improvement. Families in which there were higher levels of maternal criticism tended to do worse in CFT. On the other hand, significantly more changes were demonstrated for CFT in terms of individual psychological and family functioning.[23] Patients continued to improve after the treatment ended and at 5-year follow-up, most of them (75%) had a good outcome, 15% an intermediate outcome, and 10% had a poor outcome.[49,50]

In a design similar to these Maudsley studies, Robin and colleagues[51] in Detroit compared CFT (behavioral family systems therapy [BFST]) with ego-oriented individual therapy (EOIT) in 38 adolescents with AN. The latter comprised weekly individual sessions for the adolescent and bi-monthly collateral sessions with the parents. In describing the features of BFST, Robin and colleagues[51] pointed out the similarities with the Maudsley conjoint family therapy. That is, both treatments emphasize the parents' role in managing the eating disorder symptoms in the early stages of treatment, whereas the focus broadens in the later stages of treatment to include individual or family issues. EOIT is superficially similar to SFT, although the aims are different. SFT emphasizes helping parents to take a strong role in the management of the symptoms, whereas EOIT aims to help parents relinquish control over their daughter's eating and prepare them to accept a more assertive adolescent. Despite these differences between EOIT and SFT, the similarities between them are equally important. Both treatments provide the adolescent with regular individual therapy in which she had the opportunity to address personal and relationship issues and matters directly related to her eating difficulties. Although the parallel sessions with the parents differed in frequency and content, both treatments encouraged the parents to have an active and supportive role in their daughter's recovery and to reflect on some of the family dynamics that might have got caught up with the eating disorder.

Some notable differences between the Maudsley and Detroit studies could have had an impact on the outcome. In Robin's study, patients <75% of ideal body weight (IBW) were hospitalized at the outset of treatment (almost half the sample) and remained in the inpatient setting until they had achieved 80% IBW. In contrast, the Maudsley studies[23,48] allowed for admission only if outpatient therapy failed to arrest weight loss (4 out of 58 were admitted during the study). The duration of treatment was shorter in the Maudsley studies (6–12 months), whereas the Detroit group spent between 12 and 18 months in treatment. Finally, patients at the Maudsley appeared to have been ill for longer; the majority had had previous treatment, and a higher percentage were suffering from depression.

Posttreatment results in the Detroit study demonstrated significant improvements in both treatments with 67% of patients reaching target weight and 80% regaining menstruation. Patients continued to improve, and at 1-year follow-up, approximately 75% had reached their target weight and 85% were menstruating.[51] Physiological improvements (ie, weight and menses) were superior for patients in BFST at post-treatment and follow-up. Improvements in psychological measures (eg, eating attitudes, mood, self-reported eating-related family conflict) were comparable for the 2 groups. Robin and colleagues[24] also reported results of observational ratings of family interaction in a subsample of their study. They demonstrated a significant decrease in maternal negative communication and a corresponding increase in positive communication in BFST but not in EOIT.

A small study by Ball and Mitchell[52] in Sydney compared the outcome of behavioral family therapy and CBT in 25 13- to 23-year-olds. At the end of 1 year's treatment 72% had reached good/intermediate outcome (78%, excluding treatment dropouts) but no differences were found between treatments. The results are difficult to interpret partly because of the small sample size and partly because patients who had to be admitted to the hospital during the course of the study were excluded, potentially biasing the results.

In a recent study, Lock and colleagues[53] examined the effect of treatment dose of family therapy among 86 adolescents and found that a brief 6-month version of a manualized family therapy[28] was as effective as a year-long version. However, the longer version of this treatment was superior for those patients who came from nonintact families or presented with higher levels of obsessions and compulsions about eating. At 4-year follow-up, and regardless of the length of treatment, about two thirds of patients achieved healthy body weights and had eating disorder examination scores within the normal range.[43,48]

Summary of Family Therapy Studies in Adolescent Anorexia Nervosa

Taken together, these studies consistently show that adolescents with AN respond well to family therapy, in many instances without the need for inpatient treatment. Between 50% and 75% of adolescents are weight restored by the end of the treatment. However, most will not have started or resumed menses. At 4- to 5-year follow-up, most (60%–90%) will have fully recovered, whereas only 10% to 15% will still be seriously ill. Outpatient family therapy compares quite favorably to other treatment modalities, such as inpatient care, where full recovery rates vary between 33% and 55%.[54,55]

Given the small size and number of comparative studies, any comparisons between different kinds of family interventions ought to be interpreted with caution. Treatments that promote parents to take an active role in tackling their daughter's AN seem the most effective and may have benefits over treatments in which parents are involved in a supportive way, but are encouraged to step back from the eating problem. For instance, 1 study has shown that excluding parents from the treatment leads to a deleterious outcome and may even delay recovery to a considerable degree.[46,47] Seeing families in conjoint format seems to have an advantage in that both family and individual psychological issues are addressed. However, this form of family intervention may disadvantage families in which there are high levels of hostility or criticism.[56] Such families are perhaps more difficult to engage in family treatment,[57] a challenge that is exacerbated when the whole family is seen together. One reason for this might be that feelings of guilt and blame are increased because of criticisms or confrontations occurring during family sessions.[49] The authors' clinical experience suggests that conjoint sessions may be more useful for these families at a stage in treatment when the concerns about eating disorder symptoms have dissipated. Although there may be relative merit between different types of family interventions, these differences are small especially when compared with overall improvements in response to any of the family interventions studied.

Several reviewers recently concluded that there is compelling evidence for the effectiveness of family interventions for adolescent AN.[18,29,58] Given the status of current evidence, albeit limited, family therapy is probably the treatment of choice. Our enthusiasm for this treatment should be tempered in that the positive findings may, at least in part, be because of the lack of research on other treatments. Ego-oriented, cognitive, and psychodynamic treatments are described in the literature[51,59,60] but with the exception of ego-oriented therapy and the small RCT of CBT versus family therapy,[52] these treatments have not been systematically evaluated with adolescent AN. Likewise, there is no systematic evidence as yet for the effectiveness of multiple-family day treatment, a promising new treatment development, described in some detail later on in this article. Our knowledge of potential contraindications for the use of family treatment is limited but, clearly, caution is needed in cases in which the patient's weight is extremely low (eg, <75% IBW), where there is severe parental psychopathology, and there is evidence that where there are high levels of criticism or hostility directed at the affected offspring engaging the family in treatment is more difficult[57] and treatment outcome is worse.[23,50] However, more systematic evidence is needed to clearly delineate which families stand to benefit most from this treatment.

THEORETIC MODEL OF FAMILY INTERVENTION IN ADOLESCENT ANOREXIA NERVOSA

Although the role of the family environment in the etiology of eating disorders is unclear, there is less doubt that the presence of an eating disorder has a major impact on family life.[61] With the passing of time, food, eating, and the concomitant concerns begin to saturate the family fabric. Consequently, daily family routines and coping and problem-solving behaviors are all affected.[19] Steinglass and colleagues[62] described a similar process in families with an alcoholic member and in families coping with a wide range of chronic illnesses.[63] They proposed that families go through a stepwise reorganization in response to the challenges of the illness. In their model, the illness and its associated issues increasingly take center stage, altering the family's daily routines, their decision-making processes, and regulatory behaviors, until the illness becomes *the central organizing principle* of the family's life. Steinglass and colleagues argue that when families attempt to minimize the impact of the illness on the sufferer and other family members, they increasingly focus their attention on the present. As a result, it becomes difficult to meet the families' changing developmental needs.

The proposed model is readily applicable to eating disorders. Families trying to deal with an eating disorder often report that it feels as if time has come to a standstill and that everything in their life has come to be focused on the eating disorder.[64] The way families respond to this varies depending on the nature of the family organization, the family's style, and the particular life-cycle stage they are at when the illness occurs. What may be more predictable is the way in which the increasing emphasis on the eating disorder magnifies certain aspects of the family's dynamics while at the same time narrowing the range of their adaptive behaviors.[19]

Trying to identify which family processes may have a contributory causal effect, which are responses to the problem, or which are just incidental is difficult. Moreover, as several investigators have argued recently,[25,65] understanding mechanisms that maintain a disorder are likely to be of more usefulness for the development of effective treatments than the pursuit of etiologic explanations. From a clinical perspective this requires joining the family in an exploration of how they got caught up in the eating disorder and to help them uncover some of their strengths so that they can disentangle themselves from the problem and discover new solutions. Most crucial in the process of engaging families in treatment is to emphasize that they are part of the solution and not the problem. During treatment families may find that there are ways in which they function that they want to change. However, this is only secondary to the primary goal, which is to overcome their child's eating disorder.[19]

THE STAGES OF TREATMENT OF FAMILY INTERVENTION FOR ADOLESCENT ANOREXIA NERVOSA

The practical application of family-based treatment for adolescent AN (FBT-AN) has been well described,[19,26,27,66] the most detailed version being available now in a manualized version for clinicians.[28] In addition, a handbook to assist and guide parents through treatment has also been published.[67] This manual depicts FBT-AN as problem-focused in nature where the primary strategy is to bring about behavioral change through unified parental action. The family is held in a positive light and is seen as a significant resource in the adolescent's weight restoration and concomitant return to normal eating and health. FBT-AN does not focus on the potential origins of the disorder; in fact, it takes an agnostic stance in terms of etiology while families are reassured that they are not the cause of the eating disorder. To mobilize parents to a unified stance, and to encourage the adolescent's cooperation, this treatment aims to externalize and separate the AN pathology from the affected adolescent.[68]

FBT-AN has been described as having several distinct phases, although in practice these often overlap. The first phase of treatment is mainly concerned with supporting the parents in their effort to restore their adolescent's weight. To achieve this goal, the therapist encourages the parents to present a united front directed toward weight restoration. At first, the adolescent's food intake is under parental control with the parents monitoring meals and snacks while restricting physical activity where necessary and taking an active role in limiting purging or other behaviors that can potentially lead to weight loss. Engaging the family in this task requires the therapist to be able to convey to the parents that, however impossible the task ahead may seem to them, the therapist believes that they will eventually succeed. At the same time he or she has to show an understanding of the young person's fears while being clear that this must not deflect the parents' efforts of helping her get her life back on track, and even weight restoration has to be achieved despite frequent or considerable resistance on her part. The therapist provides liberal amounts of information to the family about the nature of eating disorders and physiologic and psychological effects of starvation, partly to help the parents gain a better understanding of the nature of the problem but also to reinforce the message that AN is a powerful illness and typically would not "allow" the sufferer to make appropriate or healthy decisions regarding food and exercise. While encouraging the parents to work together at weight restoration, the adolescent is aligned with her sibling subsystem, for example, siblings are placed in a supportive role, while the task of weight restoration is exclusively the parents' domain.

The therapist does not prescribe a particular course of action to the parents. Instead, he or she explores with the family how the parents have functioned outside of the illness context, what the particular strengths of each parent are, and how these could be used to explore weight restoration strategies best suited to their particular family. The first phase of treatment focuses almost exclusively on weight restoration and a return to healthy eating patterns. Consequently, the therapist emphasizes that this goal takes precedence over almost any other issue until the adolescent's self-starvation has been reversed.

The second phase of treatment begins at the time the patient has reached ~90% of IBW, is eating without much resistance, and the mood of the family is more upbeat. At this time the parents are guided to return responsibility over eating back to the adolescent. This process is both gradual and tailored to the age of the adolescent. Consequently, there may be a few differences between phases 1 and 2 for an 11-year-old, for whom parents are typically still very much in charge of their child's food intake. A 17-year-old, on the other hand, will be given much more responsibility and independence over her food choices. Once the parents have been able to negotiate the return of control over eating to their adolescent, topics that have been put on hold can now be explored. For instance, going to the movies with friends may now return to the agenda, but only inasmuch as the adolescent can continue to achieve a healthy weight.

The third phase of treatment usually begins around the time that the adolescent has achieved a healthy weight for age and height, one at which they are able to menstruate (for girls). This part of the treatment focuses the discussion on general issues of adolescent development and ways in which the eating disorder has affected this process. FBT-AN views the eating disorder as having taken normal progression of adolescent development off track. Once the adolescent is back on track, discussion can focus on the remaining developmental challenges and how parents can help their adolescent to navigate this process. In keeping with an age-appropriate strategy, the focus of treatment at this stage is on increased personal autonomy, relationships with peers, or getting ready to leave home for the first time. The needs of siblings and parents, which will also have been put on hold by the illness, are addressed at this stage. In the final stages of treatment issues about ending of therapy and relapse prevention strategies are also discussed.

MULTIPLE-FAMILY DAY TREATMENT FOR ADOLESCENT ANOREXIA NERVOSA

Multiple-family therapy (MFT), originally pioneered by Laqueur and colleagues[69] in the treatment of schizophrenia as a way to use the combined resources of families to improve family communication, learn by analogy, and expand their social repertoires,[70,71] has been adapted for work with various psychiatric populations,[72–76] including those with eating disorders.[77,78] The usual format of MFT is similar to most group therapies, that is, weekly or biweekly meetings, but more intensive formats have also been developed in which groups of families meet for whole days,[79] sometimes over an extended period of time, as part of a day treatment program.[80,81] This more intensive format of MFT is proving to be particularly well suited for the treatment of adolescents with eating disorders, and 2 groups in Dresden, Germany,[82] and in

London, UK,[19,83] have been developing MFT day programs that integrate the conceptual ideas of FBT-AN with those of MFT.

Bringing several families together is a powerful therapeutic resource, which helps to reduce the sense of isolation, diminish stigmatization, enhance opportunities to create new and multiple perspectives, and, above all, address the pervasive sense of helplessness that families experience when trying to deal with the AN in their daughter or son.[64,84] There are many similarities and overlaps between the individual work with families as described earlier and the multiple-family treatment approach. There are similar phases in both approaches with an early focus on helping the parents to take a strong stance against their child's anorexia while remaining sympathetic to how terrifying this is for her. Later the focus of the group shifts to include individual needs of family members and the developmental tasks that may have been put on hold by the emergence of the eating disorder. The group is both the context for joint problem solving and a source of support when things seem unbearably difficult.[85]

The MFT starts after the family has been engaged in treatment individually and they are invited to take part in a 4-day intensive workshop with up to 5 other families. The treatment continues with additional 1-day group meetings and is supplemented by individual family sessions depending on the specific need of each family.[e] The 4-day workshop provides an opportunity for a range of interventions, including whole group discussions, separate work with the adolescent group and the parent group, with a series of intervention techniques being used, including whole group discussions, role-playing, psycho-educational sessions, supported meal times, video feedback sessions, and so forth.[33]

The intensity of MFT leads to a strong sense of group cohesion from early on and a highly collaborative relationship between the families and the clinical staff. This has been contrasted with what often happens in the context of in-patient units,[86] where staff may view parents with some ambiguity because of their (staff) conscious or unconscious beliefs that the parents have failed, and are perhaps even to blame for the child's eating disorder. This is often reinforced by the parents' own sense of failure. Sometimes this can lead to the view that it is necessary to separate the adolescents from their parents to assist them in their individuation.[60] In such a situation the staff and parents can be at odds as to who is the "best" carer or, alternately, they may develop a shared belief that the hospital provides a better home. These dynamics can become easily entrenched, particularly if rapid weight loss follows discharge from an in-patient unit, which serves to confirm that hospital staff are "better" than parents, and underscore the parents' failure. Consequently, demoralized parents are keen to sanction their child's readmission to hospital eager to have her discharged later than sooner, and the chronicity of the illness is only matched by the chronicity of the evolving dynamic of the staff/family relationships. The context of MFT with its focus of using the group as the main arena for problem solving, is different, similar in some ways to a therapeutic community. One of the strengths of the MFT model is that it brings families together in a way that makes them feel empowered and allows them to draw on the expertise of the staff without needing to hand complete control over to the experts.[33]

As is the case with Maudsley family therapy approach in general[66] MFT aims to help parents rediscover their own resources and take an active role in their children's recovery. Families are encouraged to explore how it has become problematic to follow

---

[e] The MFT program developed in Dresden is somewhat different in that it has many more group follow-up days and unlike the Maudsley little individual contact with families outside of the group meetings.[86]

the normal developmental course of their family life cycle by looking at how the eating disorder and the interactional patterns in the family have become entangled. Sharing experiences among families and the intensity of this treatment program set it apart from the experience that is more typical of outpatient family therapy. In the context of MFT, the emphasis on helping families to find their own solutions is readily apparent.[33]

Each group of families develops its own unique dynamic. However, almost all groups establish an identity that evolves around discussions of their shared experience of living with AN and the effect this has on family life. Parents of a child with AN often present with a complex set of feelings such as failure, guilt, anger, fear, and embarrassment. Meeting with other families provides an opportunity to share these feelings which creates a sense of solidarity and helps families to feel less stigmatized. In MFT, family members outnumber clinicians. Consequently, this numerical advantage also has the effect of making the adolescents and their parents less central. Rather, they are members of a large group and the feeling of being constantly examined is less pronounced. This process seems to accelerate the families' ability to externalize the AN and to join forces to overcome the eating disorder.

Getting to know other families that struggle with an eating disorder also accentuates differences between them. This in turn demonstrates for families that there is no specific family structure that leads to the development of AN, which makes it easier for them to compare how other parents handle their teen's food refusal. The effect of these comparisons allows families to consider fresh perspectives on their own dilemma. The mix of joint problem solving discussions, activity techniques, and observing how other families deal with similar problems allows each family to find their own way of learning and moving on. The families are generally very respectful and supportive of each other while at the same time being willing to provide and receive feedback about each other, which generally carries considerably more weight than if it were coming from the clinician, who may be highly experienced but does not have the shared experiences around food, dieting, or hospitalization. The therapist's role is, therefore, more of a catalyst, encouraging interaction between families and creating a safe context, which enables families to make connections with one another and facilitates mutual curiosity and feedback.

Preliminary Findings

The 2 teams in London and Dresden that have been developing MFT have now had experience with several hundred adolescents with an eating disorder and their families, using this approach. In addition, several teams in the UK and also in other countries (Canada, Norway, Sweden, Denmark, the Netherlands, Switzerland, Czech Republic, Hong Kong) have taken part in MFT training and started running their own groups.[87] Feedback from both the families and the professionals who have taken part has been extremely positive, and audit data have shown low dropout rates from treatment in both centers of between 2% and 3%. In Dresden, admission rates have been reduced by 30%, while the duration of inpatient treatment has been reduced by 25%, and readmissions have been cut by half.[29,86]

Systematic follow-up data to demonstrate the effectiveness of MFT in bringing about symptomatic improvement are limited at this stage. A small study investigating the experiences of families taking part in MFT and early symptom change in 30 adolescents has been completed in London.[88] This study has shown that by 6 months (ie, half way through treatment) the average weight for height for the group was at the lower end of the normal range, with 21% of the adolescents being classified as having a good and 41% intermediate outcome on the Morgan-Russell scales.[36] The most immediate and striking change comes from the qualitative evaluation of the families' experience of the treatment and the way in which they have come to be reinvigorated in terms of their ability to help their children. For many families this discovery is accompanied by meaningful reductions in disputes around eating and replaced by a more accommodating and compassionate atmosphere between the adolescent and their families.[33]

SUMMARY

Almost all treatment models assume a specific mechanism of change (eg, cognitive restructuring, changes in interpersonal relationships) that is seen as the target of the treatment goal. However, the fact that different treatments often lead to similar outcomes would suggest that our understanding of the mechanisms of change remain limited[89] and it is likely that the actual mechanisms of change for different treatments will turn out to be different from what is assumed by theory. This is undoubtedly the case for family therapy for eating disorders, as its history clearly shows. Although the empiric evidence for the effectiveness of family therapy for adolescent AN is gaining strength, the theoretic models from which this treatment is historically derived have been shown to be wanting. Our understanding of the way in which family interventions bring about change still remains largely speculative, and our involvement with families in the more concentrated atmosphere of the MFT program has, among other things, highlighted how limited our understanding of the process of change leading to recovery is. Just as families differ in the way they respond to having a member who develops an eating disorder, so they also differ in the way they use family interventions. Some very quickly take firm charge of their daughter's eating until she returns to a healthy state, and for such families, the opportunity for parents to re-establish appropriate parental authority is the main focus around which change seems to take place. Other families step into the domain of parenting only briefly or in a more symbolic way, as if the confirmation that they could do this if necessary was all they needed. In yet other families, meeting together serves as a chance for the adolescent and the parents to start redefining the role the parents have in relation to eating and other areas of adolescent life. The commonality in these solutions seems to be that families are able to take some distance and extricate themselves from the way they have been caught up with the symptomatic behavior. In this process, many families regain their belief that they can find a way of conquering the problem, even if this may take some time.

ACKNOWLEDGMENT

The authors wish to thank James Roehrig, MA, for his contribution to this manuscript.

REFERENCES

1. Lasegue E. De L'anorexie hysterique. Archives Generales De Medecine 1873;21: 384–403 [in French].
2. Gull W. Anorexia nervosa (apepsia hysteria, anorexia hysteria). Transactions of the Clinical Society of London 1874;7:222–8.
3. Charcot JM. Clinical lectures on diseases of the nervous systems. London: New Sydenham Society; 1889.
4. Myrtle AS. Letters to the editor. Lancet 1888;1:899.
5. Playfair WS. Note on the so called anorexia nervosa. Lancet 1888;1:817.

6. Allison RS, Davies RP. The treatment of functional anorexia nervosa. Lancet 1931; 217:902–7.

7. Ryle JA. Anorexia nervosa. Lancet 1936;228:893–9.

8. Bliss EL, Branch CHH. Anorexia nervosa. New York: Hoeber; 1960.

9. Harper G. Varieties of parenting failure in anorexia nervosa: protection and parentectomy revisited. J Am Acad Child Adolesc Psychiatry 1983;22:134–9.

10. Bruch H. Perceptual and conceptual disturbances in anorexia nervosa. Psychosom Med 1962;24:187–94.

11. Bruch H. Eating disorders: obesity, anorexia nervosa, and the person within. New York: Basic Books; 1973.

12. Palazzoli MS. Self starvation: from the intrapsychic to the transpersonal approach to anorexia nervosa. London: Chaucer Publishing; 1974.

13. Minuchin S, Baker L, Rosman BL, et al. A conceptual model of psychosomatic illness in children. Family organization and family therapy. Arch Gen Psychiatry 1975;32:1031–8.

14. Minuchin S, Rosman BL, Baker L. Psychosomatic families: anorexia nervosa in context. Cambridge (MA): Harvard University Press; 1978.

15. Dare C, Eisler I, Russell GFM, et al. The clinical and theoretical impact of a controlled trial of family therapy in anorexia nervosa. J Marital Fam Ther 1990;16: 39–57.

16. Stierlin H, Weber G. Unlocking the family door. New York: Brunner/Mazel; 1989.

17. White M. Anorexia nervosa: a cybernetic perspective. Fam Ther Collections 1989; 20:117–29.

18. Kotler LA, Boudreau GS, Devlin MJ. Emerging psychotherapies for eating disorders. J Psychiatr Pract 2003;9:431–41.

19. Eisler I. The empirical and theoretical base of family therapy and multiple family day therapy for adolescent anorexia nervosa. J Fam Ther 2005;27:104–31.

20. Eisler I. Family models of eating disorders. In: Szmukler GI, Dare C, Treasure J, editors. Handbook of eating disorders: theory, treatment and research. London: Wiley; 1995. p. 155–76.

21. Kog E, Vandereycken W. Family interaction in eating disordered patients and normal controls. Int J Eat Disord 1989;8:11–23.

22. Roijen S. Anorexia nervosa families a homogeneous group? A case record study. Acta Psychiatr Scand 1992;85:196–200.

23. Eisler I, Dare C, Hodes M, et al. Family therapy for adolescent anorexia nervosa: the results of a controlled comparison of two family interventions. J Child Psychol Psychiatry 2000;41:727–36.

24. Robin AL, Siegal PT, Moye A. Family versus individual therapy for anorexia: impact on family conflict. Int J Eat Disord 1995;4:313–22.

25. Schmidt U, Treasure J. Anorexia nervosa: valued and visible. A cognitive interpersonal maintenance model and its implications for research and practice. Br J Clin Psychol 2006;45:343–66.

26. Dare C, Eisler I. Family therapy. In: Szmukler GI, Dare C, Treasure J, editors. Handbook of eating disorders; theory, treatment and research. Chichester (UK): John Wiley and Sons; 1995. p. 333–49.

27. Dare C, Eisler I, Colahan M, et al. The listening heart and the chi square: clinical and empirical perceptions in the family therapy of anorexia nervosa. J Fam Ther 1995;17:31–57.

28. Lock J, Le Grange D, Agras WS, et al. Treatment manual for anorexia nervosa: a family-based approach. New York: Guilford Press; 2001.

29. Le Grange D, Lock J. The dearth of psychological treatment studies for anorexia nervosa. Int J Eat Disord 2005;37:79–91.
30. Blitzer JR, Rollins N, Blackwell A. Children who starve themselves: anorexia nervosa. Psychosom Med 1961;23:369–83.
31. Lesser LI, Ashenden BJ, Debuskey M, et al. Anorexia nervosa in children. Am J Orthopsychiatry 1960;30:572–80.
32. Warren W. A study of anorexia nervosa in young girls. J Child Psychol Psychiatry 1968;9:27–40.
33. Eisler I, Le Grange D, Asen E. Family interventions. In: Treasure J, Schmidt U, Van Furth E, editors. Handbook of eating disorders. Chichester (UK): John Wiley and Sons; 2003. p. 291–310.
34. Martin FE. The treatment and outcome of anorexia nervosa in adolescents: a prospective study and five year follow-up. J Psychiatr Res 1985;19:509–14.
35. Herscovici CR, Bay L. Favourable outcome for anorexia nervosa patients treated in Argentina with a family approach. Eating Disorders the Journal of Treatment and Prevention 1996;4:59–66.
36. Morgan HG, Russell GF. Value of family background and clinical features as predictors of long-term outcome in anorexia nervosa: four-year follow-up study of 41 patients. Psychol Med 1975;5:355–71.
37. Dare C. Family therapy for families containing an anorectic youngster. Ohio (OH): Ross Laboratories; 1983.
38. Mayer RD. Family therapy in the treatment of eating disorders in general practice. MSc Dissertation. Birkbeck College, University of London; 1994.
39. Stierlin H, Weber G. Anorexia nervosa: lessons from a follow-up study. Fam Syst Med 1987;7:120–57.
40. Le Grange D, Gelman T. The patient's perspective of treatment in eating disorders: a preliminary study. S Afr J Psychol 1998;28:182–6.
41. Wallin U, Kronwall P. Anorexia nervosa in teenagers: change in family function after family therapy at 2-year follow-up. Nordic J Psychiatry 2002;56:363–9.
42. Le Grange D, Binford R, Loeb K. Manualized family-based treatment for anorexia nervosa: a case series. J Am Acad Child Adolesc Psychiatry 2005;44:41–6.
43. Lock J, Couturier J, Agras WS. Comparison of long term outcomes in adolescents with anorexia nervosa treated with family therapy. J Am Acad Child Adolesc Psychiatry 2006;46:666–72.
44. Loeb KL, Walsh BT, Lock J, et al. Open trial of family-based treatment for full and partial anorexia nervosa in adolescence: evidence of successful dissemination. J Am Acad Child Adolesc Psychiatry 2007;46:792–800.
45. Lock J, Le Grange D, Fordsburg S, et al. Is family therapy effective for children with anorexia nervosa? J Am Acad Child Adolesc Psychiatry 2006;45:1023–8.
46. Russell GFM, Szmukler GI, Dare C, et al. An evaluation of family therapy in anorexia nervosa and bulimia nervosa. Arch Gen Psychiatry 1987;44:1047–56.
47. Eisler I, Dare C, Russell GFM, et al. Family and individual therapy in anorexia nervosa. A 5-year follow-up. Arch Gen Psychiatry 1997;54:1025–30.
48. Le Grange D, Eisler I, Dare C, et al. Evaluation of family treatments in adolescent anorexia nervosa: a pilot study. Int J Eat Disord 1992;12:347–57.
49. Squire-Dehouck B. Evaluation of conjoint family therapy versus family counselling in adolescent anorexia nervosa patients: a two year follow-up study dissertation. Kings College, University of London; 1993.
50. Eisler I, Simic M, Russell GFM, et al. Family therapy for adolescent anorexia nervosa: a five year follow-up study of a controlled comparison of two family interventions. J Child Psychol Psychiatry 2007;41:552–60.

51. Robin AL, Siegal PT, Moye A, et al. A controlled comparison of family versus individual therapy for adolescents with anorexia nervosa. J Am Acad Child Adolesc Psychiatry 1999;38:1482–9.
52. Ball J, Mitchell P. A randomized controlled study of cognitive behaviour therapy and behavioural family therapy for anorexia nervosa patients. Eating disorders. J Treat Prevent 2004;12:303–14.
53. Lock J, Agras WS, Bryson S, et al. A comparison of short and long term family therapy for adolescent anorexia nervosa. J Am Acad Child Adolesc Psychiatry 2005;44:632–9.
54. Gowers S, Clark A, Roberts C, et al. Clinical effectiveness of treatments for anorexia nervosa in adolescents: randomised controlled trial. Br J Psychiatry 2007;191:427–35.
55. Steinhausen H, Grigoroiu-Serbanescu M, Boyadjieva S, et al. Course and predictors of rehospitalization in adolescent anorexia nervosa in a multisite study. Int J Eat Disord 2008;41:29–36.
56. Le Grange D, Eisler I, Dare C, et al. Family criticism and self-starvation: a study of expressed emotion. J Fam Ther 1992;14:177–92.
57. Szmukler GI, Eisler I, Russell GFM, et al. Anorexia nervosa, parental 'expressed emotion' and dropping out of treatment. Br J Psychiatry 1985;147:265–71.
58. Carr A. The effectiveness of family therapy and systemic intervention for adult focused problems. J Fam Ther, in press.
59. Bowers WA, Evans K, Van Cleve L. Treatment of adolescent eating disorders. In: Reinecke MA, Dattilio FM, editors. Cognitive therapy with children and adolescents: a casebook for clinical practice. New York: Guilford Press; 1996. p. 247–80.
60. Jeammet P, Chabert C. A psychoanalytic approach to eating disorders: the role of dependency. In: Esman AH, editor. Adolescent psychiatry: developmental and clinical studies, Annals of the American Society for Adolescent Psychiatry. Vol. 22. Hillsdale (NJ): The Analytic Press, Inc; 1998. p. 59–84.
61. Bara-Carril N, Nielsen S. Family, burden of care and social consequences. In: Treasure J, Schmidt U, Van Furth E, editors. Handbook of eating disorders. Chichester (UK): John Wiley and Sons; 2003. p. 191–206.
62. Steinglass P, Bennett LA, Wolin SJ, et al. The alcoholic family. New York: Basic Books; 1987.
63. Steinglass P. Multiple family discussion groups for patients with chronic medical illness. Fam Syst Health 1998;16:55–70.
64. Whitney J, Eisler I. Theoretical and empirical models around caring for someone with an eating disorder: the reorganization of family life and interpersonal maintenance factors. J Mental Health 2005;14:575–85.
65. Shafran R, de Silva P. Cognitive-behavioural models. In: Treasure J, Schmidt U, Van Furth E, editors. Handbook of eating disorders. Chichester (UK): Wiley; 2003. p. 121–38.
66. Dare C, Eisler I. Family therapy for anorexia nervosa. In: Garner DM, Garfinkel PE, editors. Handbook of psychotherapy for anorexia nervosa and bulimia. 2nd edition. New York: Guilford press; 1997. p. 307–24.
67. Lock J, Le Grange D. Help your teenager beat an eating disorder. New York: Guilford Press; 2004.
68. White M, Epston D. Narrative means to therapeutic ends. New York: Norton; 1990.
69. Lacquer HP, La Burt HA, Morong E. Multiple family therapy: further developments. Int J Soc Psychiatry 1964;10:69–80.

70. Lacquer HP. Mechanisms of change in multiple family therapy. In: Sager CJ, Kaplan HS, editors. Progress in group and family therapy. New York: Bruner/Mazel; 1972.

71. Lacquer HP. Multiple family therapy: questions and answers. In: Bloch D, editor. Techniques of family psychotherapy. New York: Grune and Stratton; 1973.

72. Gonsalez S, Steinglass P, Reisse D. Putting the illness in its place: discussion groups for families with chronic medical illnesses. Fam Process 1989;28:69–87.

73. Kaufman E, Kaufman P. Multiple family therapy with drug abusers. In: Kaufman E, Kaufman P, editors. Family therapy of drug and alcohol abuse. New York: Gardner; 1979.

74. Asen E, George E, Piper R, et al. A systems approach to child abuse: management and treatment issues. Child Abuse Negl 1989;13:45–57.

75. Lemmens GM, Wauters S, Heireman M, et al. Beneficial factors in family discussion groups of a psychiatric day clinic: perceptions by the therapeutic team and the families of the therapeutic process. J Fam Ther 2003;25:41–63.

76. Lemmens GMD, Eisler I, Migerode L, et al. Family discussion group therapy for major depression: a brief systemic multi-family group intervention for hospitalized patients and their family members. J Fam Ther 2007;29:49–68.

77. Slagerman M, Yager J. Multiple family group treatment for eating disorders: a short term program. Psychiatr Med 1989;7:269–83.

78. Wooley S, Lewis K. Multi-family therapy within an intensive treatment program for bulimia. In: Harkaway J, editor. Eating disorders: the family therapy collections, 20. Rockville (MD): Aspen Publications; 1987.

79. Anderson CM, Hogarty GE, Reiss DJ. Family treatment of adult schizophrenic patients: a psycho-educational approach. Schizophr Bull 1980;6:460–505.

80. Asen E, Stein R, Stevens A, et al. A day unit for families. J Fam Ther 1982;4:345–58.

81. Cooklin A, Miller A, McHugh B. An institution for change: developing a family day unit. Fam Process 1983;22:453–68.

82. Scholz M, Asen KE. Multiple family therapy with eating disordered adolescents. Eur Eat Disord Rev 2001;9:33–42.

83. Dare C, Eisler I. A multi-family group day treatment programme for adolescent eating disorder. Eur Eat Disord Rev 2000;8:4–18.

84. Poser M. Anorexia nervosa—a parent's perspective. J Fam Ther 2005;27:144–6.

85. Poser M. Anorexia nervosa—my story. J Fam Ther 2005;27:142–3.

86. Scholz M, Rix M, Scholz K, et al. Multiple family therapy for anorexia nervosa: concepts, experiences and results. J Fam Ther 2005;27:132–41.

87. Fairbairn P, Eisler I. Intensive multiple family day treatment: clinical and training perspectives. In: Cook S, Almosnino A, editors. Therapies multifamiliales des groupes comme agents therapeutiques (multiple family therapy: groups as therapeutic agents). Paris: Editions Eres.

88. Salaminiou E. Families in multiple family therapy for adolescent anorexia nervosa. Response to treatment, treatment experience and family and individual change. [Unpublished PhD Thesis]. Kings College, University of London; 2005.

89. Asay TP, Lambert MJ. The empirical case for the common factors in therapy: quantitative findings. In: Hubble MA, Duncan BL, Scott DM, editors. The heart and soul of changeWhat works in therapy. Washington, DC: APA; 1999. p. 33–56.

Pharmacotherapy for Eating Disorders and Obesity

Pauline S. Powers, MD*, Heidi Bruty, MD

KEYWORDS

- Pharmacotherapy • Anorexia nervosa • Bulimia nervosa
- Obesity

Eating disorders are significant problems most commonly occurring among late adolescent and young women. These are often chronic, relapsing conditions associated with psychiatric comorbidity and medical sequelae. Most of the literature over the past several decades has focused on anorexia nervosa (AN) and bulimia nervosa (BN). Other clinically significant eating disturbances, such as binge eating disorder, night eating syndrome, and sleep-related eating disorder, have recently been recognized, especially because of the risk for obesity associated with these disorders and the increase in obesity within the population. Despite the prevalence of eating disorders in the population, there is a relative dearth of evidenced-based support and little guidance from the literature regarding pharmacologic approaches for treating eating disorders. This, however, is not the case regarding the treatment of obesity. For the treatment of eating disorders in children and adolescents, the literature is essentially non-existent. With little guidance, clinicians attempt to apply the strategies suggested for the treatment of eating disorders in adult patients to children and adolescents, resulting in off-label use of medications in children and adolescents. There is no guidance for the appropriate dosing for this population and little knowledge exists regarding the effect of these medications on growth and development.

PHARMACOTHERAPY FOR ANOREXIA NERVOSA

Currently, no medications are approved by the Food and Drug Administration (FDA) for the treatment of AN. Evidence-based support for the effectiveness of pharmacotherapy as a first-line strategy in the treatment of underweight or weight-restored patients with AN is lacking. Current pharmacotherapy strategies focus on either reducing anxiety or alleviating mood symptoms, which may facilitate re-feeding, increase hunger, or induce weight gain as a side effect of a particular agent or treat a medical

College of Medicine, University of South Florida, 3515 East Fletcher Avenue, Tampa, FL 33613, USA
* Corresponding author.
E-mail address: ppowers@health.usf.edu (P.S. Powers).

Child Adolesc Psychiatric Clin N Am 18 (2008) 175–187
doi:10.1016/j.chc.2008.07.009
1056-4993/08/$ – see front matter © 2008 Elsevier Inc. All rights reserved.

complication.[1] None of these strategies is completely effective and there is currently no drug that specifically targets the core features of the disorder, such as body image distortion, extreme perfectionism, obsessional thoughts, and anticipatory anxiety regarding eating. Treatment of this disorder is also complicated by the fact that treatments that may prove to be useful in one phase of treatment, for example, the weight restoration phase, may not be useful during another phase, for example, the weight maintenance phase.

Because patients with AN commonly demonstrate significant comorbid psychopathology, such as obsessive-compulsive, depressive, or anxiety symptoms, the role of antidepressants, particularly selective serotonin reuptake inhibitors (SSRIs), has been explored for both acutely ill and weight-restored patients with AN. However, there are no published controlled trials of outpatient treatments with SSRIs in patients with a low body mass index (BMI). Clinical reports and studies suggest that extremely low-weight patients are unresponsive to the antidepressant, anti-obsessional, and anxiolytic effects of SSRIs.[1] This is likely owing to the fact that significantly starved patients remain in a relative hyposerotonergic state in the brain secondary to the nutritional effects of a diet low in tryptophan. Studies have shown that SSRIs are not effective for depression when patients without an eating disorder undergo dietary restriction.[2] Thus, without any serotonin substrate to act on, SSRIs cannot work effectively.

Although SSRIs are not efficacious during the weight restoration phase of AN, there is evidence that supports the role of SSRIs during the maintenance phase of treatment, particularly in preventing relapse. In 1 study, fluoxetine in dosages of up to 60 mg/d was associated with decreased relapse episodes, better maintenance of weight, and fewer symptoms of depression.[3] It is important to note that this study had a small sample size and a high dropout rate. For weight-restored AN patients receiving cognitive-behavioral therapy to help prevent relapse, adding fluoxetine to the treatment does not further decrease the risk for relapse.[4] This suggests that even weight-restored patients may be resistant to the effects of SSRIs. Weight-restored patients who have significant comorbid depression, anxiety, or obsessive-compulsive disorder often benefit from the use of SSRIs but as an adjunctive treatment to psychotherapy and a nutritional rehabilitation program.

Malnourished patients are much more prone to the side effects of medications. Thus, at the time of initiating pharmacotherapy, it is recommended to use the lowest initial doses. Because this patient population is usually reluctant to take medications, starting at low doses to minimize side effects and closely monitoring for early manifestations of troublesome side effects will help avoid noncompliance. Starting at low doses and increasing slowly will also help avoid nausea and diarrhea, which are commonly associated with the use of SSRIs and can worsen eating behaviors and prevent weight gain. At the time of treating children, particularly with antidepressants, the FDA black box warning (indicating a possible serious side effect) regarding suicidal behaviors must be included in the informed consent with patients and their families. Likewise, patients started on antidepressants must be monitored closely for any significant agitation or suicidal behavior after the initiation of medication and after any increase in dosage.

There are no published data supporting the use of serotonin norepinephrine reuptake inhibitors (SNRIs) for AN. Bupropion is contraindicated for this disorder secondary to the increased risk for seizures among eating disorder patients. Although mirtazapine has been known to increase appetite, it is associated with neutropenia and is not recommended for this patient population, which may already be at risk for blood disorders. Tricyclic antidepressants (TCAs) should be avoided in AN patients secondary to the risk for hypotension and cardiac arrhythmias (particularly prolongation of QTc interval) in this patient population.

Second-generational antipsychotics (atypical antipsychotics) can be useful during the weight-restoration phase or in the treatment of other associated symptoms of AN, particularly severe obsessions, anxiety, limited insight, and near delusional thinking regarding body image. Several case studies of inpatients treated with olanzapine at a dosage of 5 to 10 mg/d reported weight increases, decreased fear of fatness, reduced agitation, and reduced resistance to treatment.[5,6] Other open label uncontrolled trials and case reports have supported the use of olanzapine, not only in promoting weight gain but also countering the associated symptoms of AN.[7,8] In a recent double-blind placebo-controlled study[9] with olanzapine, results indicated that pharmacologic therapy, by modifying specific brain biochemical alternations, may improve certain, but not all, aspects of AN. The study confirmed the results of previous open label trials with olanzapine, suggesting that the medication has positive effects on associated symptoms of the disorder, such as depression, anxiety, obsessivity-compulsivity, and aggressiveness, than on the commonly considered typical anorexic symptoms. In the study, there was increased BMI in the patients but no significant difference existed between the effects of the 2 treatment groups on statistical analysis. When the AN patients were stratified according to type, the increase in BMI was significantly greater in the binge–purge type of AN patients than in the restrictive type. A recent double-blind placebo-controlled trial of olanzapine among 34 adult women with AN attending a day treatment program for eating disorders has been reported.[10] Compared to placebo, olanzapine resulted in a greater increase in weight gain, earlier achievement of target BMI, and a greater rate of decrease in obsessive symptoms. Adverse effects were similar in the two groups. Other atypical antipsychotics, such as quetiapine, aripiprazole, ziprasadone, and risperidone, have not been as extensively studied as olanzapine.

For antipsychotic medications, the risk for developing metabolic disturbances, such as insulin resistance and hyperlipidemia, should be disclosed during the informed consent process and monitored with routine blood work. In addition, the emergence of extrapyramidal symptoms, especially in underweight and debilitated patients, should be considered and assessed routinely with appropriate movement scales. Because ziprasadone may be associated with QT prolongation, this medication should not be used in AN patients with low body weight or abnormal electrolytes. The known association of weight gain with the use of atypical antipsychotics frequently causes noncompliance in AN patients who are resistant to treatment.

There is no evidence to support the efficacy of mood stabilizers for the symptoms of AN. In the presence of bipolar disorder, lithium should be used cautiously with AN patients, who are commonly dehydrated and have impaired renal functioning, which may lead to lithium toxicity.

There are other medications used to address the associated features and medical complications. For example, AN patients report early satiety and abdominal bloating especially during re-feeding which may be secondary to gastroparesis. The use of pro-motility agents, such as metoclopramide, may assist with alleviating abdominal complaints during re-feeding; however, there is the risk for extra-pyramidal symptoms, especially in underweight AN patients, and this should be monitored closely. In a small double-blind placebo-controlled crossover study, erythromycin (200 mg) administered by slow intravenous infusion, markedly accelerated the gastric emptying of a semisolid meal in all the AN patients studied.[11] Based on evidence of its potent gastroprokinetic properties, it offers an alternative treatment for impaired gastric motor functioning. The alleviation of severe constipation associated with long-term use of laxatives or their withdrawal may require the use of stool softeners, such as Colace.

In addition to the above, AN is associated with a high prevalence of osteoporosis and osteopenia, presumably related in part to estrogen deficiency and hypercortisolism associated with starvation. In patients with prolonged amenorrhea, hormone replacement therapy, in the form of oral contraceptive pills, is commonly prescribed to improve patients' bone mineral density. However, there is no evidence that this intervention is effective. In a randomized, placebo-controlled trial of adults with AN, estrogen replacement had no effect on bone mineral density.[12] Furthermore, 2 additional studies[13,14] examined the role of estrogen–progestin oral contraceptives in adolescent outpatients. Despite some weight gain in patients in both of these studies, there was no effect of the estrogen–progestin on bone mineral density. In addition to the lack of usefulness in the prevention of bone loss, hormone replacement therapy is not recommended because it usually induces monthly menstrual bleeding in AN patients, obscuring the major sign that indicates weight normalization in women and providing a false sense of reassurance to patients with ongoing symptoms. Furthermore, estrogen should not be given to girls before their growth is complete as it can cause premature fusion of the epiphyses.[13] There is no indication for the use of biphosphonates, such as alendronate or risendronate, in patients with AN nor are they approved for use in premenopausal women.[1] These medications are teratogenic, may be stored in bone for years posttreatment, and pose a significant risk in female patients of childbearing age. At this point, the recommended treatment for low bone mineral density includes weight gain and calcium with vitamin D supplementation.[13]

PHARMACOTHERAPY FOR BULIMIA NERVOSA

The pharmacotherapy of BN has been extensively studied in the literature. Unlike AN, there have been various medications found to have greater efficacy than placebo in treating BN, such as the TCAs, SSRIs, serotonin norepinephrine reuptake inhibitors, and other antidepressant medications.[15] In addition, other agents, such as serotonin receptor antagonists and anticonvulsant medications, particularly topiramate, have been helpful.

The efficacy of antidepressants in BN is attributable to 2 concurrent effects: they contribute to reductions in the core symptoms of binge eating and vomiting and improve the mood and anxiety components that accompany this disorder.[16] The efficacy of antidepressants has been consistently demonstrated in various randomized, double-blind placebo-controlled BN treatment trials. However, the relapse rates with these agents are very high, with close to one third of patients relapsing.[17] Thus, it is recommended that patients continue antidepressant therapy for at least 9 months to 1 year. Although TCAs and monoamine oxidase inhibitors (MAOIs) have literature supporting their efficacy in the treatment of BN, their current clinical application in the treatment of this disorder has been replaced by the SSRI medications. This is due to the fact that SSRIs have proven efficacy in the treatment of BN, there is FDA indication for the use of an SSRI (fluoxetine) in this disorder, and SSRIs have a markedly better side effect profile. Due to their toxicity and potential lethality in overdose, TCAs can be problematic in BN patients who have comorbid depression and suicidal tendencies. In addition, patients with electrolyte imbalances related to purging behaviors may be more at risk for cardiac side effects on this class of medication. Managing the restricted diet required for the use of MAOIs can be problematic in BN patients who have careless binge eating behaviors, thus placing them at risk for a hypertensive episode.

The SSRI antidepressant fluoxetine is the only medication that has FDA approval for the treatment of BN at a dosage of 60 mg/d. The only other SSRI shown to be effective is sertraline, which was studied in a small randomized controlled trial.[18] The dosages of SSRIs effective in the treatment of BN are typically higher than the doses used in the treatment of depression. For example, in the report of the Fluoxetine Bulimia Nervosa Collaborative Study Group,[19] which was instrumental in leading to FDA approval of fluoxetine for the treatment of this disorder, patients who received fluoxetine at 60 mg/d demonstrated the greatest reduction in binge eating frequency and vomiting episodes. Fluoxetine has also been demonstrated as safe and effective at 60 mg/d in treating BN in the adolescent population.[20] One antidepressant, bupropion, is contraindicated for use in the treatment of BN because it has been associated with an increased risk for seizures in this patient population.[21]

In prescribing antidepressant medications, especially to children and adolescents, clinicians must provide appropriate informed consent to patients and their families, including the black box warning regarding suicidal behaviors associated with antidepressant medications in children. In addition, because SSRI medications are usually titrated to higher doses for the treatment of BN, patients may experience more side effects, and a thorough review of potential side effects should be provided to patients, particularly side effects that may interfere with compliance and management of the disorder. For example, higher doses of SSRIs may cause more constipation, and stool softeners can be used to help manage this side effect. Other common side effects that may occur at high doses include insomnia, nausea, asthenia, and sexual side effects.[19]

Topiramate has been demonstrated to be a useful alternative treatment.[22,23] In a 2-site double-blind placebo-controlled study, subjects with BN who were between the ages of 16 and 50 years were randomly assigned to 10 weeks of treatment with placebo or a titrated dose of topiramate up to a maximum dosage of 400 mg/d. Patients in the topiramate group demonstrated a 44.8% reduction in mean weekly number of binge/purge days versus a 10.7% reduction in the placebo group. In this study, the topiramate-treated patients also had a decrease in mean body weight of 1.8 kg.[23] A more recent study supported the effectiveness of topiramate in reducing binge–purge episodes and also in reducing body weight.[24] Due to its association with weight loss, caution should be used in normal- to lower-weight patients with BN. Other common side effects, such as word-finding difficulties, somnolence, dizziness, and paresthesias, should be monitored, as these have been reported by patients in clinical practice.

The peripherally active 5-hydroxytriptamine 3 (5-HT3) antagonist ondansetron has been demonstrated as a potential treatment for BN in reducing binge–vomit frequency in 2 small studies, 1 open label trial and 1 randomized double-blind trial.[25,26] Based on the high cost of this medication, it is not usually a feasible treatment option.

For patients with BN who have comorbid bipolar disorder or other conditions that may warrant the use of a mood stabilizer, the use of lithium carbonate and valproic acid is problematic. Lithium has not been shown to be effective in the treatment of BN.[27] In addition, maintaining an appropriate therapeutic lithium level may be challenging in a patient with bingeing and purging episodes, which may lead to shifts in fluids and electrolytes. Both lithium and valproic acid lead to weight gain, which limits compliance. Similarly, the weight gain associated with atypical antipsychotics interferes with the acceptability and adherence to this class of medication in patients with BN. Methylphenidate may be helpful for BN patients with attention-deficit hyperactivity disorder.[28] Because this medication is known to cause appetite suppression and potential weight loss, the abuse of this medication to induce weight loss may occur.

OBESITY
Definitions and Diagnoses

Use of BMI for children is complicated by growth and development differences between boys and girls at different ages. To address these issues, the Centers for

Disease Control and Prevention (CDC) use growth charts with age and BMI that are different for boys and girls. Children between age 2 and 19 years with a BMI between the 85th and 95th percentile are described as "at risk of overweight," and those at or above the 95th percentile are described as "overweight" (http://www.cdc.gov). The term obese is not used by the CDC to describe these children.

Several eating disorders associated with overweight begin in adolescence, including binge eating disorder (BED), night eating syndrome (NES), and sleep-related eating disorder (SRED). Early recognition may decrease the future likelihood and severity of overweight problems. **Table 1** lists several of the most important differences between these 3 disorders.

Etiology of Obesity

An important causative factor in the increase in obesity may be that the drive to consume available calories (whether or not this is healthy in the long run) is "hard-wired" in the hypothalamus, which has connections with a wide variety of systems that control hunger, satiety, and mood. Attempts to change these well-developed systems are likely to meet significant physiologic barriers, which may also partially explain why many weight loss drugs have been problematic, including amphetamine (which has a high abuse potential), fenfluramine, and dexfenfluramine (both associated with valvular heart disease), and now complications with depression have been seen with the drug rimonabant (currently approved in the European Union but not by the FDA).

FOOD AND DRUG ADMINISTRATION: CURRENT RECOMMENDED TREATMENTS

The FDA approves weight loss drugs for short- and long-term use. Drugs approved for short-term use (12 weeks) include phentermine, benzphetamine, mazindol, diethylpropion, and phendimetrazine. These drugs have the potential for adverse cardiovascular side effects; and are not approved for use in children and adolescents. By long-term use, the FDA means up to 2 years. The problem with this definition is that overweight in children and adolescents can become a chronic condition, and longer-term use of medications may be needed. No medications are currently approved for children younger than 12 years, and only 2 (sibutramine and orlistat) are approved for long-term use in adolescents.

Table 1
Characteristics distinguishing bulimia nervosa (BN), binge eating disorder (BED), night eating syndrome (NES), and sleep-related eating disorder (SRED)

Clinical Characteristic	BN	BED	NES	SRED
Morning anorexia	No	No	Yes	Yes
Evening hyperphagia	No	No	Yes	No
Eating pattern	Binges	Binges	Snacks	Snacks, unusual items
Compensatory behavior	Yes	No	No	No
Awareness of eating	Yes	Yes	Yes	No
Polysomnography	Normal	Normal	Low sleep efficiency	Sleep disorder
Treatment	CBT	CBT	Sertraline	Treat sleep disorder
	SSRIs	SSRIs	Relaxation therapy	Dopamine agonists

Abbreviation: CBT, cognitive behavior therapy.

Data from Cloak NL, Powers PS: Beating obesity: help patients control binge eating disorder and night eating syndrome. Current Psychiatry 2006;5:26; with permission.

Summary of Effects of Sibutramine and Orlistat

The benefits of currently recommended treatments are modest. For example, a recent meta-analysis[29] of 80 studies of adults completing a minimum 1-year weight management intervention found an average weight loss of 5% to 8% during the first 6 months for interventions involving a reduced-energy diet or weight loss medications (orlistat or sibutramine). Weight losses in the range of 3% to 6% were maintained at 48 months, and none of the groups had weight regain to baseline. There was slightly greater improvement in the studies that included medication, and the groups that were advice-only and exercise-only had minimal weight loss at any time point. Among the 80 studies there was an attrition rate of 29% at the 1-year follow-up, and the overall attrition rate at the end of the study (irrespective of the length of the study) was 31%. High dropout rates are an important problem in obesity studies because patients who drop out from obesity studies may do so because they have been unsuccessful in achieving weight loss. In this thoughtful meta-analysis the investigators studied only patients who completed the intervention, because most of the reported 80 studies did not provide information on participants who left the study early.

For children younger than 12 years, data on the results of pharmacotherapy are scant, and no weight-loss medications are FDA approved. Rather than the use of medications, the usual recommendation is weight maintenance followed by a slow rate of weight loss of approximately 0.45 kg/mo. The method for children is typically behavioral and family-oriented dietary change, often using strategies such as the Stoplight Diet.[30]

For adolescents, behavioral weight-loss programs with or without medications (sibutramine or orlistat) have been best studied. Orlistat, a medication that inhibits lipase and thus decreases absorption of fat, has been approved by the FDA for patients between 12 and 16 years of age. Orlistat is available as a prescription drug, and in 2007 it was approved by the FDA as an over-the-counter non-prescription drug in a lower dosage than the prescription medication. Sibutramine is the only anorectic agent approved for long-term use in obese adolescents 16 years and older.

Sibutramine

Several placebo-controlled randomized studies have evaluated the effectiveness of sibutramine in adolescents and found that sibutramine with behavior therapy is more effective than either behavior therapy or sibutramine alone.[31,32] The side effects are usually a minimal increase in blood pressure, which may be offset by a reduction in BMI.[33] However, some individuals may show a more pronounced increase in blood pressure, which should be monitored at the time of taking sibutramine. The typical dose has been 10 mg/d; when discontinued there has usually been a modest regain of weight (although not to baseline) during the ensuing year. Weight losses over 6 to 12 months of drug treatment have averaged between 6 to 9 kg (13–20 lb) compared with 2 to 3 kg (4.4–6.6 lb) in the behavior groups. In the studies of adolescents, premature discontinuation of treatment (where reported) has typically been high for both the behavior group and medication group. For example, in one of the best-designed studies by Berkowitz and colleagues (2006), 24% dropped out of the medication plus behavior therapy group and (38%) prematurely discontinued treatment in the behavior therapy only group.

The response to sibutramine has been compared between obese African American and white adolescents and found to be significantly greater in the white group than in the African American group.[34] A small study among obese Mexican adolescents found that sibutramine results in a mean loss of 7 kg (15 lb).[35] Sibutramine is only FDA approved for adolescents 16 years or older, although studies similar to those that resulted in approval by the FDA for this age have been completed for adolescents between ages 12 and 16 years.

Orlistat

Orlistat is an FDA-approved drug for long-term use in adolescents between 12 and 16 years of age; orlistat is a reversible inhibitor of gastric and pancreatic lipase and results in decreased dietary fat absorption. Approval for adolescents was based on 6 clinical trials (see Dunican and colleagues, 2007[36] for a review), 5 of which showed statistically significant reductions in mean BMI ranging from 0.55 to 4.09 kg/m^2; 1 small study did not show benefit in weight loss. The studies varied greatly in terms of design, length of follow-up, and reported data. For example, 2 studies in the review showed a small increase in weight among patients on placebo compared with those on orlistat, but differences in age group studied (some of whom were probably in their adolescent growth spurt) and reported data (weight change versus BMI) complicate interpretation. As with sibutramine, the beneficial effect on weight loss is less among adult African Americans than among white adults.[37] In adults, orlistat has been shown to improve cardiovascular risk factors, including reduction in cholesterol and improvements in waist circumference and insulin sensitivity.[38] The most common adverse events are gastrointestinal, including frequent fatty oily stools, inability to control stools, and oily leakage from the rectum. A second concern has been the possibility that orlistat may decrease absorption of fat soluble vitamins A, D, E, and K or affect the pharmacokinetics of highly lipophilic drugs. These risks have not been fully elucidated, and the usual recommendation is that patients take a multiple vitamin pill and that the possibility of interference with lipophilic drugs (such as warfarin and thyroxine) be considered when these lipophilic medications are prescribed. The usual prescription dose of orlistat in adolescents is 120 mg 3 times daily with meals.

In 2007, the FDA approved orlistat (in a lower dose, 60 mg. 3 times daily with meals and 1 daily multiple vitamin pill) as an over-the-counter drug for weight loss in adults 18 years and older. There has been significant concern over the possibility of abuse of this drug, because many patients with eating disorders use over-the-counter diet products to control weight and suppress appetite.[39] There have also been case reports of misuse of orlistat among eating disorder patients even when it was only available by prescription.[40]

DRUGS NOT APPROVED BY THE FOOD AND DRUG ADMINISTRATION FOR OBESITY TREATMENT

Rimonabant was approved for use in the European Union in 2006 but has not been approved by the FDA. It is an endocannabinoid antagonist and acts in the central nervous system by increasing satiety and altering patterns of eating. The drug results in about a 5 kg (11 lbs) greater weight loss than placebo.[41] It also has peripheral effects in the liver, adipose tissue, and skeletal muscles and is associated with improvements in triglycerides, HDL cholesterol, and hemoglobin A1c in diabetics. The major adverse effects are on mood, and among patients with depression, rimonabant is contraindicated. This side effect contributed to the unanimous decision by the FDA not to approve the drug.

The early onset of obesity is 1 of several factors contributing to the increased likelihood of impaired glucose tolerance and subsequent development of type 2 diabetes mellitus in adolescents. Metformin is an oral antidiabetic agent that decreases hepatic glucose production and is approved by the FDA for type 2 diabetes mellitus in patients 10 years and older. It has been shown to be beneficial in young patients with type 1 or 2 diabetes mellitus and in girls at risk for the polycystic ovarian syndrome, and it may moderate the weight gain effect of certain antipsychotic medications. It has been proposed that metformin might prevent the development of type 2 diabetes mellitus in at-risk obese children and adolescents.[42] Two studies[43,44] comparing metformin to placebo in at-risk adolescents have shown significant weight losses with metformin and improved fasting glucose levels, but the effect on insulin sensitivity was equivocal. Although metformin is not currently approved for the treatment of obesity in adolescents, it may eventually prove to be useful to those adolescents at risk for type 2 diabetes mellitus. Side effects include the rare development of lactic acidosis and poor renal clearance in patients with impaired kidney function.

INVESTIGATIONAL TARGETS FOR TREATMENT OF OBESITY

The recognition that we are on the verge of an obesity epidemic and associated illnesses has led to a search for more effective medication treatments. New developments in understanding the various factors that influence hunger and satiety have led to new investigational drugs. The targets of these drugs have been described by Bays[45] as generally falling into 4 categories: (1) central nervous system agents that affect neurotransmitters (eg, bupropion); (2) leptin/insulin/central nervous system pathway agents; (3) gastrointestinal neural pathway agents (eg, agents that decrease ghrelin activity); (4) agents that increase metabolic rate (eg, thyroid receptor agonists); and (5) a variety of other more diverse agents. It has been recognized that the various receptors that respond to hunger and satiety signals are also related to cognitive, emotional, sensory, and motor functions. The interactions between these various functions are being conceptualized as "molecular networks"[46] and may help explain why the history of antiobesity drugs is associated with serious adverse physiologic and psychologic consequences. That is to say, the receptors that modulate hunger and satiety are embedded within and embed the receptors that control emotions and cognition.

MEDICATIONS AND WEIGHT CHANGE

Many medications can affect weight and most cause weight gain. Most of the medications that cause weight gain are used for psychiatric or neurologic conditions. Weight change does not seem to be a simple class effect. For example, some antiepileptic drugs used as mood stabilizers cause weight gain (eg, valproate) but others are either weight neutral (eg, tegretol) or cause weight loss (eg, lamotrigine). **Table 2** lists commonly prescribed medications that can result in weight change.

Because many patients with eating disorders have other comorbid psychiatric disorders, the possibility of weight change needs to be carefully considered when prescribing medications for these comorbid conditions or for the eating disorder. There have been case reports of patients developing AN after a medication that can cause weight loss was prescribed, or BN may develop when a medication that can cause weight gain is prescribed. It is recommended that the following steps be undertaken when a medication is prescribed for a patient with an eating disorder. First, consider the potential for weight change in the risk/benefit assessment before prescription. Second, when possible, consider weight-neutral drugs in patients at normal weight. Third, a discussion with the patient is advisable before use of a medication that can cause weight change. Fourth, monitor weight and eating disorder symptoms closely after weight-altering medications are initiated or doses are changed. Fifth, carefully consider if adherence to the medication regimen has been affected by the possibility of weight gain.

Table 2
Weight effects of some commonly used prescription medications

	Weight Gain	Weight Loss	Weight Neutral
Antidepressants	Mirtazapine	Bupropion	Most SSRIs
	Paroxetine		Nefazodone
	Tricyclic antidepressants		Tranylcypromine
	Phenelzine		Venlafaxine
	Isocarboxazid		
Mood stabilizers	Valproate		Lamotrigine
	Lithium		
	Carbamazepine		
Anticonvulsants	Valproate	Topiramate	Tiagabine
	Carbamazepine	Zonisamide	Lamotrigine
	Pregabalin	Felbamate	
	Vigabatrin		
	Gabapentin		
Antipsychotics	Most typical agents	Molindone	Ziprasidone
	Clozapine		Aripiprazole
	Olanzapine		
	Risperidone		
	Quetiapine		
Other psychotropics	Cyproheptadine	Amphetamine	Buspirone
		Modafinil	Benzodiazepines
		Methylphenidate	

Data from Powers PS, Cloak NL. Medication-related weight changes: Impact on treatment of eating disorder patients. In: Yager J, Powers PS. Editors. Clinical Manual of Eating Disorders. Washington, D.C.: American Psychiatric Publishing, Inc.: 2007. p. 270; with permission.

SUMMARY

Although only fluoxetine has been approved by the FDA for adults with BN, many medications are used both for symptoms of eating disorders and for common comorbid conditions. No medication has been approved for adolescents with either AN or BN. One medication (orlistat) has been approved for long-term use for overweight adolescents or those at risk for overweight (see earlier comment as to the precise indication for these drugs) 12 years and older; use of sibutramine has been approved for those 16 years and older. However, there are very few randomized clinical trials on the effects of obesity drugs on children and adolescents and little is known of their use outside of clinical trials. Careful consideration should be given to prescription of off-label medications for adolescents with eating disorders who may be at particular risk for side effects because of the physiologic complications of semi-starvation and metabolic abnormalities from purge behavior.

REFERENCES

1. Kaplan AS, Noble S. Management of anorexia nervosa in an ambulatory setting. In: Yager J, Powers PS, editors. Clinical manual of eating disorders. Washington, DC: American Psychiatric Publishing, Inc.; 2007. p. 127–47.

2. Delgado PL, Miller HL, Salomon RM, et al. Tryptophan-depletion challenge in depressed patients treated with desipramine or fluoxetine: implications for the role of serotonin in the mechanism of antidepressant action. Biol Psychiatry 1999; 46(2):212–20.

3. Kaye W, Nagata T, Weltzin TE, et al. Double-blind placebo-controlled administration of fluoxetine in restricting type anorexia nervosa. Biol Psychiatry 2001;49(7):644–52.

4. Walsh BT, Kaplan AS, Attia E, et al. Fluoxetine after weight restoration in anorexia nervosa: a randomized, placebo-controlled trial. JAMA 2006;295(22):2605–12.

5. Hansen L. Olanzapine in the treatment of anorexia nervosa. [letter]. Br J Psychiatry 1999;175(87):592.

6. La Via MC, Gray N, Kaye WH. Case reports of olanzapine treatment of anorexia nervosa. Int J Eat Disord 2000;27(3):363–6.

7. Powers PS, Santana CA, Bannon YS. Olanzapine in the treatment of anorexia nervosa: an open label trial. Int J Eat Disord 2002;32(2):146–54.

8. Barbarich NC, McConaha CW, Gaskill J, et al. An open trial of olanzapine in anorexia nervosa. J Clin Psychiatry 2004;65(11):1480–2.

9. Brambilla F, Garcia C, Fassino S, et al. Olanzapine therapy in anorexia nervosa psychobiological effects. Int J Eat Disord 2007;22(4):197–204.

10. Bissada H, Tasca GA, Barber AM, et al. Olanzapine in the treatment of low body weight and obsessive thinking in women with anorexia nervosa: A randomized, double-blind, placebo-controlled trial. Am J Psychiatry 2008;165:1281–8.

11. Stacher G, Peeters TL, Bergmann H, et al. Erythromycin effects on gastric emptying, antral motility and plasma motilin and pancreatic polypeptide concentrations in anorexia nervosa. Gut 1993;34(2):166–72.

12. Klibanski A, Biller BM, Schoenfeld DA, et al. The effects of estrogen administration on trabecular bone loss in young women with anorexia nervosa. J Clin Endocrinol 1995;80:898–904.

13. Golden NH. Osteopenia and osteoporosis in anorexia nervosa. Adolesc Med 2003;14(1):97–108.

14. Munoz MT, Morande G, Garcia Centenera JA, et al. The effects of estrogen administration on bone mineral density in adolescents with anorexia nervosa. Eur J Endocrinol 2002;146(1):45–50.

15. Mitchell JE, Steffen KJ, Roerig JL. Management of bulimia nervosa. In: Yager J, Powers PS, editors. Clinical manual of eating disorders. American Psychiatric Publishing, Inc.; 2007. p. 171–93.

16. Mitchell JE, Peterson CB, Myers T, et al. Combining pharmacotherapy and psychotherapy in the treatment of patients with eating disorders. Psychiatr Clin North Am 2001;24(2):315–23.

17. Agras W, Rossiter E, Arnow B, et al. Pharmacologic and cognitive-behavioral treatment for bulimia nervosa: a controlled comparison. Am J Psychiatry 1992; 149(1):82–7.

18. Milano W, Petrella C, Sabatino C, et al. Treatment of bulimia nervosa with sertraline: a randomized controlled trial. Adv Ther 2004;21(4):232–7.

19. Fluoxetine in the treatment of bulimia nervosa: a multi-center, placebo-controlled double-blind trial. Fluoxetine Bulimia Nervosa Collaborative Study Group. Arch Gen Psychiatry 1992;49(2):139–47.

20. Kotler LA, Devlin MJ, Davies M, et al. An open trial of fluoxetine for adolescents with bulimia nervosa. J Child Adolesc Psychopharmacol 2003;13(3):329–35.

21. Horne RL, Ferguson JM, Pope HG Jr, et al. Treatment of bulimia with bupropion: a multicenter controlled trial. J Clin Psychiatry 1988;49(7):262–6.

22. Hedges DW, Reimherr FW, Hoopes SP, et al. Treatment of bulimia nervosa with topiramate in a randomized, double-blind, placebo-controlled trial, part 2: improvement in psychiatric measures. J Clin Psychiatry 2003;64(12):1449–54.

23. Hoopes SP, Reimherr FW, Hedges DW, et al. Treatment of bulimia nervosa with topiramate in a randomized, double-blind, placebo-controlled trial, part 1: improvement in binge purge measures. J Clin Psychiatry 2003;64(11):1335–41.

24. Nickel C, Tritt K, Muehlbacher M, et al. Topiramate treatment in bulimia nervosa patients: a randomized, double-blind, placebo-controlled trial. Int J Eat Disord 2005;38(4):295–300.

25. Hartman BK, Faris PL, Kim SW, et al. Treatment of bulimia nervosa with ondansetron. Arch Gen psychiatry 1997;54(10):969–70.

26. Faris PL, Kim SW, Meller WH, et al. Effect of decreasing afferent vagal activity with ondansetron on symptoms of bulimia nervosa: a randomized, double-blind trial. Lancet 2000;355(9206):792–7.

27. Hsu LK, Clement L, Santhouse R, et al. Treatment of bulimia nervosa with lithium carbonate: a controlled study. J Nerv Ment Dis 1991;179(6):351–5.

28. Schweickert LA, Strober M, Moskowitz A. Efficacy of methylphenidate in bulimia nervosa comorbid with attention-deficit hyperactivity disorder: a case report. Int J Eat Disord 1997;21(3):299–301.

29. Franz M, VanWormer J, Crain A, et al. Weight-loss outcomes: a systematic review and meta-anaysis of weight-loss clinical trials with a minimum 1-year follow-up. J Am Diet Assoc 2007;107(10):1755–67.

30. Epstein L, Squires S. The Stoplight Diet for children. New York: Little Brown & Co.; 1988.

31. Berkowitz R, Wadden T, Tsershakovec A, et al. Behavior therapy and sibutramine for the treatment of adolescent obesity. JAMA 2003;289(14):1805–12.

32. Berkowitz R, Fujioka K, Daniels S, et al. Effects of sibutramine treatment in obese adolescents. Ann Intern Med 2006;145(2):81–91.

33. Daniels S, Long B, Crow S, et al. Cardiovascular effects of sibutramine in the treatment of adolescents: results of a randomized, double-blind, placebo-controlled study. Pediatrics 2007;120(1):e147–57.

34. Budd G, Hayman L, Crump E, et al. Weight loss in obese African American and Caucasian adolescents. J Cardiovasc Nurs 2007;22(4):288–96.

35. Garcia-Morales L, Berber A, Macias-Lara C, et al. Use of sibutramine in obese Mexican adolescents: a 6-month, randomized, double-blind, placebo-controlled parallel-group trial. Clin Ther 2006;28(5):770–82.

36. Dunican K, Desilets A, Montalbano J. Pharmacotherapeutic options for overweight adolescents. Ann Pharmacother 2007;41(9):1445–55.

37. McDuffie J, Calis K, Uwaifo G, et al. Efficacy of orlistat as an adjunct to behavioral treatment in overweight African American and Caucasian adolescents with obesity-related co-morbid conditions. J Pediatr Endocrinol Metab 2004;17(3): 307–19.

38. Krempf M, Louvet J, Allanic H, et al. Weight reduction and long-term maintenance after 18 months treatment with orlistat for obesity. Int J Obes Relat Metab Disord 2003;27(5):591–7.

39. Cumella E, Hahn J, Woods B. Weighing Allis's impact. Eating disorder patients might be tempted to abuse the first FDA-approved nonprescription diet pill. Behav Healthc 2007;27(6):32–4.

40. Fernandez-Aranda F, Amor A, Jiminez-Murcia S, et al. Bulimia nervosa and misuse of orlistat: two case reports. Int J Eat Disord 2001;30(4):458–61.

41. Curioni C, André C. Rimonabant for overweight or obesity. Cochrane Database Syst Rev 2006;4:CD006. 10.1002/14651858.CD006162.pub2.
42. Freemark M. Pharmacologic approaches to the prevention of type 2 diabetes in high risk pediatric patients. J Clin Endocrinol Metab 2003;88(1):3–13.
43. Srinivasan S, Ambler G, Baur L, et al. Randomized, controlled trial of metformin for obesity and insulin resistance in children and adolescents: Improvement in body composition and fasting insulin. J Clin Endocrinol Meta 2006;91(6): 2074–80.
44. Freemark M, Bursey D. The effects of metformin on body mass index and glucose tolerance in obese adolescents with fasting hyperinsulinemia and a family history of type 2 diabetes. Pediatrics 2001;107(4):e55.
45. Bays H. Current and investigational antiobesity agents and obesity therapeutic treatment targets. Obes Res 2004;12(6):1197–211.
46. Myslobodsky M. Molecular network of obesity: what does it promise for pharmacotherapy. Obes Rev 2008;9:236–45.

Evidence-Based Behavioral Treatment of Obesity in Children and Adolescents

Laura Stewart, PhD, RD[a],*, John J. Reilly, PhD[b], Adrienne R. Hughes, PhD[c]

KEYWORDS

• Obesity • Overweight • Children • Adolescents • Treatment

Obesity is the most common childhood disease and is widely acknowledged as having become a global epidemic.[1,2] There are well-recognized health consequences of childhood obesity, both during childhood and adulthood, affecting health and psychological and economic welfare.[3,4] The importance of finding effective strategies for the management of childhood obesity has international significance with the publication of various expert reports and evidence-based guidelines in recent years.[3,5–7] However, these guidelines and reports have all concluded that there is a lack of high-quality published research on effective childhood obesity treatment strategies.[8,9] Although systematic reviews and guidelines indicate that there is a lack of high-quality published research on effective management of pediatric obesity, the literature provides some guidance on how to treat pediatric obesity. This review aims to provide a summary of successful approaches to help manage childhood and adolescent obesity, identified by systematic reviews and evidence-based clinical guidelines.

All of the evidence-based clinical guidelines[3,5–7,10,11] have concluded that treatment programs should be multicomponent, targeting changes in diet, physical activity, and sedentary behavior (in particular television [TV] viewing and other forms of screen-based media use). The use of behavioral change strategies is recommended consistently in evidence-based guidance on treatment, and these should be family-based, age-appropriate, and tailored to individual needs.[3,6,7,10,11] **Table 1** summarizes the major principles of childhood weight management and outlines the main sources of evidence-based guidance on treatment. However, while the evidence-based guidelines have recommended behavioral approaches to treatment, they generally do not

[a] The Children's Weight Clinic PO Box 28533, Edinburgh EH4 2WW, Scotland, UK
[b] Division of Developmental Medicine, University of Glasgow, 1st Floor Tower Block QMH, Yorkhill Hospitals, Glasgow G3 8SJ, Scotland, UK
[c] Department of Sports Studies, University of Stirling, FK9 4LA, Scotland, UK
* Corresponding author.
E-mail address: laura@childrensweightclinic.com (L. Stewart).

Child Adolesc Psychiatric Clin N Am 18 (2008) 189–198
doi:10.1016/j.chc.2008.07.014
childpsych.theclinics.com
1056-4993/08/$ – see front matter © 2008 Elsevier Inc. All rights reserved.

Table 1
Principles of treatment of obesity in children and adolescents derived from evidence-based treatment guidelines

Principles of Treatment	Internet-Based Sources of Evidence
Treatment should be commenced only when the parents are ready and willing to make lifestyle changes.	Evidence-based review & management guidance (Scotland); SIGN 69 www.sign.ac.uk
Treatment should be family based, with at least 1 of the parents involved.	English guidelines NICE 43 (2006) www.nice.org.uk/guidance/CG43/guidance
Lifestyle changes in diet, physical activity, and sedentary behaviors should be targeted.	USA Expert committee report on management (Barlow 2007) www.pediatrics.org/cgi/content/full/120/supplement_4/S164
Behavioral change techniques should be an integral part of any treatment program	Evidence-based review & management guidance (Australia); www.obesityguidelines.gov.au
Weight maintenance is an acceptable goal of treatment for most patients, with height increasing and the BMI decreasing over time	Review of systematic reviews (Canada); www.caphc.org/partnerships/obesity.html
For children older than 7 y, weight loss of not >0.5 kg/mo may be advised.[3,6,7,10]	Cochrane reviews of prevention and treatment (Summerbell et al); www.nelh.nhs.uk

describe how to implement/deliver these strategies with obese children and their families. The remainder of the present review, therefore, expands on the issue of how to incorporate behavioral approaches into treatment interventions, which is lacking from current guidelines.

ROLE OF HEALTH PROFESSIONALS IN TREATMENT

Most parents, and many health professionals, are unaware of the impact of obesity in childhood and adolescence and many parents may be unaware that their own son or daughter is obese.[12] Evidence-based guidance[3,5–7] indicates that a fundamental role of the health professional is to educate the child and family on the consequences of obesity and the lifestyle changes necessary to treat obesity, to help motivate families to make and sustain lifestyle changes, and to facilitate positive behavioral changes. Several health professionals may undertake management of childhood obesity either as individuals or in a multidisciplinary team, for example, physicians, dietitians, clinical psychologists, and health coaches. All health professionals involved must have knowledge of diet, physical activity, and sedentary behavior components of a healthy lifestyle, be skilled in the use of behavior change techniques, and understand the importance of interacting with the child and family in a positive, empathetic, and non-judgmental manner.[13] The qualities and skills required by health professionals for behavioral treatment of childhood and adolescent obesity are outlined in **Table 2**.

Successful treatment of obesity demands a sustained commitment and effort from the whole family, and the health professional must endeavor to maintain a positive attitude and help motivate the child and family toward weight control. For parents, the support and attitude of the health professional have been shown to be of vital importance to them continuing with the program and also in their perception of the outcome of the treatment.[13,14] Because obesity is a chronic condition, a parent's

Table 2	
Qualities and skills required for optimal treatment by health professionals[15]	
Qualities of Health Professional	**Skills Required of the Health Professional**
• Acceptance • Genuineness • Empathy	• Appropriate use of questions (open questions) • Active listening (mirroring, paraphrasing, and reflecting) • Affirmation • Summarizing

perceptions of the last health professional to treat their child could be important to whether they are likely to engage in further treatment episodes.

Health professionals may be office-based, working with individual children and their families.[15] Others may hold group sessions, where it is not uncommon for separate sessions for children and parents.[16,17] Most studies using group-based interventions have also included physical activity sessions as an integral part of the treatment program.[16,18] Although good evidence exists on the behaviors to target (ie, diet, physical activity, and sedentary behavior) and how to modify these behaviors (ie, employ behavioral techniques and involve families), there is a lack of evidence on the most effective setting (eg, community, primary care, secondary care) and delivery mode (eg, group, individual, or both) to implement these components.[6,8] However, it seems appropriate to suggest that an integrated pathway of care should incorporate both group work and individual office-based programs to allow choice of the most suitable program for a child and family.

The optimal intensity and length of successful weight management programs, including length of each session, number of sessions, and over what period of time, remain unclear. However, systematic reviews have concluded that greatest impacts on weight status have been achieved by programs that have frequent sessions (weekly or biweekly) and that have included long-term monitoring of participants' progress for up to 12 months.[16,19] It is widely believed that greater "intensity" of treatment leads to greater effects on weight status. For example, the recent Bright Bodies intervention reported by Savoye and colleagues[16] involved twice weekly sessions of exercise and nutrition/behavior modification for 6 months and then biweekly sessions for 6 months, with a scheduled patient contact time of approximately 110 hours. At 12 months, those undertaking the Bright Bodies intervention had a mean increase in weight of 0.3 kg. In the recent low- to moderate-intensity Scottish Childhood Overweight Treatment Trial (SCOTT; scheduled patient contact time 5–6 hours), individual families visited an office-based dietitian for nutrition and behavior modification of 8 sessions over 6 months. At the end of the 6-month treatment, those undertaking the intervention treatment had a median weight increase of 3.2 kg.[20] Even intense interventions achieve relatively modest changes in weight status; therefore, although successful management of obese children is achievable, success represents fairly modest changes in weight status for most patients.

ROLE OF THE PARENTS IN TREATMENT

Evidence-based guidance has repeatedly emphasized the importance of involving the whole family in making the necessary lifestyle changes.[3,5–7,10] The role of the parents is pivotal and consideration of their parenting styles is necessary for successfully engaging in childhood obesity management, and health professionals should have an understanding of these issues.[10,21,22] There are 4 recognized parenting styles, and these are briefly outlined in **Table 3**.

The authoritative parenting style has been shown to have a positive effect on healthy weight status, with the parents giving the children boundaries while supporting them to make healthy choices within these boundaries.[21] Indeed, some studies have successfully targeted childhood weight management exclusively through parent groups, where, alongside education on healthy family lifestyle changes, positive parenting skills and attitudes were taught.[19,23] There are several simple pieces of advice that can be given to parents and other adults in the family that can ensure positive support for the child in lifestyle changes. The following list has been adapted from the evidence-based treatment guidelines published by the Scottish Intercollegiate Guidelines Network (SIGN) in 2003, guideline number 69 (www.sign.ac.uk).[3]

- be a role model to your child and family;
- follow the same healthy eating plan; buy more healthy foods and less high-sugar/high-fat snacks;
- offer a treat to reward behavioral changes/ achievement of lifestyle goals (trip to the cinema or the park; book/toy/comic; friend to stay overnight);
- have regular family meal times;
- teach children to eat only when they are hungry and not to fill up on snacks all day;
- discourage eating when doing other activities, such as watching TV or doing schoolwork.

USE OF BEHAVIORAL MODIFICATION TECHNIQUES

The use of behavioral change techniques, such as decisional balance charts, goal setting, self-monitoring, problem-solving barriers, and rewards, have been shown to be successful in managing lifestyle changes in children and have been recommended in recent evidence-based guidelines.[6,7] Behavioral change techniques are now considered to be central to behavioral treatment of obesity.[24–26] Most of these techniques are employed within lifestyle change programs to assist the child and family in raising their awareness and focus on aspects of their lifestyles that require change, to motivate the child and family to make lifestyle changes, and then to monitor those changes. To help readers consider the appropriate use of these techniques, those most commonly employed are described in brief in the following section.

Decisional Balance (Exploring Readiness to Change)

Decisional balance involves comparing the perceived pros (benefits) and cons (costs) of making lifestyle changes. This process involves asking the child and the parents to consider the personal benefits of making lifestyle changes and "slimming down"

Table 3 Parenting styles[21]	
Authoritative (respect for child's opinion, but maintains clear boundaries)	**Permissive** (indulgent, without discipline)
Authoritarian (strict disciplinarian)	**Neglectful** (emotionally uninvolved and does not set rules).

Data from Rhee KE, Lumeng JC, Appugliese DP, et al. Parenting styles and overweight status in first grade. Pediatr 2006;117(6):2047–54.

(eg, be able to wear fashionable clothes, not be bullied at school, or be able to run faster) and the perceived cons (costs) of changing behavior (eg, do not like playing outside when it is raining, or do not want to give up sweets or watching TV).[15] The aim of the decisional balance is to help the family realize that the pros outweigh the cons, which in turn helps motivate them to change behavior.[27]

Problem-Solving Barriers

Encouraging families to identify barriers preventing behavior change and exploring ways to overcome these barriers is a useful strategy to promote behavior change and increase motivation to change lifestyle.[24,25]

Self-Monitoring of Lifestyle

The recording of lifestyle by the child or family (for example the amount of TV viewing) is regarded by evidence-based guidelines[6,7] as being a key component of behavioral change, which enhances motivation to change lifestyle by increasing self-awareness.[24,28,29] Monitoring the child's diet, activity, and sedentary behavior in a diary raises awareness of his or her current lifestyle; this can be used to identify changes that could be made to the child's current lifestyle and allows the family to monitor progress toward their goals.

Goal Setting by the Client

Goal setting is frequently used in lifestyle programs to increase and maintain the child and family's motivation for behavior change. Goal setting involves allowing the child to take responsibility for identifying the lifestyle changes he or she feels able to make and setting goals for these behavior changes.[24,27] However evidence-based guidance suggests that it is important for the health professional and the parents to assist with goal setting by ensuring that the goals are SMART—small, measurable, achievable, recorded, and timed.[15,30]

Evidence-based guidelines and expert committee statements[3,5–7] have repeatedly recommended that families should be encouraged to make small, progressive changes to behavior that are realistic and achievable to enhance confidence and ensure success (eg, gradually reduce TV viewing from 4 hours/day to 3 hours/day, finally to 2 hrs/d). The goals agreed on should be written down and a copy given to the child and parents to take away. The child and parents should be taught the principles of goal setting so that they can continue with goal setting in the long-term once the program is finished.

Contracting

The signing of a "contract" between the child, parents, and health professional may help to reinforce the commitment to meeting the lifestyle change goals that the child and parents have set in the allotted time period.[24,25,29]

Rewards for Reaching Goals

Allowing the child to choose a reward for achieving the agreed lifestyle change goals has been found to be helpful as a positive reinforcement to both the setting and attainment of goals.[24,25,29] Rewards should be inexpensive and not food related, such as a book, a magazine, or a family excursion.

Environmental/Stimulus Control

Environmental/stimulus control involves controlling stimuli or cues that encourage or sustain the unhealthy behavior and providing cues that support/promote the new necessary lifestyle changes. For example, the parent avoids buying and bringing into the home high-sugar/high-fat snacks, or the child avoids walking home from school past a local sweet shop.[25]

Preventing Relapse

Relapse prevention involves helping the child and family to identify possible high-risk situations in which sticking to goals could be difficult, for example, holidays, parties, and wet weather, and then helping them to develop strategies to cope with these high-risk situations (eg, participating in an indoor activity during wet weather). This may be performed as a paper exercise or as simulation and role play.[24,25] Relapse prevention is particularly important at the end of the program to ensure that the child and family maintain behavior/lifestyle changes in the long-term. Planning ahead for difficult situations and continuing with or returning to goal setting and self-monitoring would be useful.[25]

DIETARY CHANGE

As previously noted, all evidence-based guidelines and expert committee statements on treatment suggest that dietary change is an essential element of treatment. Positive, healthy changes in dietary habits that incorporate a nutritionally balanced diet in conjunction with a decrease in energy intake have been recommended consistently.[6,7,10,11] Manipulation of certain macronutrients, such as dietary fat and carbohydrates, have been suggested by some authors but systematic reviews have concluded that there is little or no high-quality evidence at present to recommend these approaches for childhood weight management.[6,7,10] When reviewing the child's dietary intake, the health professional needs to, in particular, consider intakes of sugary drinks, high-fat foods, snacks, meals eaten outside the house, and portion sizes.[7] Necessary dietary changes should include decreasing high-energy snacks while replacing these with, for example, fruit or vegetables, having regular meal times and more family meal times. Discussing portion sizes of snacks and meals can be important, as many children and their parents have little understanding of the concept of age-appropriate portion sizes. The use of particular dietary education techniques, such as a "traffic light" system, may be helpful in facilitating dietary change.[15,20,29]

It is important to ensure that normal growth occurs when dietary intake is restricted. Therefore, any dietary advice should ensure an adequate intake of protein, vitamins, and minerals, although with modest dietary changes that aim for weight maintenance, nutrient deficiency is unlikely.

CHANGE IN PHYSICAL ACTIVITY AND SEDENTARY BEHAVIOR

Changes in physical activity levels and sedentary behavior are recommended consistently as essential components of treatment in all of the current evidence-based guidelines and systematic reviews of treatment.[3,6,7,10,11] There is a widespread agreement in evidence-based guidance on a target to increase physical activity of at least moderate intensity to at least 1 hr/d, and emphasis in the guidelines listed in **Table 1** has been on increasing lifestyle activities rather than structured or prescribed aerobic or resistance exercise. Research has shown that placing the treatment emphasis on increasing lifestyle activities, such as walking, can be particularly effective in controlling weight on a long-term basis.[29]

There is also widespread agreement around the recommendation to decrease sedentary behavior (screen time) to no more than 2 hrs/d or 14 hrs/wk.[6,7,10] Screen time behavior might be more measurable and more modifiable than changes in physical activity in obese children and may be helpful in treatment by encouraging increases in physical activity and/or decreases in energy intake.

There is still some debate around the actual amount, intensity, or type of physical activity that should be undertaken by children and adolescents for weight management.[10] Evidence from recent studies that have used objective methods to measure physical activity levels and levels of sedentary behaviors suggests that obese children spend much less time than recommended in moderate- to vigorous-intensity physical activity and much more time than is recommended in a sedentary state.[20,31]

CLINICAL OUTCOMES OF TREATMENT
Dropout/Noncompliance with Treatment

The health professional should be aware that a high dropout rate and high nonattendance rate are to be expected, with loss of up to 50% of patients referred to pediatric weight management clinics.[32,33] Continued engagement with treatment seems to have a positive effect on weight outcomes;[34] although evidence is limited, it appears that nonattendance at treatment or remaining on a waiting list for treatment appears to be associated with continuing increase in the degree of obesity as indicated by increases in body mass index (BMI) Z score.[18]

Weight Status as an Outcome

Most evidence-based treatment guidelines recommend that weight maintenance with a continued growth in height is an appropriate clinical outcome.[3,6,35] The extent to which patients typically achieve weight maintenance is unclear, but most recent obesity treatment randomized controlled trials suggest that most patients do not achieve weight maintenance over the medium- to long term (6–12 months). In the reporting of research, BMI centiles or Z scores are often used to quantify weight-based outcomes.[36,37]

At present the magnitude of the change in either weight or BMI required to produce clinically meaningful changes for obese children is unclear due to lack of evidence. Reinehr and Andler (2004) have suggested that a decrease in BMI Z score greater than 0.5 is required to modify cardiovascular risk factors.[38] In older children and adolescents with extreme obesity, particularly with more severe comorbidities, a steady weight loss may be an appropriate goal of therapy.[7] Assessing the extent to which treatment programs have affected weight status is difficult because of differences in study designs, patients groups, and methods of quantifying weight and BMI change,[8,9] but it is likely that most of the fairly low- to moderate-intensity behavioral treatment programs in Europe [18,20,39] typically achieve changes in BMI Z score of less than 0.3 over 6 to 12 months. Such modest effects on weight status suggest that treatment should continue for prolonged periods, perhaps years. More intensive, but therefore less generalizable, treatments may achieve greater effect on weight-based outcomes.[16]

Psychosocial Outcomes

Recent qualitative studies have begun to suggest that changes in weight outcomes are not as important to parents as a positive change in their child's quality of life, self-esteem, and self-worth.[13,14] These changes should be given serious consideration by health professionals. Recent evidence also suggests that, despite modest impact on weight status, even low- to moderate-intensity treatment programs are associated with positive changes in measures of psychosocial health and well-being, such as quality of life.[17,31,40]

RADICAL AND NOVEL THERAPIES

Obese adults, usually those with morbid obesity, are often offered what are described as radical treatments. The term "radical treatments" encompasses use of drug therapy, liquid meal replacements, and surgery. Some of these treatments have now been recommended for adolescents with extreme obesity, though evidence-based guidelines have consistently avoided recommending such treatments for patients with less severe obesity.[6] Drugs such as Orlistat taken in combination with diet, lifestyle intervention, and behavioral modifications have been shown to have a modest additive effect in teenagers.[6,41]

Other relatively new modes of treatment for children and adolescents, such as residential treatment[42] and surgery,[6] have also shown some promise. However, systematic reviews and evidence-based management guidelines have concluded consistently that the evidence on these treatments is limited in both quality and quantity at present and they may be more appropriate for adolescent patients with more extreme obesity and with serious comorbid conditions.

SUMMARY

The evidence base suggests that treatment of child and adolescent obesity should be directed at motivated families who perceive obesity as a problem and have indicated a willingness to make lifestyle changes. The evidence suggests that management should involve the whole family and focus on changes in sedentary behavior, physical activity, and diet.

Management should only be undertaken by health professionals who have had the necessary training and are motivated. They should be skilled in the appropriate use of behavioral change techniques, notably assessing readiness to change, self-monitoring, goal setting, rewards, contracting, stimulus control, problem solving, and preventing relapse.

The intensity and length of the ideal treatment program are still unclear. However, even low-intensity treatments are likely to have modest benefits for weight status (compared with no treatment) and marked benefits for other outcomes, such as quality of life.

REFERENCES

1. World Health Organization. Obesity: preventing and managing the global epidemic. World Health Organ Tech Rep Ser 2000;894:16.
2. Lobstein T, Baur L, Uauy R, for the IASO International Obesity Task Force. Obesity in children and young people: a crisis in public health. Obes Rev 2004;5(Suppl 1): 4–85.
3. Scottish Intercollegiate Guideline Network (SIGN). Management of Obesity in children and young people. SIGN 69. Edinburgh (UK): SIGN; 2003.
4. Reilly JJ, Methven E, McDowell ZC, et al. Health consequences of obesity. Arch Dis Child 2003;88:748–52.
5. Gibson P, Edmonds L, Haslam DW, et al. An approach to weight management in children and adolescents (2–18 years) in primary care (RCPCH). J Fam Health Care 2002;12(4):108–9.
6. National Institute for Health and Clinical Excellence. Obesity guidance on the prevention, identification, assessment and management of overweight and obesity in adults and children. NICE clinical guidelines 2006;43.

7. Barlow SE, The Expert Committee. Expert committee recommendations regarding the prevention, assessment and treatment of child and adolescent overweight and obesity: summary report. Pediatrics 2007;120:S164–92.
8. Summerbell CD, Ashton V, Campbell KJ, et al. Interventions for treating obesity in children. [Cochrane Review]. The Cochrane Library 2003;(3):CD001872.
9. Collins CE, Warren J, McCoy P, et al. Measuring effectiveness of dietetic interventions in child obesity: a systematic review of randomized trials. Arch Pediatr Adolesc Med 2006;160(9):906–22.
10. National Health and Medical Research Council. Clinical practice guidelines for the management of overweight and obesity in children and adolescents. 2003 Commonwealth of Australia.
11. Raine KD. Overweight and obesity in Canada. A population health perspective. Ontario (Canada), Canadian Institute for Health Information; 2004.
12. Baur L. Childhood obesity: practically invisible. Int J Obes 2005;29:351–2.
13. Stewart L, Chapple J, Hughes AR, et al. Parents' journey through treatment for their child's obesity: qualitative study. Arch Dis Child 2008;93:35–9.
14. Dixey R, Rudolf MC, Murtagh J. WATCH IT: obesity management of children: a qualitative exploration of the views of parents. International Journal of Health Promotion and Education 2006;44:131–7.
15. Stewart L, Houghton J, Hughes AR, et al. Dietetic management of pediatric overweight: development of a practical and evidence-based behavioral approach. J Am Diet Assoc 2005;105:1810–5.
16. Savoye M, Shaw M, Dziura J, et al. Effects of a weight management program on body composition and metabolic parameters in overweight children. a randomized controlled trial. JAMA 2007;297(24):2697–704.
17. Edwards C, Nicholls D, Croker H, et al. Family-based behavioural treatment of obesity: acceptability and effectiveness in the UK. Eur J Clin Nutr 2006;60: 587–92.
18. Rudolf MCJ, Christie D, McElhone S, et al. WATCH IT: a community based programme for obese children and adolescents. Arch Dis Child 2006;91:736–9.
19. Golley RK, Magarey AM, Baur LA, et al. Twelve-month effectiveness of a parent-led, family-focused weight-management program for prepubertal children: a randomized controlled trial. Pediatrics 2007;119:517–25.
20. Hughes AR, Stewart L, Chapple J, et al. Randomized, controlled trial of a best-practice individualized behavioral program for treatment of childhood overweight: Scottish childhood overweight treatment trial (SCOTT). Pediatrics 2008; 121(3):e539–46.
21. Rhee KE, Lumeng JC, Appugliese DP, et al. Parenting styles and overweight status in first grade. Pediatrics 2006;117(6):2047–54.
22. Dietz WH, Robinson TN. Overweight children and adolescents. N Engl J Med 2005;352(20):2100–9.
23. Golan M. Parents as agents of change in childhood obesity–from research to practice. Int J Pediatr Obes 2006;1(2):66–76.
24. Stark LJ. Can nutrition counseling be more behavioural? Lessons learned from dietary management of cystic fibrosis. Proc Nutr Soc 2003;62:793–9.
25. Robinson TN. Behavioural treatment of childhood and adolescent obesity. Int J Obes 1999;23(Suppl 2):S52–7.
26. Lask B. Motivating children and adolescents to improve adherence. J Pediatr 2003;143:430–3.
27. Rollnick S, Mason P, Butler C. Health behavior change. A guide for practitioners. Edinburgh: Churchill Livingstone; 1999.

28. Foreyt JP, Paschali AA. Behaviour therapy. In: Kopleman P, editor. The management of obesity and related disorders. London: Martin Dunitz; 2001. p. 165–78.

29. Epstein LH, Wing RR, Valoski AM. Childhood obesity. Pediatr Clin North Am 1985; 32(2):363–79.

30. Hunt P. Dietary counseling: theory into practice. Journal of the Institute of Health Education 1995;33(1):4–8.

31. Hughes AR, Henderson A, Ortiz-Rodriguez V, et al. Habitual physical activity and sedentary behaviour in a clinical sample of obese children. Int J Obes 2006;30: 1494–500.

32. Stewart L, Deane M, Wilson DC. Failure of routine management of obese children: an audit of dietetic intervention. Arch Dis Child 2004;89(suppl 1):A13–6.

33. Quattrin T, Liu E, Shaw N, et al. Obese children who are referred to the pediatric endocrinologist: characteristics and outcomes. Pediatrics 2005;115:348–51.

34. Denzer C, Reithofer E, Wabitsch M, et al. The outcome of childhood obesity management depends highly upon patient compliance. Eur J Pediatr 2004;163: 99–104.

35. Barlow SE, Dietz WH. Obesity evaluation and treatment: expert committee recommendations. Pediatrics 1998;102(3):1–11.

36. Cole TJ, Faith MS, Pietrobelli A, et al. What is the best measure of adiposity change in growing children: BMI, BMI %, BMI z-score or BMI centile? Eur J Clin Nutr 2005;59:419–25.

37. Hunt LP, Ford A, Sabin MA, et al. Clinical measures of adiposity and percentage fat loss: which measure most accurately reflects fat loss and what should we aim for? Arch Dis Child 2007;92:399–403.

38. Reinehr T, Andler W. Changes in the atherogenic risk factor profile according to degree of weight loss. Arch Dis Child 2004;89:419–22.

39. Flodmark CE, Lissau I, Moreno LA, et al. New insight into the field of children and adolescents' obesity: the European perspective. Int J Obes 2004;28:1189–96.

40. Daley AJ, Copeland RJ, Wright NP, et al. Exercise therapy as a treatment for psychopathologic conditions in obese and morbidly obese adolescents: a randomized controlled trial. Pediatrics 2006;118:2126–34.

41. Chanoine JP, Hampl S, Jensen C, et al. Effect of orlistat on weight and body composition in obese adolescents. JAMA 2005;293(23):2873–83.

42. Gately PJ, Cooke CB, Barth JH, et al. Children's residential weight loss camps can work. Pediatrics 2005;116:73–7.

Preventing Eating Disorders

Heather Shaw, PhD[a],*, Eric Stice, PhD[a], Carolyn Black Becker, PhD[b]

KEYWORDS

- Eating disorders • Prevention
- Meta-analysis • Dissonance interventions

Eating pathology (EP) is characterized by chronicity and relapse, results in impaired psychosocial functioning, and is related to elevated risk for suicide.[1,2] EP also increases the risk for future depressive disorders, anxiety disorders, substance abuse, health problems, and obesity.[3,4] Moreover, EP remains challenging to treat and the effects have been limited.[1,2] As a result, considerable efforts have been devoted to developing effective prevention programs. This article reviews eating disorder (ED) prevention programs that have been evaluated in controlled trials. In particular, the authors identify the sample, intervention, and design features that produced larger intervention effects, review programs that appear particularly promising, and offer suggestions for future prevention efforts.

Early ED prevention programs produced limited effects.[5] In an attempt to improve outcomes, researchers now target well-established risk factors underlying EP, an approach that has proved to be more successful. Presently, little is known about the risk factors specific to anorexia nervosa, bulimia nervosa, or binge ED. Well-established risk factors for EP, more generally, that are supported by multiple independent prospective studies, include elevated perceived pressure to be thin, internalization of the thin-ideal standard of female beauty, body mass, body dissatisfaction, and negative affect.[6,7] Randomized experiments reducing thin-ideal internalization, body dissatisfaction, and negative affect also resulted in reductions in ED symptoms,[8,9] suggesting that these may be causal risk factors. Dieting was previously thought to be a well-established risk factor for EP because it predicted future EP in prospective studies.[10] More rigorous controlled experiments, however, have found that assignment to a low-calorie weight loss diet resulted in decreased bulimic symptoms in normal weight young women, overweight women, obese binge-eating women, and women with threshold and subthreshold bulimia nervosa.[11–14] Although it is possible that bulimic symptoms could increase over time, 1 study found that random

This work was supported by the National Institutes of Health grant MH/DK 61957.
[a] Oregon Research Institute, 1715 Franklin Boulevard, Eugene, OR 97403, USA
[b] Deptartment of Psychology, Trinity University, One Trinity Place, San Antonio, TX 78212-7200, USA
* Corresponding author.
E-mail address: hshaw@ori.org (H. Shaw).

Child Adolesc Psychiatric Clin N Am 18 (2008) 199–207
doi:10.1016/j.chc.2008.07.012

childpsych.theclinics.com

assignment of body-dissatisfied adolescent girls to a weight maintenance diet intervention resulted in reduced EP at 3-year follow-up,[15] which is the longest follow-up for a study of this kind to date. Some have argued that the prospective studies relied on invalid dietary restraint measures, which may explain the inconsistent findings.[16]

META-ANALYSIS OF EATING DISORDER PREVENTION PROGRAMS: DEFINING SUCCESSFUL PROGRAMS

Meta-analyses are ideal for elucidating participant, intervention, and research design features associated with the strongest intervention effects on ED risk factors and symptoms and the optimal conditions for prevention efforts. Understanding the characteristics of successful ED programs is essential for continuing to refine interventions to reduce the prevalence of EP. Accordingly, this article is organized around key findings from the authors' recent meta-analytic review of ED prevention programs that point to successful program features.

Because only key findings of the meta-analysis are summarized in this article, readers are referred to the work of Stice and colleagues.[17] for methodological details, specific hypotheses, and results. Overall, the results showed that 51% of the prevention programs included in the meta-analysis resulted in significant reductions in at least 1 established EP risk factor, 29% of the prevention programs resulted in significant reductions in EP, and some interventions reduced extant EP and prevented increases in EP that were observed in control groups. The overall percentage of prevention programs that produced positive effects with regard to EP is comparable to results showing changes in body mass index in obesity prevention programs (21%)[18] and results showing changes in condom use in HIV prevention programs (22%).[19] These results are encouraging, particularly given that early ED programs were typically unsuccessful at reducing ED or EP risk factors. Outcome variables examined in the meta-analysis were body mass, thin-ideal internalization, body dissatisfaction, dieting, and negative affect because these factors were identified in prospective risk factor studies as predictors of subsequent onset of EP.[20] Average effect sizes for the outcomes ranged from 0.10 to 0.18 at termination and from 0.04 to 0.13 at follow-up. Although these average effect sizes are small in magnitude, individual effect sizes from prevention trials ranged from nonexistent to large, and several factors associated with larger effects were identified by the moderation analyses. Based on prior research, potential moderators of intervention effects included in the analyses were participant features (risk status [selective or universal], sex, and age), design features (use of validated measures and length of follow-up), and intervention features (session format [interactive or didactic], type of interventionist [professional interventionist or endogenous provider], number of sessions, and program content). Here, the program features that emerged as important moderators of intervention effects are highlighted.

FEATURES OF SUCCESSFUL EATING DISORDER PREVENTION PROGRAMS

The meta-analysis pointed to several important features of ED prevention programs that moderated effect sizes and also to particularly promising prevention programs. More specifically, several moderators emerged as being important in producing strong intervention effects. First, selected programs targeting high-risk individuals produced larger effects than did universal programs for most outcomes. One possible reason for the improved effects with selected programs is that high-risk participants may be more motivated to participate in programs to reduce current distress from elevated risk factors, such as body dissatisfaction or negative affect. In fact, only selected interventions prevented future increases in EP observed in control groups, suggesting that the effects did not just result from an initial decrease in eating disturbances. Several universal prevention programs were also more effective for subgroups of high-risk participants than for the full sample.[21–25] Three studies not included in the meta-analysis, however, found that a dissonance-based program produced similar results for low- and high-risk subgroups.[26–28] This program, explained in detail later in the article, attempts to induce cognitive dissonance in participants by having them argue against the culturally prescribed thin-ideal beauty standard, which is thought to lead to a shift in attitudes and to produce behavioral change. Indeed, some researchers have argued for universal programs based on the notion that they can effectively challenge the broader sociocultural environment thought to contribute to the development and persistence of EDs.[29] Furthermore, Becker has found in her work that sororities rejected a selected approach in favor of a universal approach because they felt that the program should be mandatory for all members.

Participant age was also an important moderator of intervention effects. Programs with older adolescents (older than 15 years) had larger effects, perhaps because interventions are more effective when delivered during the peak risk period when EP emerges. Younger adolescents also may have limited insight and ability to apply the principles of the intervention. In addition, low levels of EP during early adolescence may lead to floor effects. Interactive interventions also produced stronger effects, which is consistent with other prevention research that has found that didactic psychoeducational interventions are less effective than interactive interventions.[30] Interactive interventions are probably more engaging, which facilitates internalizing important concepts and promotes attitudinal and behavioral change.

The type of interventionist was also important because interventions delivered by trained interventionists were more effective than those delivered by endogenous providers (eg, teachers, nurses, and counselors). Effects may be smaller for endogenous providers because they have competing demands, such as teaching or other full-time job responsibilities, which make it difficult to deliver the prevention program with fidelity. Endogenous providers may also receive less training, supervision, and practice in delivering the intervention compared with trained interventionists. However, as efforts to disseminate efficacious programs continue, further research will need to investigate factors that may increase the effectiveness of programs when they are delivered by endogenous providers because endogenous providers are often more economically viable, an important consideration in determining sustainability of programs in natural settings.

Intervention content was also an important moderator of effect sizes. Consistent with prior research,[30] interventions with psychoeducational content produced weaker effects. Body acceptance interventions were more effective than programs without this focus, possibly because body dissatisfaction increases the risk for a host of other disturbances, such as unhealthy dieting, negative affect, and ED behavior (eg, vomiting for weight control). Thus, reducing body dissatisfaction can also decrease these disturbances. Dissonance-induction interventions also produced larger effects for thin-ideal internalization, body dissatisfaction, dieting, and negative affect, and EP than programs without this content. Interventions with sociocultural content and a stress and coping focus had limited effects. The 15 programs that produced effects for EP varied considerably and included programs aimed at enhancing self-esteem, stress management skills, body acceptance, healthy weight control behaviors, and critical analysis of the thin ideal. This implies that EP prevention can occur through a variety of methods or that nonspecific factors explain some of the intervention effects. Thus, it is also important to examine the specific programs that produced the strongest, most persistent effects.

SUCCESSFUL EATING DISORDER PREVENTION PROGRAMS

The meta-analytic review identified several prevention programs that have successfully reduced current and future ED symptoms and several that have also reduced the risk for onset of threshold or subthreshold EDs,[16,31] which has been difficult to achieve. In this section, some of the more successful, promising programs that were highlighted by the meta-analysis are briefly discussed.

DISSONANCE-INDUCTION INTERVENTIONS: THE BODY PROJECT

The Body Project is an intervention based on the social psychological principle of cognitive dissonance. The main theory behind this intervention is that by encouraging girls and women to take an active stance in arguing against the culturally mandated thin ideal, they will experience cognitive dissonance and shift their belief systems to align with this anti–thin-ideal stance. Body Project is a highly interactive and brief (3- and 4-session versions) intervention that has been replicated by 5 independent laboratories and outperformed alternative interventions and thus considered efficacious or empirically established (see Shaw and Stice[32] for a review of this program). This intervention has successfully reduced the risk for future onset of both ED symptoms and obesity and resulted in improved psychosocial functioning and reduced mental health care use at 1-year follow-up in a self-selected sample of young women with body dissatisfaction.[8] Furthermore, a follow-up article[15] reported that relative to assessment-only controls, dissonance participants had significantly lower thin-ideal internalization, body dissatisfaction, negative affect, bulimic symptoms, and psychosocial impairment by 2- to 3-year follow-up. Importantly, the dissonance intervention reduced the risk for onset of threshold and subthreshold anorexia nervosa, bulimia nervosa, and binge-eating disorder through a 3-year follow-up compared with assessment-only controls (6% versus 15%), which represents a 60% reduction in the number of expected cases that would have theoretically emerged without this intervention. Results suggest that for every 100 young women who complete the dissonance intervention, approximately 9 or fewer show the onset of EP.

SORORITY BODY IMAGE PROGRAM

Becker and colleagues[26] developed a 2-session version of the dissonance intervention and successfully applied it to sororities. Their results suggested that the intervention produced significantly greater reductions in thin-ideal internalization, body dissatisfaction, and dieting compared with those in a waitlist control at 1-month follow-up in sorority members and that the intervention also produced significant reductions in EP.[26] Becker has also found that this program can be successfully implemented by peer leaders in effectiveness trials[27,33] and produces significant effects at 8-month follow-up. Demonstrating the effectiveness of such a brief intervention applied to a broader social system suggests that this program can be widely adapted and easily disseminated.

HEALTHY WEIGHT INTERVENTION

The healthy weight intervention was originally included as a control group in a study testing the dissonance program and was also found to reduce the future onset of both ED symptoms and obesity and result in improved psychosocial functioning and reduced mental health care use at 1-year follow-up.[8] Furthermore, this intervention was also found to produce true prophylactic effects and reduced the onset of EDs at 3-year follow-up.[15] What differentiates this program from other psychoeducational interventions is that it aims to teach participants how to achieve and maintain a healthy weight through making small, gradual changes in diet and exercise. The program also incorporates social psychological principles, such as motivational interviewing and public commitments to change, which is novel. It is a brief 4-session intervention and seems to be easily disseminated by endogenous providers and professional interventionists.

GIRL TALK

Girl Talk is an interactive, 6-session intervention that consists of a peer-support group that is centered on promoting critical media use, body acceptance, healthy weight control behaviors, and stress management skills.[34] In an effectiveness trial of a 10-session version of this program delivered by public health nurses in a school,[35] participation in the intervention led to increases in weight-related esteem and decreases in dieting at post-test and 3-month follow-up among middle schools girls compared with the control group. A subsequent evaluation of this intervention delivered across different schools, however, failed to replicate these positive findings.[36]

STUDENT BODIES

Student Bodies[37] is an 8-week computer-administered ED prevention program based on cognitive-behavioral body-dissatisfaction interventions.[38] This intervention provides information on ED, healthy weight control behaviors, and nutrition and includes an unstructured e-mail support interchange, which allows participants to express their emotional reactions to the intervention. This program has successfully reduced ED risk factors, such as body dissatisfaction,[39] and positive results have been replicated in multiple trials conducted by the same laboratory. Other researchers[40] tested the long-term effectiveness of Student Bodies and whether the participants depended on clinically moderated online discussion groups that were included in previous trials. They found that overall, participants using the program without a clinical moderator for the online discussion had the best outcomes. More specifically, at post-test, this group showed significantly lower bulimic pathology and lower body dissatisfaction at 8-month follow-up than the control groups. More recently, Taylor and colleagues[31] tested whether this intervention, which included a moderated online discussion group, could prevent the onset of EDs in at-risk college women. They found that the program significantly reduced ED risk factors (weight and shape concerns), and notably reduced the onset of EDs in participants with elevated body mass index and in participants with baseline compensatory behaviors.

WEIGH TO EAT

Another intervention that is psychoeducational but incorporates social-cognitive principles for behavior change is Weigh to Eat, developed by Neumark-Sztainer and colleagues.[40] Weigh to Eat is a school-based program aimed at changing knowledge, attitudes, and behaviors related to nutrition and weight control, improving body and self-image, and promoting greater self-efficacy in approaching social pressures regarding excessive eating and dieting.[40] In an effectiveness trial of this 10-session intervention implemented by a health educator, it produced significant improvements in knowledge, healthy weight control behaviors, dieting, and binge eating at 6-month follow-up, although only the effects for binge eating remained significant at the 2-year follow-up. No significant changes were observed for body dissatisfaction and negative affect at either of the follow-up assessments.

ADDITIONAL PROMISING PROGRAMS

A couple of other psychoeducation-based interventions have proved to be successful, despite the overall finding that in general these types of programs are not effective. For example, Stice and colleagues,[41] in a replication of a preliminary trial of a 15-week psychoeducational college course on EDs, found that, compared with a matched control group, participants showed significantly greater reductions in thin-ideal internalization, body dissatisfaction, dieting, and ED symptoms as well as less weight gain at post-test and 6-month follow-up.

Similarly, Stewart and colleagues[23] also found positive effects from a psychoeducational program that can also be characterized as a body acceptance program, addressing not only sociocultural pressures to be thin and body dissatisfaction but also changes associated with puberty, development of EDs, self-esteem, and dieting. Their results showed that the intervention produced a small reduction in dietary restraint and attitudes to shape and weight at post-test, although the change did not persist through the 6-month follow-up.

SUMMARY

This review highlighted that researchers in the ED field have developed several prevention programs that have successfully decreased current EP and the risk for future increases in EP, and that many programs have successfully decreased the risk factors for ED. Furthermore, when the content of the interventions that produced effects is examined, it seems as though a range of intervention methods and features can successfully reduce ED risk factors and symptoms. Several prevention approaches appear to be promising, but interventions that decreased attitudinal risk factors and promoted healthy weight control behaviors were particularly effective. Some interventions appeared to be superior to minimal-intervention control conditions and some produced effects that persisted for up to 2 years. Selected (versus universal), interactive (versus didactic), multisession (versus single-session) programs, offered to participants older than 15 years (versus younger participants) and delivered by professional interventionists (versus endogenous providers), produced larger intervention effects. Larger effects were also observed for interventions with body acceptance and dissonance-induction foci and without psychoeducational content.

In interpreting the meta-analytic findings, establishing the relation between a moderator and an effect size does not establish causality. It could be that an effect is a result of some other variable that was not modeled (eg, prevention programs for those younger than 15 years could be less effective because they do not target causal risk factors). In addition, theoretic considerations, rather than empiric evidence, guided some of the authors' conclusions regarding the moderators. For example, there is no empiric evidence supporting the speculation that the success of selected programs is a result of the distress of high-risk samples causing them to more effectively engage in the program content. Finally, many programs that have produced promising effects have not included long-term follow-up periods, which makes it difficult to discern the persistence of the effects.

Although many programs produced positive effects, they could be larger and more persistent. In fact, the average effects in the meta-analysis overall were relatively small, ranging from nonexistent to large. Furthermore, researchers should build on successful content and design features suggested by the meta-analysis. More researchers should also examine mediators of intervention effects, which is necessary to understand the effects of the nonspecific factors that likely explained why some interventions did not produce stronger effects than minimal-intervention control conditions. Examining the moderators of intervention effects is also vital in identifying the types of participants who best respond to particular prevention programs and in suggesting how to design programs that benefit more participants.

To better understand the role of various etiologic ED risk factors, more randomized experimental trials of prevention programs are also needed. Such trials are the only way to isolate the role of a risk factor on EP. Furthermore, many trials did not include a control group, making it impossible to separate the intervention effects from the effects of the passage of time, regression to the mean, or measurement artifacts. More trials also need to incorporate placebo or alternative intervention control groups, which helps to isolate intervention effects from those arising from nonspecific factors, demand characteristics, or expectancies. Several trials did not include a measure of ED symptoms or diagnoses, which limits what can be learned, and few effectiveness trials assess whether an intervention works when recruitment and delivery are performed by endogenous providers rather than professional interventionists. Finally, many researchers failed to report effect sizes, making it difficult to interpret the findings, and few researchers examined differential change in outcomes across conditions, which is essential for the proper interpretation of effects.

Researchers should use these results as a foundation for developing future ED prevention interventions. The most efficacious interventions should be refined and tested in effectiveness trials to enhance cost-effectiveness and identify possible barriers to wide dissemination of these programs. Independent replications of the most promising prevention trials need to be conducted, and moderators and mediators need to be further examined. General prevention techniques that build on successful content features, such as incorporating social psychological principles—such as dissonance and strategic presentation to combat risk factors—should be developed. Finally, clinical preventionists who have limited resources for research should attempt to implement existing efficacious programs and report on their clinical experiences, as opposed to using new untested programs that may have little effect. Finally, the authors hope that the findings from the summary of the literature can be used to help researchers continue to conduct methodologically rigorous and programmatic studies to help refine and improve prevention programs aimed at reducing the risk for and prevalence of ED and EP and also to help clinicians implement programs that are more likely to produce beneficial results.

REFERENCES

1. Wilson GT, Becker CB, Heffernan K. Eating disorders. In: Mash EJ, Barkley RA, editors. Child psychopathology. 2nd edition. New York: Guilford; 2003. p. 687–715.
2. Stice E, Bulik CM. Eating disorders. In: Beauchaine PP, Hinshaw SP, editors. Child and adolescent psychopathology. Hoboken (NJ): Wiley & Sons; 2008. p. 643–69.
3. Johnson JG, Cohen P, Kasen S, et al. Eating disorders during adolescence and the risk for physical and mental disorders during early adolescence. Arch Gen Psychiatry 2002;59:545–52.
4. Stice E, Cameron R, Killen JD, et al. Naturalistic weight reduction efforts prospectively predict growth in relative weight and onset of obesity among female adolescents. J Consult Clin Psychol 1999;67:967–74.
5. Pearson J, Goldklang D, Striegel-Moore R. Prevention of eating disorders: challenges and opportunities. Int J Eat Disord 2002;31:233–9.

6. Stice E. A prospective test of the dual pathway model of bulimic pathology: mediating effects of dieting and negative affect. J Abnorm Psychol 2001;110: 124–35.

7. Wertheim EH, Koerner J, Paxton S. Longitudinal predictors of restrictive eating and bulimic tendencies in three different age groups of adolescent girls. J Youth Adolesc 2001;30:69–81.

8. Stice E, Shaw H, Burton E, et al. Dissonance and healthy weight eating disorder prevention programs: a randomized efficacy trial. J Consult Clin Psychol 2006;74: 263–75.

9. Burton EM, Stice E, Bearman SK, et al. An experimental test of the affect-regulation model of bulimic symptoms and substance use: an affective intervention. Int J Eat Disord 2008;40:27–36.

10. Field AE, Camargo CA, Taylor CB, et al. Relation of peer and media influences to the development of purging behaviors among preadolescent and adolescent girls. Arch Pediatr Adolesc Med 1999;153:1184–9.

11. Burton EM, Stice E. Evaluation of a healthy-weight treatment program for bulimia nervosa: a preliminary randomized trial. Behav Res Ther 2006;44:1727–38.

12. Goodrick GK, Poston WS, Kimball KT, et al. Nondieting versus dieting treatments for overweight binge-eating women. J Consult Clin Psychol 1998;66:363–8.

13. Klem ML, Wing RR, Simkin-Silverman L, et al. The psychological consequences of weight gain prevention in healthy, premenopausal women. Int J Eat Disord 1997;21:167–74.

14. Presnell K, Stice E. An experimental test of the effect of weight-loss dieting on bulimic pathology: tipping the scales in a different direction. J Abnorm Psychol 2003;112:166–70.

15. Stice E, Marti N, Spoor S, et al. Dissonance and healthy weight eating disorder prevention programs: long-term effects from a randomized efficacy trial. J Consult Clin Psychol 2008;76:329–40.

16. Stice E, Fisher M, Lowe MR. Are dietary restraint scales valid measures of acute dietary restriction? Unobtrusive observational data suggest not. Psychol Assess 2004;16:51–9.

17. Stice E, Shaw H, Marti CN. A meta-analytic review of eating disorder prevention programs: progress at last. Annu Rev Clin Psychol 2007;3:233–57.

18. Stice E, Shaw H, Marti CN. A meta-analytic review of obesity prevention programs for children and adolescents: the skinny on interventions that work. Psychol Bull 2006;132:667–91.

19. Logan TK, Cole J, Leukefeld C. Women, sex, and HIV: social and contextual factors, meta-analysis of published interventions, and implications for practice and research. Psychol Bull 2002;128:851–85.

20. Stice E. Risk and maintenance factors for eating pathology: a meta-analytic review. Psychol Bull 2002;128:825–48.

21. Buddeberg-Fischer B, Klaghofer R, Gnam G, et al. Prevention of disturbed eating behaviour: a prospective intervention study in 14- to 19-year old Swiss students. Acta Psychiatr Scand 1998;98:146–55.

22. Killen JD, Taylor CB, Hammer L, et al. An attempt to modify unhealthful eating attitudes and weight regulation practices of young adolescent girls. Int J Eat Disord 1993;13:369–84.

23. Stewart DA, Carter JC, Drinkwater J, et al. Modification of eating attitudes and behavior in adolescent girls: a controlled study. Int J Eat Disord 2001;29:107–18.

24. Stice E, Fisher M, Martinez E. Eating disorder diagnostic scale: additional evidence of reliability and validity. Psychol Assess 2004;16:60–71.

25. Weiss K, Wertheim EH. An evaluation of a prevention program for disordered eating in adolescent girls: examining responses of high and low risk girls. Eat Dis: J Treat Prev 2005;14:265–85.
26. Becker CB, Smith L, Ciao AC. Reducing eating disorder risk factors in sorority members: a randomized trial. Behav Ther 2005;36:245–54.
27. Becker CB, Bull S, Schaumberg K, et al. Effectiveness of peer-led eating disorder prevention: a replication trial. J Consult Clin Psychol 2008;76:347–54.
28. Green M, Scott N, Diyankova I, et al. Eating disorder prevention: an experimental comparison of high level dissonance, low level dissonance, and no-treatment control. Eat Disord 2005;13:157–69.
29. Levine MP, Smolak L. The prevention of eating problems and eating disorders: theory, research, and practice. Mahwah (NJ): Lawrence Erlbaum; 2006.
30. Larimer ME, Cronce JM. Identification, prevention, and treatment: a review of individual-focused strategies to reduce problematic alcohol consumption by college students. J Stud Alcohol 2002;s14:148–63.
31. Taylor CB, Bryson S, Luce KH, et al. Prevention of eating disorders in at-risk college-age women. Arch Gen Psychiatry 2006;63:881–8.
32. Shaw H, Stice E. Preventing eating disorders: a school-based dissonance program. In C LegCroy, editor. Handbook of prevention and intervention programs for adolescent girls. Hoboken, NJ: Wiley; 2008.
33. Becker CB, Smith L, Ciao AC. Peer-facilitated eating disorders prevention: a randomized effectiveness trial of cognitive dissonance and media advocacy. J Couns Psychol 2006;53:550–5.
34. McVey GL, Davis R. A program to promote positive body image: a 1-year follow-up assessment. J Early Adolesc 2002;22:96–108.
35. McVey G, Lieberman M, Voorberg N, et al. School-based peer support groups: a new approach to the prevention of disordered eating. Eat Disord 2003;11: 169–85.
36. McVey G, Lieberman M, Voorberg N, et al. Replication of a peer support program designed to prevent disordered eating: is a life skills approach sufficient for all middle school students? Eat Disord 2003;11:187–95.
37. Winzelberg AJ, Eppstein D, Eldredge KL, et al. Effectiveness of an internet-based program for reducing risk factors for eating disorders. J Consult Clin Psychol 2000;68:346–50.
38. Butters JW, Cash TF. Cognitive-behavioral treatment of women's body-image dissatisfaction. J Consult Clin Psychol 1987;55:889–97.
39. Low KG, Charanasomboon S, Lesser J, et al. Effectiveness of a computer-based interactive eating disorder prevention program at long-term follow-up. Eat Disord 2006;14:17–30.
40. Neumark-Sztainer D, Butler R, Palti H. Eating disturbances among adolescent girls: evaluation of a school-based primary prevention program. J Nutr Educ 1995;27:24–31.
41. Stice E, Orjada K, Tristan J. Trial of a psychoeducational eating disturbance intervention for college women: a replication and extension. Int J Eat Disord 2006;39: 233–9.

Obesity Prevention in Children and Adolescents

Boyd Swinburn, MB, ChB, FRACP, MD

KEYWORDS

- Obesity • Childhood • Adolescence • Prevention
- Community • Policy

In the high-income countries of the world (Western Europe, North America, and Australasia), the childhood obesity epidemic started to increase rapidly over the 1980s and 1990s.[1] In middle-income countries, the epidemic started more recently and even in some of the poorer countries, it is overtaking undernutrition in prevalence rates.[2] The epidemic travels through population subgroups in a relatively consistent fashion, accelerated versions of which are being seen in transition countries.[3,4] In the early stages of the epidemic, the effects are seen predominantly in middle-aged people, women, urban dwellers, and the higher socioeconomic status (SES) groups. Children are relatively unaffected. As time passes (and the population's economic prosperity increases), the obesity prevalence rates in men increase to match those in women and children.[1] The SES gradient reverses (especially in women) as lower-income people gain access to the "obesogenic" forces in the environment and education about the need for healthy eating and regular physical activity slows the rate of weight gain in the higher SES groups.[5,6]

Specific obesogenic factors that may be driving childhood obesity include the marketing of energy-dense foods and beverages in general, but also specifically, to children; concerns about the safety of neighborhoods; both parents (or the solo parent) working so that children spend their after-school time inside the house; and electronic and computer games. A recent review showed only some parallels between children's physical activity patterns and the rise in obesity.[7] There have been no discernible trends of decreasing physical activity levels or increasing television (TV) viewing (in developed countries) in children, but there is a clear pattern of reduced walking and cycling for transport and a recent increase in electronic games use, especially in boys.[7] On the other hand, food marketing has changed remarkably and globally over the past 30 years, and children in the United States alone are the target population for an estimated $10 billion of food marketing.[8] The increase in food consumption

School of Exercise and Nutrition Sciences, Deakin University, 221 Burwood Highway, Melbourne 3125, Australia
E-mail address: boyd.swinburn@deakin.edu.au

Child Adolesc Psychiatric Clin N Am 18 (2008) 209–223
doi:10.1016/j.chc.2008.07.015
1056-4993/08/$ – see front matter © 2008 Elsevier Inc. All rights reserved.

childpsych.theclinics.com

since the 1970s is also evidence that increasing energy intake is driving the obesity epidemic.[9] Indeed, the known positive relationship between body weight and total energy expenditure (consisting mainly of resting metabolic rate and the energy cost of physical activity) suggests that any potential declines over the past 30 years in the energy cost of physical activity have been more than overtaken by the increases in resting metabolic rate secondary to higher body weights.[10,11] The evidence pointing toward energy intake as the dominant driver of the epidemic comes from a range of different research and analysis directions.[9–13]

Obesity can be considered an inevitable consequence of the commercial successes of industries creating an overconsumption of food and labor-saving devices.[14] Contemporary market forces heavily favor behaviors that satisfy people's short-term preferences (eg, eating the food available) over long-term preferences (ie, healthy weight), and this is especially true for children. Hence, if the market, as the main mechanism for determining choices, results in outcomes that make our children worse off, then the market has failed to sustain and promote social and individual goals.[14] This is a serious market failure and demands government intervention.

PARADIGMS FOR THE PREVENTION OF CHILDHOOD OBESITY

Obesity is a societal, rather than a medical, problem, so there are several lenses through which to view the issues of prevention. Each of these paradigms has its validity, and probably the combination of all of them will provide the best chance to reduce childhood obesity.

The Clinical Approach

Reducing the burden of disease through the clinical approaches of screening for people at risk and treating them individually is effective where there are well-proven, effective clinical interventions available. The treatment of elevated blood pressure and hyperlipidemia to prevent cardiovascular diseases is a classic example. Most of the costs of obesity occur in later adulthood and many of the obesity-related diseases, such as diabetes, can be partially prevented through screening and intensive management programs.[15] Therefore, weight management programs for at-risk adults represents an attractive, albeit expensive, strategy for tackling obesity because it could potentially have quite rapid effects on reducing the health consequences of obesity in a population. The problem with this approach is that the effectiveness of all obesity treatment programs (except bariatric surgery) wears off over time, and often people return to their original weight (or more) after a few years,[16] and there is limited evidence on how to avoid this.[17] The evidence on the effectiveness of weight management of obese children is fairly limited with only 18 trials included in the Cochrane review of the topic.[18] Many of the trials were in tertiary care institutions, and the studies, overall, had small numbers and were of mixed quality. The reviewers did not draw any direct conclusions from their review, apart from the need to build more quality evidence.

Public Health Approach

A public health approach would be to try to prevent unhealthy weight gain in the first place, and this could either occur in children and adolescents or in young adults, because peak weight occurs in middle-aged adults. Because children are still growing and there is good access to settings such as schools for health promotion, they make a better priority group to target than young adults. In addition, society has a responsibility to protect children, and therefore, public and political pressure is greater to prevent unhealthy weight gain in children. However, the major pay-off in terms of

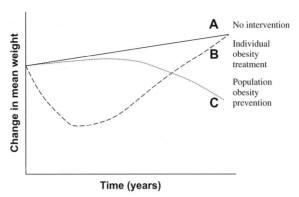

Fig. 1. Schematic diagram of the patterns of weight change from individual and population approaches. Line A (——) represents the gradual increase in body weight in adults followed longitudinally and children followed serial cross-sectionally without any interventions (ie, the control condition). Line B (————) represents the typical weight change pattern of a group of overweight adults with maximum early effects, which wane over time. Line C (......) represents the likely response of a population of children exposed to a whole-of-community program and measured in a serial cross-sectional manner (to avoid the complicating effects of growth on weight change).

reduced health care costs, even with successful programs, is many decades into the future. **Fig. 1** shows a schematic illustration of the weight change patterns for both types of approaches. With no intervention, the mean weight of a cohort of overweight adults (followed longitudinally) or a population of children in a community (followed serial cross-sectionally) gradually increases over time. There is a large body of evidence on the pattern of weight loss interventions in adults—the impact is realized early in the intervention, it tends to be at its maximum within 6 to 12 months, and over subsequent years, weight tends to return to that of an untreated group.[16,19] There is little evidence on the long-term impact of a community program on the prevention of unhealthy weight gain in children, but the reported changes in a demonstration project in 2 villages in Northern France[20] follow the pattern one might expect—a gradual flattening of the trajectory of weight gain to a plateau, and then a reduction as healthier eating and physical activity patterns become the new norms. Public health approaches are discussed in detail later.

"Free" Market Approach

In orthodox economic theory, the (perfectly) competitive market results in "efficiency" and there is no need for government intervention. Well-informed individuals make rational choices based on their personal preferences. These choices maximize their utility; that is, individuals satisfy their preferences in the best possible way for themselves. For parents who make choices for their children, their preferences extend to what is the best for them and their children. Markets, in turn, respond to the public's revealed preferences by allocating more resources to the preferred activities. Thus, the market would "self-correct" by providing the healthy foods that people demand because they want to avoid unhealthy weight gain. While this process will hold to some extent for the better educated and wealthier sections of the population (thus increasing health inequalities), the profits to be made from encouraging overconsumption are too great and a lower consumption would probably mean lower commercial returns.

A continued reliance on the marketplace as a self-correcting mechanism to reduce obesity is likely to be a recipe for continued increasing obesity and inequalities.

Human Rights Approach

Three sets of declared human rights apply to childhood obesity: the Convention on the Rights of the Child,[21] the right to adequate food,[22] and the right to health.[23] There is a clear responsibility for society to minimize the obesogenic environmental forces that impinge on children and to provide, and promote, healthy food and recreational opportunities for them. If society fulfilled these responsibilities, childhood obesity would be greatly reduced because children's (and to a large degree, adolescents') behaviors are closely determined by their environments. These are now being articulated into the concept that children have a right to be free from obesity.[24]

Risks/Benefits Approach

An alternate view of managing childhood obesity in its societal context is to balance the risks and benefits of any action on all players. For example, the UK Food Standards Agency undertook a risk assessment in relation to its proposed actions to reduce food marketing to children.[25] However, it is a difficult and controversial task to measure and compare the likely improvements in children's health versus the likely reductions in corporate profits from marketing restrictions. A risk-benefit approach is intrinsically more favorable to the case for commercial interests, whereas a rights-based approach is intrinsically more favorable to the case for children. Because children suffer the consequences of targeted marketing of energy-dense foods and beverages without having any powers to change it, a risk-benefit approach is the least helpful in preventing childhood obesity, where the ground is heavily contested.

OVERVIEW OF POPULATION-BASED STRATEGIES

As societies develop their strategies to tackle the epidemic of obesity in children, they will be able to draw on the types of strategies, policies, and programs that have worked to control other epidemics. The usual comparison epidemic is smoking,[26] and although critics state that the comparison is unfair because food is needed for life but tobacco is not, there are many parallels in relation to the approaches taken by governments, the public, and private vested interests. The most powerful interventions for tobacco control have been taxation, legislation, and, particularly in the United States, lawsuits, and these have been supported by prominent, ongoing social marketing campaigns and support services such as Quitlines. There are also many parallels with how the tobacco and food sectors have responded to the moves for public health action by denying the evidence, promoting uncertainty in the evidence, political lobbying, "buying" opinions of experts, public relations initiatives, such as supporting education programs, and so on. There are also common lessons from the control of epidemics other than tobacco, such as road injuries, HIV AIDS, skin cancer, and cardiovascular diseases.[27] One of the key lessons is that, in general, education-dominated strategies are weak compared with policy/legislative approaches, environmental change, or fiscal instruments.[28] This is because most of the risk behaviors do not occur as a result of a knowledge deficit. Therefore, adding more knowledge is unlikely to change those behaviors unless it is backed by other strategies, especially policies targeting the environments to make healthy food and activity choices easier.

Many countries have already developed national plans of action on obesity.[29–31] A comprehensive framework for action would cover all the main settings and sectors (eg, health care, schools, pre-schools, transport, urban planning, and the food sector) and ensure that support actions (eg, monitoring, capacity building, research, and social marketing) are included. The main strategy options under each of those headings usually include policies/regulations, programs, and social marketing and education strategies. In general, countries can get to this stage of developing a plan relatively easily—the implementation of the plan is the problem. The 4 ingredients to achieve implementation are political leadership; supportive policies; ongoing, substantial funding for programs and social marketing; and robust population monitoring, program evaluation, and research.[32]

POLITICAL LEADERSHIP

It has taken a long time for the data on the rise of the obesity epidemic to become converted into political and public awareness. In many countries, the epidemic was discernible in the 1980s, but it took another 20 years before it found its way into the popular media in any meaningful way.[33] This awareness of the problem has, in a few places, converted into true political leadership, where concrete policies and regulations have been developed and ongoing funding streams have been secured. An example in the United States has been the action in Arkansas, spearheaded by the then-Governor Mike Huckabee. The Arkansas Child and Adolescent Obesity Initiative included legislation (Act 1220) that, among other things, established the annual body mass index (BMI) check for all children, with the information conveyed to parents through a Health Report Card.[34,35] The legislation seems to have triggered multiple responses in districts, schools, and homes, and the prevalence of childhood obesity in Arkansas (one of the states where obesity is most prevalent in the United States) now seems to have flattened off.[36]

Singapore is another place where there has been a strong political commitment to action on childhood obesity for many years. In response to a steady increase in obesity prevalence (defined as greater than 120% of median weight-for-height) from 2% in 1976 to 15% in 1992, the Ministry of Education, in close collaboration with the Health Promotion Board (Ministry of Health), established the Trim and Fit (TAF) program to increase physical fitness and reduce obesity among school children.[37] TAF was part of a National Healthy Lifestyle program implemented nationwide that backed up a multi-sectoral and multi-pronged approach to lowering the population's risk of non-communicable disease with political commitment and support. At the school level, TAF integrated nutrition education into the school curriculum, controlled the types of foods and beverages available at school, conducted annual fitness tests, boosted opportunities for physical activity, provided information to parents and students, and ran clinics for obese children. The prevalence of obesity fell from 1994 to 2003 by 2% to 3% (even allowing for a change in definitions).[37] Although this evaluation points to the success of the program, there were several components of it, such as the after-school programs for overweight children, that could increase stigmatization, and the program has since been stopped.

SUPPORTIVE POLICIES

The "soft paternalism" approaches of social marketing and health promotion programs need to be supported by the "hard paternalism" options of laws, regulations, enforceable policies, and fiscal instruments[38] if there is to be any hope of countering the powerful obesogenic commercial forces. The softer instruments are preferred by most governments, but there are growing calls for the law to use the "harder" instruments to help tackle obesity.[39] In addition, the "softer" interventions, such as health education, may increase health inequalities if they are picked up more by higher-income families than lower-income families. Laws and regulations, on the other hand, tend to be applied across the board, so policies banning vending machines in schools should, at least, not increase inequalities and, in fact, may reduce inequalities, if the schools in poorer areas had more vending machines in the first place. Knowing the population impact of any obesity prevention intervention is difficult at this stage because of the lack of empiric evidence. Individual and population impacts have, however, been modeled for children and adolescents,[40] and the range of estimated population impacts is wide. The point estimate for the lowest impact initiative (the 'walking school bus' program of parent-supervised walking groups to school) was 30 disability-adjusted life years (DALYs) saved per year compared with the highest impact intervention modeled (bans on food marketing to children) of 37,000 DALYs saved per year. The uncertainty and sensitivity analyses provided a degree of robustness around the ranking of the 13 modeled interventions; nevertheless, it was clear that no single intervention by itself was nearly powerful enough to turn the childhood obesity epidemic around.

For some health issues, such as road injuries, workplace safety, tobacco control, and illicit drugs, governments have created laws and regulations that require certain behaviors of their citizens. However, requiring certain eating and physical activity behaviors to prevent obesity or chronic diseases is highly unlikely to happen—all foreseeable laws and regulations are targeted at the environment (making healthy choices easier), not at individuals. A few examples of potential policy initiatives are outlined in the following section.

Food and Beverage Marketing to Children

This is the touchstone issue of childhood obesity—it is difficult to see how this epidemic could be reversed in the face of tens of billions of dollars being spent each year by the food industry to encourage children to eat obesogenic foods. Such marketing is inherently exploitative, because young children are incapable of discerning its commercial intent,[8] whereas children of all ages are susceptible to its influence. Several evidence reviews have concluded that marketing clearly influences food preferences, positive beliefs, food purchases, and consumption.[8,41,42] The Province of Quebec, Canada, has the most stringent regulations protecting children from the marketing of any products,[43] and Sweden, Norway, and, now, the United Kingdom also have substantive regulations in place that provide some protection to children from broadcast food marketing at specific times.[44] However, the food and advertising industries readily circumvent such piecemeal regulations by broadcasting across borders or using a myriad of marketing techniques, such as competitions, sponsorship of children's sport, Internet games, direct marketing, and so on. The International Obesity Taskforce has undertaken a global consultation on a set of principles (the Sydney Principles) to guide action on reducing food and beverage marketing to children.[45] These are outlined in **Box 1**. Of the 7 principles, only the third one (that regulations must be statutory) is opposed by the food and advertising industries but it has been well described that the alternative of self-regulation by the industry itself provides little or no protection for children.[46] National and international pressure for regulations to ban, or severely limit, commercial marketing of obesogenic foods to children is increasing from public health and consumer groups.

Food Service Policies

Governments can show their commitment to childhood obesity prevention in ways that have potentially important impact and cost little. They can take an organizational

Box 1
The Sydney Principles. Guiding principles for achieving a substantial level of protection for children against the commercial promotion of foods and beverages

Actions to reduce commercial promotions to children should

1. Support the rights of children

   Regulations need to align with and support the United Nations Convention on the Rights of the Child and the Rome Declaration on World Food Security, which endorse the rights of children to adequate, safe, and nutritious food.

2. Afford substantial protection to children

   Children are particularly vulnerable to commercial exploitation, and regulations need to be sufficiently powerful to provide them with a high level of protection. Child protection is the responsibility of every section of society—parents, governments, civil society, and the private sector.

3. Be statutory in nature

   Only legally enforceable regulations have sufficient authority to ensure a high level of protection for children from targeted marketing and the negative impact that this has on their diets. Industry self-regulation is not designed to achieve this goal.

4. Take a wide definition of commercial promotions

   Regulations need to encompass all types of commercial targeting of children (eg, TV advertising, print, sponsorships, competitions, loyalty schemes, product placements, relationship marketing, Internet) and be sufficiently flexible to include new marketing methods as they develop.

5. Guarantee commercial-free childhood settings

   Regulations need to ensure that childhood settings such as schools, child care, and early childhood education facilities are free from commercial promotions that specifically target children.

6. Include cross-border media

   International agreements need to regulate cross-border media such as Internet, satellite and cable TV, and free-to-air TV broadcast from neighboring countries.

7. Be evaluated, monitored, and enforced

   The regulations need to be evaluated to ensure that the expected effects are achieved, independently monitored to ensure compliance, and fully enforced.

role model approach and have healthy eating and physical activity policies within their own departments, and they can institute food service policies not only within their own departments but also in institutions and agencies under their jurisdiction, such as schools, hospitals, pre-school settings, and government-funded agencies. Such policies, which have been mainly studied in schools and pre-schools,[47–49] cannot only influence the quality of the food served in those settings but also act as "lighthouse interventions" that spread the "light" to areas beyond their boundaries.

Urban Planning and Transport Policies

While there is considerable cross-sectional evidence linking the built environment with active transport and recreational physical activity,[50,51] there is limited experience in using planning regulations to achieve outcomes of increased physical activity, although these options exist in theory.[52] There are likely to be much more powerful drivers of changes to urban planning and transport policies—these include reducing congestion, reducing greenhouse gas emissions, increasing livability, and reducing injuries. Obesity prevention measures in the built environment substantially overlap with these more potent drivers of change, and thus obesity prevention advocacy needs to be closely linked with the environmental, sustainability, and livability movements.

SCHOOL AND COMMUNITY-BASED PROGRAMS

Systematic reviews of the effectiveness of school- or community-based interventions to prevent childhood obesity are somewhat discouraging.[53,54] In these reviews, there were only 20 to 30 published studies included, and on the whole, their impact was slight or non-existent. A broader review that tried to synthesize the evidence into "best practice" recommendations[55] was a little more optimistic, although it found substantial research gaps in intervention research with pre-school children, new immigrants to wealthy countries, targeting homes, whole communities, and focused on "upstream" interventions. Most interventions were short term, and they had some effect on preventing unhealthy weight gain without causing any negative effects, such as disordered eating patterns. Since these reviews, more optimistic results have started to emerge from whole-of-community projects in various countries including the United States,[56] New Zealand,[57] Chile,[58] Australia,[59] and the Netherlands.[60] These programs used a variety of approaches, and it is not yet clear what the optimal mix of strategies should be.

Community Capacity-Building Approach

In the community-based programs that the author and his group have been evaluating in Australia, New Zealand, Fiji, and Tonga,[61] the approach taken has been a community capacity-building one.[59,62] This approach does not bring specific programs or interventions to a community but rather brings the support systems to help the community organizations build their own capacity to promote healthy eating and physical activity—ensuring that the leadership, organizational structure, resources, and skills are created to maximize relevance and sustainability.[63] Given the wide variety of contexts for community-based obesity prevention (different age groups, localities, ethnicities, levels of disadvantage, and existing activities), a structured, yet flexible system is needed, because designing a one-size-fits-all program is not possible. This, however, has several practical consequences: external funding needs to come with sufficient flexibility for its use with decision making ceded to the local level; the processes need rigor so that building partnerships, skills, action plans, and so on, can be done in a quality way; and evaluation across the different portfolios of community interventions (as defined by each community) can be a challenge.

"Safety" of Community Programs

There is an understandable concern about school or community programs potentially doing some harm by stimulating children to go on diets, reducing their self-esteem, promoting distorted body size perceptions, or triggering teasing or bullying about body size. In the childhood obesity prevention program evaluated in the Victorian rural town of Colac, in Australia (population 11,000), several "safety indicators" in the intervention community and the comparison population were assessed.[59] Changes from baseline to follow-up were not significantly different between the groups (n = 2162) for the following indicators: prevalence of thinness/underweight, self-reported level of children's "unhappiness" with their body size, proportion not feeling good about themselves, attempts to lose weight in the previous 12 months, and frequency of teasing about weight. Close monitoring of clinical and community intervention programs for potential negative impacts continues to be important at this early stage of our knowledge of the risks and benefits of interventions. However, active, sensitive programs to promote healthy eating and reduce obesity seem more likely to reduce disordered eating patterns than increase them. This is because the potentially distorting messages from the fashion world can be countered and, if unhealthy weight gain can be prevented through population approaches, the driving forces for unhealthy eating patterns can be diminished.

Scaling Up Community Action

The shift from intervening in demonstration communities to the whole childhood population to reduce obesity will take a shift in thinking from "projects" to "systems." Systems are, of course, much more complex and are often under the control of different sectors. In Australia, for example, monitoring systems for childhood obesity and related behaviors are under the control of states and territories, but information feedback systems to change agents (eg, parents, primary care, schools, and local government) are either non-existent or inconsistent, and systems for training, skill development, and program support are shared between many different federal, state, or local government agencies and professional organizations. Add to that the fact that evaluation of processes and outcomes is generally weak because neither program funders nor research funding agencies consider it a high priority.

The program with the most experience in large-scale childhood obesity prevention is the Ensemble prévenons l'obésité des enfants (EPODE) program in France.[64] The program's origins were with a small demonstration project in two towns in Northern France,[20] which, over a period of 12 years (1992–2004), showed promising reductions in the prevalence of overweight and obesity. This was followed by a scale of up to 10 further communities in France in 2004, then a further rolling expansion (about 130 communities, mainly in France but also in Belgium and Spain by 2008), and an emerging EPODE European Network.[64] The EPODE system is structured to build community capacity by ensuring community leadership (committed mayors nominate their communities for the program and join the EPODE Mayors' Club), resource allocation (about half from local government for implementation and half from various sources for the core support services of training, social marketing development, and evaluation), suitable structures (usually through local government structures), and skills development (coordinated training, standard manuals, and regular network meetings). The paradigms needed to make this scale of an enterprise successful will require a thorough understanding of the systems as they grow, ongoing evaluation of the processes and outcomes, and building in continuous quality improvement mechanisms. This requires an entirely different skill set compared with that needed to develop and evaluate a time-limited, well-controlled demonstration project in a single, closely defined location, such as a small town.

Social Marketing

A critical strategy for community (and broader) attempts to prevent childhood obesity is social marketing, which is defined as the application of marketing concepts, tools, and techniques to any social issue.[65] It is more than just a bag of advertising and promotional tools; it is both a philosophy and a set of principles about how to achieve mutually satisfying exchanges between marketers and consumers. Marketing, and therefore social marketing, relies on a comprehensive and fully integrated approach to achieving campaign objectives. The concept of "exchanges" is important to grasp because identifying the "product" being gained and the "cost" being paid is critical to developing the appropriate messages. Take, for example, developing messages to parents about ensuring that their children eat a healthy breakfast before school. The "product" or benefit they stand to gain that means the most to them may be improved concentration at school and better grades. The "cost" may be getting themselves and their child up a bit earlier in the morning to have the time to prepare and eat breakfast. The communication messages would then focus on how to overcome the barriers to getting up earlier (ie, minimizing the costs) and enhancing the awareness of the potential gains in better school concentration (ie, maximizing the benefits). Such messages would have greater resonance than ones that say parents should get their children to eat a healthy breakfast for some potential, far-off health gains for them. The development of social marketing messages requires substantial formative evaluation of the final messages for preventing childhood obesity and these messages are likely to focus predominantly at the behavioral or attitudinal antecedents to unhealthy weight gain[66] whereas, for preventing or managing adult obesity, body weight or obesity itself may form part of the message.[67]

Comparing Effectiveness and Cost-Effectiveness of Interventions

Ideally, decision makers should be making evidence-based decisions on policy and allocation of resources. However, evidence on effectiveness and cost-effectiveness of various options for preventing childhood obesity is very limited.[53] Until firmer empiric evidence comes to hand, modeled estimates (and accompanying uncertainty estimates) can be made using the best available evidence. We have used the Assessing Cost-Effectiveness (ACE) methodologies for doing this for 13 specified interventions to reduce childhood and adolescent obesity.[40] The ACE approach is to undertake technical analyses for estimating intervention costs (in steady state), population impact (in terms of reduced mean BMI or reduced DALYs), and cost-effectiveness ratios in parallel with due process with a working group of end-users including government policy advisors. The 13 interventions included policies (eg, banning food advertisements targeting children), programs (eg, school interventions, walking school bus), and clinical interventions (eg, primary care treatment for overweight children and gastric-banding surgery for morbidly obese adolescents). The modeled estimates showed wide variation across the interventions with often 100-fold differences in population impact and cost-effectiveness (eg, about 37,000 DALYs saved and $300 m[illion] saved per year for banning TV food advertisements to children vs. about 30 DALYs saved at a cost of $22 m/y for the walking school bus).[40] Some interventions, such as banning food advertisements targeting children, had a small impact per child, but the wide reach meant it had a substantial population impact. Conversely, gastric-banding surgery obviously applied to only a small number of adolescents, but its large impact per person meant that the overall population impact in terms of reduced DALYs was important.

ADDRESSING INEQUALITIES IN CHILDHOOD OBESITY

Reducing inequalities in obesity is as important a goal as reducing obesity itself, and this has major implications for the implementation of childhood obesity prevention. There is good evidence that, in wealthy countries, children from more disadvantaged or lower-income families have a higher risk of overweight and obesity than their more advantaged peers.[68,69] In addition, certain ethnic groups consistently have a high prevalence of childhood obesity,[70,71] which reflects a mix of cultural, socioeconomic, and migration factors, producing a predisposition to unhealthy weight gain.

Interventions need to take this distribution into account. Some strategies have the potential to increase this gradient and others have the potential to reduce the gradient. A market forces approach favors the wealthy since they are more able to afford healthier places to live in (eg, closer to amenities and less crime) and healthier foods. In addition, people in wealthier neighborhoods are more likely to be successful in lobbying to keep fast food outlets in the neighborhood to a minimum, to have better amenities in local parks, and healthier food in school canteens. Similarly, information, education, and some social marketing strategies may favor the more advantaged sections of the community because they tend to be more literate, more receptive to messages about health, and more future-oriented. Specific targeting of social marketing messages to disadvantaged segments of the population may help to overcome this intrinsic problem of communication-based approaches. Similarly, if programs (such as after-school activity programs) are offered in a non-targeted manner, they could be preferentially picked up by the more advantaged populations.

On the other hand, policy-based interventions of environmental changes tend to affect a wider spectrum of the population and, in general, are more equitable.[72,73] Whole-of-community programs may also help to reduce the socioeconomic gradient with obesity. The Be Active Eat Well community project in Colac, Victoria, Australia, which the author and his group supported and evaluated over 3 years of intervention, showed no significant relationships between socioeconomic status and weight gain in the intervention children, whereas in the comparison population, virtually all analyses showed that the children from lower socioeconomic backgrounds gained more weight than their more advantaged peers.[59]

SUMMARY

The burgeoning obesity epidemic in children and adolescents needs a serious public health response. The commercial drivers of increased energy intake and sedentary activities are so powerful that government policy leadership is needed to change the "rules," the culture, and price structures around food, transport, and recreation so that healthy choices become the easy, default choices. The marketplace, as currently structured, has clearly failed to deliver the best outcomes for children. Regulations to substantially reduce food and beverage marketing to children is a policy priority, and scaling up community capacity to create healthy environments and promote healthy food and activity choices for children is a funding priority. Obesity prevention interventions that are well funded, follow established public health principles, and are properly evaluated should not only reduce childhood and adolescent obesity prevalence but also reduce the inequalities associated with obesity. These interventions, coupled with population reductions in unhealthy weight gain, may also have the potential to reduce disordered eating patterns and body image in children and adolescents.

ACKNOWLEDGMENTS

The work of my collaborators and colleagues on obesity prevention projects is gratefully acknowledged, especially that of Jean Michel Borys, Andrea Sanigorski, Colin Bell, Peter Kremer, Rob Carter, Marj Moodie, Robert Scragg, Jan Pryor, Elizabeth Waters, Mark Lawrence, and Gary Sacks.

REFERENCES

1. Lobstein T, Baur L, Uauy R. Obesity in children and young people: a crisis in public health. Obes Rev 2004;5(Suppl 1):4–104.
2. World Health Organisation. Obesity: preventing and managing the global epidemic. Report of a WHO consultation. Geneva (Switzerland): World Health Organisation; 2000. WHO Technical Report Series 894.
3. Popkin BM. The nutrition transition in low-income countries: an emerging crisis. Nutr Rev 1994;52(9):285–98.
4. Monteiro CA, Benicio MHD'A, Conde WL, et al. Shifting obesity trends in Brazil. Eur J Clin Nutr 2000;54(4):342–6.
5. Ball K, Crawford D. Socioeconomic status and weight change in adults: a review. Soc Sci Med 2005;60(9):1987–2010.
6. Armstrong J, Dorosty AR, Reilly JJ, et al. Coexistence of social inequalities in undernutrition and obesity in preschool children: population based cross sectional study. Arch Dis Child 2003;88(8):671–5.
7. Katzmarzyk PT, Baur LA, Blair SN, et al. International conference on physical activity and obesity in children: summary statement and recommendations. Int J Pediatr Obes 2008;3(1):3–21.
8. Institute of Medicine. Food marketing to children and youth. Threat or opportunity?. Washington, DC: National Academy of Sciences; 2006.
9. Bleich S, Cutler D, Murray C, et al. Why is the developed world obese? Annu Rev Public Health 2008;29:273–95.
10. Swinburn BA, Jolley D, Kremer PJ, et al. Estimating the effects of energy imbalance on changes in body weight in children. Am J Clin Nutr 2006;83(4):859–63.
11. Goris AHC, Westerterp KR. Physical activity, fat intake and body fat. Physiol Behav 2008;94(2):164–8.
12. Putnam J, Allshouse J, Scott Kantor L. US per capita food supply trends: more calories, refined carbohydrate, and fats. Food Review 2002;25(4):2–15.
13. Cook P, Coles-Rutishauser IHE, Seelig M. Comparable data on food and nutrient intake and physical measurements from the 1983, 1985 and 1995 National Nutrition Surveys. Brisbane (Australia): Australian Food and Nutrition Monitoring Unit; 2001.
14. Moodie R, Swinburn B, Richardson J, et al. Childhood obesity - a sign of commercial success but market failure. Int J Pediatr Obes 2006;1(3):133–8.
15. Knowler WC, Barrett-Connor E, Fowler SE, et al. Reduction in the incidence of type 2 diabetes with lifestyle intervention or metformin. N Engl J Med 2002; 346(6):393–403.
16. Swinburn BA, Metcalf PA, Ley SJ. Long term (5 year) effects of a reduced-fat diet intervention in individuals with glucose intolerance. Diabetes Care 2001;24: 619–24.
17. Harvey EL, Glenny AM, Kirk SF, et al. An updated systematic review of interventions to improve health professionals' management of obesity. Obes Rev 2002; 3(1):45–55.
18. Summerbell CD, Ashton V, Campbell KJ, et al. Interventions for treating obesity in children. Cochrane Database Syst Rev 2003;(3):CD001872.
19. Tsai AG, Wadden TA. Systematic review: an evaluation of major commercial weight loss programs in the United States. Ann Intern Med 2005;142(1): 56–66.
20. Borys JM. A successful way of preventing childhood obesity: the Fleurbaix-Laventie Study. Paper presented at: Proceedings of the 18th International

Congress of Nutrition: nutrition safari for innovative solutions; 19–23 September, 2005; Durban, South Africa.

21. United Nations. Convention on the Rights of the Child. Available at: http://www2. ohchr.org/english/law/crc.htm. Accessed September 2008.

22. United Nations. International Covenant on Economic, Social and Cultural Rights. General Comment 12 on the Right to Adequate Food 1966. Available at: http:// www.inhchr.ch/tbs/doc.nsf/(Symbol)/3d02758c70731d58025677f003b73b9?Open document. Accessed September 2008.

23. United Nations. International covenant on economic, social and cultural rights. General comment 11 on the right to the highest attainable standards of health. Available at: http://www.unhchr.ch/tbs/doc.nsf/0/3d02758c707031d58025677f003b73b9? Opendocument. Accessed September 2008.

24. United Nations System Standing Committee on Nutrition. Joint working groups statement on 'The human right of children and adolescents to adequate food and to be free from obesity and related diseases: the responsibilities of food and beverage corporations and related media and marketing industries' issued by the Working Groups on nutrition throughout the life cycle and nutrition, ethics and human rights, Rome (Italy), February 26–March 5, 2007. Available at: http://www.unsystem.org/ scn/Publications/AnnualMeeting/SCN34/34_humanrights.htm. Accessed September 2008.

25. Office of Communications (Ofcom) United Kingdom. Television Advertising of Food and Drink Products to Children, Final statement. 2007. Available at: http://www. ofcom.org.uk/consult/condocs/foodads_new/statement/. Accesses September 2008.

26. Chopra M, Darnton-Hill I. Tobacco and obesity epidemics: not so different after all? BMJ 2004;328(7455):1558–60.

27. Swinburn B. Sustaining dietary changes for preventing obesity and diabetes: lessons learned from the successes of other epidemic control programs. Asia Pac J Clin Nutr 2002;11(Suppl 3):S598–606.

28. Casswell S. Population level policies on alcohol: are they still appropriate given that "alcohol is good for the heart'? Addiction 1997;92(Suppl 1):S81–90.

29. National Obesity TaskForce. Healthy weight 2008-Australia's Future. Canberra (Australia): Department of Health & Ageing; 2003.

30. Tonga Ministry of Health. A national strategy to prevent and control non-communicable diseases in Tonga. Nuku'alofa, Tonga Ministry of Health; 2003.

31. Ministry of Health New Zealand. Healthy eating - healthy action, oranga pumau - oranga kai. Wellington, New Zealand: Ministry of Health; 2002.

32. WHO. Global strategy on diet, physical activity and health: a framework to monitor and evaluate implementation. Geneva (Switzerland): World Health Organisation; 2006.

33. International Food Information Council. Trends in obesity related media coverage. Available at: http://www.ific.org/research/obesitytrends.cfm. Accessed September 2008.

34. Ryan KW, Card-Higginson P, McCarthy SG, et al. Arkansas fights fat: translating research into policy to combat childhood and adolescent obesity. 2006/07. Health Affairs 2006;25(4):992–1004.

35. Denehy J. Health report cards: an idea whose time has come? J Sch Nurs 2004; 20(3):125–6.

36. University of Arkansas for Medical Sciences. Year three evaluation: Arkansas Act 1220 of 2003 to combat childhood obesity. Little Rock (AR): Fay W. Boozman College of Public Health; 2005. 2006.

37. Toh CM, Cutter J, Chew SK. School based intervention has reduced obesity in Singapore. BMJ 2002;324:427.
38. Milio N. Nutrition and health: patterns and policy perspectives in food-rich countries. Soc Sci Med 1989;29(3):413–23.
39. Gostin LO. Public health law in a new century: part I: law as a tool to advance the community's health. JAMA 2000;283(21):2837–41.
40. Haby MM, Vos T, Carter R, et al. A new approach to assessing the health benefit from obesity interventions in children and adolescents: the assessing cost-effectiveness in obesity project. Int J Obes (Lond) 2006;30(10):1463–75.
41. Hastings G, Stead M, McDermott L, et al. Review of the research on the effects of food promotion to children. Glasgow (United Kingdom): Centre for Social Marketing, University of Strathclyde; 2003.
42. Dalmeny K, Hanna E, Lobstein T. Broadcasting bad health: why food marketing to children needs to be controlled. Washington, DC: The International Association of Consumer Food Organizations; 2003.
43. Office de la Protection du Consommateur Quebec. Consumer Protection Act, Section 248. Available at: http://www2.publicationsduquebec.gouv.qc.ca/dynamicSearch/telecharge.php?type=2&;file=/P_40_1/P40_1_A.html. Accessed September 2008.
44. Hawkes C. Marketing food to children: the global regulatory environment. Geneva: World Health Organisation; 2004.
45. Swinburn B, Sacks G, Lobstein T, et al. The 'Sydney Principles' for reducing the commercial promotion of foods and beverages to children. Public Health Nutrition 2008;11:881–6.
46. Hawkes C. Self-regulation of food advertising: what it can, could and cannot do to discourage unhealthy eating habits among children. Nutrition Bulletin 2005;30:374–82.
47. Vereecken CA, Bobelijn K, Maes L. School food policy at primary and secondary schools in Belgium-Flanders: does it influence young people's food habits? Eur J Clin Nutr 2005;59(2):271–7.
48. Lissau I, Poulsen J. Nutrition policy, food and drinks at school and after school care. Int J Obes (Lond) 2005;29(Suppl 2):S58–61.
49. Story M, Kaphingst KM, French S. The role of child care settings in obesity prevention. Future Child 2006;16(1):143–68.
50. Handy SL, Boarnet MG, Ewing R, et al. How the built environment affects physical activity: views from urban planning. Am J Prev Med 2002;23(2 Suppl):64–73.
51. Frank LD, Andresen MA, Schmid TL. Obesity relationships with community design, physical activity, and time spent in cars. Am J Prev Med 2004;27(2):87–96.
52. Hayne CL, Moran PA, Ford MM. Regulating environments to reduce obesity. J Public Health Policy 2004;25(3–4):391–407.
53. Summerbell C, Waters E, Edmunds L, et al. Interventions for preventing obesity in children. Cochrane Database Syst Rev 2005;(3):CD001871.
54. Doak CM, Visscher TLS, Renders CM, et al. The prevention of overweight and obesity in children and adolescents: a review of interventions and programmes. Obes Rev 2006;7:111–36.
55. Flynn MAT, McNeil DA, Maloff B, et al. Reducing obesity and related chronic disease risk in children and youth: a synthesis of evidence with â€˜best practiceâ€™ recommendations. Obes Rev 2006;7:7–66.

56. Economos CD, Hyatt RR, Goldberg JP, et al. A community intervention reduces BMI z-score in children: shape up Somerville first year results. Obesity (Silver Spring) 2007;15(5):1325–36.
57. Taylor RW, McAuley KA, Barbezat W, et al. APPLE project: 2-y findings of a community-based obesity prevention program in primary school age children. Am J Clin Nutr 2007;86(3):735–42.
58. Kain J, Uauy R, Albala C, et al. School-based obesity prevention in Chilean primary school children: methodology and evaluation of a controlled study. Int J Obes Relat Metab Disord 2004;28(4):483–93.
59. Sanigorski A, Bell A, Kremer P, Cuttler R, et al. Reducing unhealthy weight gain in children and its related gradient with socio-economic status through community capacity building: results of a quasi-experimental intervention program (Be Active Eat Well). International Journal of Obesity 2008;32:1060–7
60. Singh AS, Paw Chin A, Maidy MJ, et al. Short-term effects of school-based weight gain prevention among adolescents. Arch Pediatr Adolesc Med 2007;161(6):565–71.
61. Swinburn B, Pryor J, McCabe M, et al. The Pacific OPIC project (Obesity Prevention in Communities): objectives and design. Pacific Health Dialog 2007;14:139–46.
62. Labonte R, Bell Woodard G, Chad K, et al. Community capacity building: a parallel track for health promotion programs. Can J Public Health 2002;93(3):181–2.
63. Hawe P, King L, Noort M, et al. Indicators to help with capacity building in health promotion. NSW Department of Health and the Australian Centre for Health Promotion, Department of Public Health and Community Medicine, University of Sydney; 2000.
64. EPODE. Ensemble prevenons l'obesite des enfants. Available at: www.epode.fr.
65. Donovan R, Henley N. Social marketing: principles and practices. Melbourne (Australia): IP Publishing; 2003.
66. Bellows L, Anderson J, Gould SM, et al. Formative research and strategic development of a physical activity component to a social marketing campaign for obesity prevention in preschoolers. J Community Health 2008;33(3):169–78.
67. Wammes B, Oenema A, Brug J. The evaluation of a mass media campaign aimed at weight gain prevention among young Dutch adults. Obesity (Silver Spring) 2007;15(11):2780–9.
68. Lobstein T, Millstone E. Context for the PorGrow study: Europe's obesity crisis. Obes Rev 2007;8(Suppl 2):7–16.
69. Wake M, Hardy P, Canterford L, et al. Overweight, obesity and girth of Australian preschoolers: prevalence and socio-economic correlates. Int J Obes (Lond) 2004;31:1044–51.
70. Waters E, Ashbolt R, Gibbs L, et al. Double jeopardy: the influence of ethnicity over sociodemographic status on childhood overweight and obesity: findings from an inner urban population of primary school children. Int J Pediatr Obes, 2008; in press.
71. Ogden CL, Carroll MD, Curtin LR, et al. Prevalence of overweight and obesity in the United States, 1999–2004. JAMA 2006;295(13):1549–55.
72. Swinburn B, Egger G. Influence of obesity-producing environments. In: Bray GA, Bouchard C, editors. Handbook of obesity—clinical applications. 2nd editon. New York: Marcel Dekker, Inc; 2004. p. 97–114.
73. Swinburn B, Egger G. Preventive strategies against weight gain and obesity. Obes Rev 2002;3(4):289–301.

Outcome of Eating Disorders

Hans-Christoph Steinhausen, MD, Dipl.Psych., PhD

KEYWORDS

- Anorexia nervosa • Bulimia • Nervosa • Course
- Outcome • Follow-up

Studies in the long-term development of eating disorders are of considerable interest because the etiology of these disorders is not known precisely, and interventions are of limited success in a sizeable proportion of these patients. In the recent past, there has been a remarkable increase in scientific studies of various facets of eating disorders including a notable number of outcome studies. Most of the outcome studies have dealt with anorexia nervosa because it has been recognized as a clinical entity for a more than a century in comparison to bulimia nervosa, which was described and first defined only in 1979 by Russell.[1]

The literature available on the prognosis and outcome of eating disorders is rich in terms of the number of studies, the varying sizes of samples, the outcome parameters, and the conclusions that can be drawn from these studies. As will be shown later in this chapter, less is known about the natural, that is, untreated course, and despite a small number of controlled intervention studies, there is hardly any knowledge as to the long-term effects of intervention.

In this article, separately for anorexia nervosa and bulimia nervosa, a review will be provided first on the limited knowledge of the natural course and the effects of intervention studies. This will be followed by a summarizing review of the various studies on the outcome and prognosis for eating disorders. For anorexia nervosa, it can also be possible to report specifically on the course of the disorder in patients with adolescent onset. Given the larger body of studies addressing these issues in anorexia nervosa rather than in bulimia nervosa, this chapter is thus divided into 2 major but unequal parts, with each providing some major conclusions at the end.

ANOREXIA NERVOSA
Studies of Natural Course

There are only a few studies addressing the natural history of eating behavior, attitudes, and disorders. Most of these studies are based on questionnaires that deal with eating attitudes and behavior; only a few have assessed eating disorders that

Department of Child and Adolescent Psychiatry, University of Zurich, Neumünsterallee 9, Postfach, CH-8032 Zurich, Switzerland
E-mail address: hc.steinhausen@kjpd.uzh.ch

Child Adolesc Psychiatric Clin N Am 18 (2008) 225–242
doi:10.1016/j.chc.2008.07.013
1056-4993/08/$ – see front matter © 2008 Elsevier Inc. All rights reserved.

childpsych.theclinics.com

fulfill clinical criteria of diagnoses and assessment. Among the latter, more information is provided on the natural course of bulimia nervosa than on anorexia nervosa. In conjunction with other studies on eating attitudes and behavior, they provide some limited evidence that a substantial percentage of subjects at risk and untreated cases remain stable with regard to their condition across a considerable time span.[2] Findings from two population studies, namely, the Victorian Adolescent Health Cohort Study in Australia[3] and from Oregon in the United States,[4] show that by young adulthood 11% and 30% of subjects, respectively, had a persistent eating disorder, including partial and full syndromes.

Outcomes

The most exhaustive review of the outcome of anorexia nervosa in the 20th century has been provided by the author.[5] In this review, a total of 119 study series, covering 5,590 patients, that were published in the literature in English and German were analyzed with regard to mortality, global outcome, and other psychiatric disorders at follow-up. A precise description of the review methodology is beyond the scope of this article and can be retrieved in published articles.

In this article, the 4 major outcome parameters of mortality, recovery, improvement, and chronicity and the other psychiatric disorders were analyzed in various ways. First, descriptive means and standard deviations were calculated as shown in **Table 1**. Given the rather wide standard deviations with extreme ranges across the studies and the varying sizes of the patient groups, the means in this table reflect only a central trend.

The mean crude mortality rate amounted to 5.0%. In the surviving patients, on average, full recovery was found in only less than half of the patients, whereas 33% improved, and 20% developed a chronic course of the disorder. Outcome was slightly better for the core symptoms, with normalization of weight occurring in almost 60% of the patients, normalization of menstruation in 57%, and normalization of eating behavior in 47%. However, these slightly higher rates of normalization of the core symptoms, compared with the global outcome rating, may be largely due to the similar total group sizes. Nevertheless, this gap remained, even after adaptation for group size (when only the studies that reported both global outcomes ratings and normalization of the core symptoms were considered).

Additional psychiatric disorders were seen in a large proportion of anorectic patients at follow-up. Frequent diagnoses were neurotic disorders, including anxiety disorders and phobias, affective disorders, substance use disorders, obsessive-compulsive disorder (OCD), and unspecified personality disorders, including borderline states. A few studies reported a high rate of OCD, and a less pronounced rate of histrionic personality disorder and schizophrenia was only rarely observed at follow-up.

The analyses of the data also controlled for 3 major effect variables that might have affected the outcome. Only the 4 major outcome parameters and studies that reported these variables were considered for these analyses. The 3 major effect variables included duration of follow-up (<4 years, 4–10 years, >10 years), age at onset of the disorder (adolescence only vs. mixed samples with onset in adolescence and adulthood), and time period of study (1950–1979; 1980–1989; 1990–1999).

Findings for duration of follow-up are shown in **Table 2**. As one can see, all 4 outcome parameters were significantly affected by duration of follow-up, and all 4 effect sizes were large. With increasing duration of follow-up, mortality rates also increased. In the surviving patients, there was a strong tendency toward recovery with increasing

Table 1
Outcome of anorexia nervosa based on 119 patient series (N = 5,590)

Outcome Variable	Group Size (N)	Rate of Outcome (%)		
		Mean	SD	Range
Mortality	5,334	5.0	5.7	0–2
Recovery	4,575	46.9	19.7	0–92
Improvement	4,472	33.5	17.8	0–75
Chronicity	4,927	20.8	12.8	0–79
Symptom normalization				
Weight	2,245	59.6	15.3	15–92
Menstruation	2,719	57.0	17.2	25–96
Eating behavior	1, 980	46.8	19.6	0–97
Affective disorder	1,972	24.1	16.3	2–67
Neurotic or anxiety disorder	1.478	25.5	14.9	4–61
Obsessive-compulsive disorder	992	12.0	6.4	0–23
Schizophrenia	1,097	4.6	5.7	1–28
Personality disorder				
Unspecified or borderline	1,115	17.4	16.8	0–69
Histrionic	308	16.6	19.9	0–53
Obsessive-compulsive disorder	202	31.4	25.1	0–76
Substance abuse disorder	627	14.6	10.4	2–38

Data from Steinhausen H-C. The outcome of anorexia nervosa in the 20th century. Am J Psychiatry 2002;159:1284–93.

duration of follow-up. The rate of recovery increased whereas the rates of improvement and chronicity declined.

The mortality rate was much lower in the group of younger patients than that in the group with a much wider age at onset of illness, as shown in **Table 3**. The rates of recovery, improvement, and chronicity were more favorable in the group with the younger patients. However, in each instance, in addition to duration of follow-up, the interactions between duration of follow-up and each outcome variable were significant, as shown in **Fig. 1**. The interaction effects showed that the differences between

Table 2
Outcome of anorexia nervosa in 119 patient series by duration of follow-up (N = 3,147)

	Percent of Subjects, by Duration of Follow-up							
	≤4 Years (N = 577)		4–10 Years (N = 2,132)		>10 Years (N = 438)		Analysis	
Outcome Variable	Mean	SD	Mean	SD	Mean	SD	P	Effect Size (%)
Mortality	0.9	2.0	4.9	4.3	9.4	8.3	<0.001	20.4
Recovery	32.6	23.4	47.0	15.7	73.2	16.2	<0.001	30.5
Improvement	32.7	12.7	32.4	14.1	8.5	9.5	<0.001	28.0
Chronicity	34.4	18.5	19.7	10.6	13.7	8.7	<0.001	21.7

Data from Steinhausen H-C. The outcome of anorexia nervosa in the 20th century. Am J Psychiatry 2002;159:1284–93.

Table 3
Outcome of anorexia nervosa in 119 patient series by age at onset (N = 3,099)

Outcome Variable	Adolescents Only (N = 784)		Adolescents and Adults (N = 2,315)		Percent of Subjects, by Age of Subjects			Effect Size (%)		
					F Test					
	Mean	SD	Mean	SD	Effect of Age at Onset	Effect of Duration of Follow-up (df = 2)	Interaction (df = 2)	Age at Onset, y	Duration of Follow-up, y	Interaction
Mortality	1.8	2.5	5.9	5.7	***	***	***	6.6	3.9	3.7
Recovery	57.1	15.0	44.2	21.8	***	***	***	0.6	3.0	0.1
Improvement	25.9	16.7	30.7	16.6	*	***	***	0.02	3.8	0.5
Chronicity	16.9	7.5	23.5	14.9	***	***	***	1.1	2.6	1.2

*$P<0.05$; ***$P<0.001$.
Data from Steinhausen H-C. The outcome of anorexia nervosa in the 20th century. Am J Psychiatry 2002;159:1284–93.

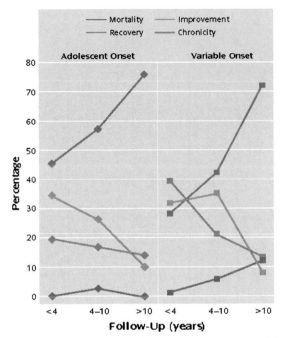

Fig. 1. Outcome of anorexia nervosa in 119 patient series by duration of follow-up and age at onset. A total of 577 patients had less than 4 years of follow-up, 2,132 had 4 to 10 years of follow-up, and 438 had more than 10 years of follow-up. (*From* Steinhausen H-C. The outcome of anorexia nervosa in the 20th century. Am J Psychiatry 2002;159:1284–93; with permission.)

the subgroups with different onsets of illness were wider or narrower or even inverted for the 4 outcome measures, depending on the duration of follow-up. A comparison of the 2 effect sizes, as shown in **Table 4**, indicates that the effect of age at onset was stronger for mortality, whereas the effect of duration of follow-up was stronger for recovery, improvement, and chronicity.

Mortality showed a complex pattern of time trends (**Fig. 2**; see **Table 2**). It was absent both for short and extended study courses in the early studies (with only 1 study each), from 1950 through 1979, whereas it increased linearly in the studies from 1980 to 1989 and from 1990 to 1999, with the highest rate for the most extended studies reported for 1980–1989. There were few differences between the studies for 1980–1989 and the studies for 1990–1999 on the other outcome measures—recovery, improvement, and chronicity—whereas the studies from 1950 through 1979 primarily stood out because of high recovery rates and low rates of improvement and chronicity during short-term courses (<4 years). For all 4 outcome measures, the effect sizes for duration of follow-up were markedly stronger than those for time period.

Prognostic Factors

Not all, but a considerable number of outcome studies also provided some information on prognosis. However, there was a large variability as to the type and number of prognostic factors considered for analysis in the various studies. A summary of

Table 4
Outcome of anorexia nervosa in 119 patient series by time period of study (N = 3,147)

Outcome Variable	Percent of Subjects by Time Period						F Test			Effect Size (%)		
	1950–1979 (N = 256)		1980–1989 (N = 979)		1990–1999 (N = 1,912)		Effect of Time Period	Effect of Duration of Follow-up	Interaction	Time Period, y	Duration of Follow up, y	Interaction
	Mean	SD	Mean	SD	Mean	SD						
Mortality	4.7	5.9	5.2	5.0	4.6	5.4	***	***	***	1.0	6.1	4.6
Recovery	47.0	26.3	49.9	19.5	47.2	20.7	***	***	***	0.1	13.0	14.9
Improvement	28.7	14.5	29.1	15.2	29.3	16.1	n.s.	***	***	—	1.2	1.1
Chronicity	22.2	17.1	20.7	8.7	22.0	15.3	***	***	***	0.3	2.3	1.4

***$P<0.001$.
Data from Steinhausen H-C. The outcome of anorexia nervosa in the 20th century. Am J Psychiatry 2002;159:1284–93.

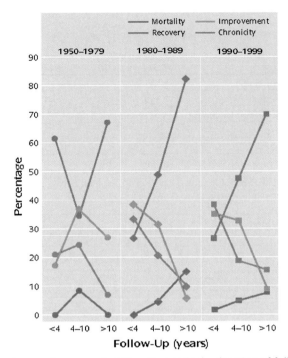

Fig. 2. Outcome of anorexia nervosa in 119 patient series by duration of follow-up and time period of study. A total of 577 patients had less than 4 years of follow-up, 2,132 had 4 to 10 years of follow-up, and 438 had more than 10 years of follow-up. (*From* Steinhausen H-C. The outcome of anorexia nervosa in the 20th century. Am J Psychiatry 2002;159:1284–93; with permission.)

findings across all studies is given in **Table 5**, containing the frequency of studies with identified prognostic factors.

For most of the prognostic factors, the findings were considerably heterogeneous. Most obviously, this interpretation applies to the ambiguous findings regarding age at onset of illness. In addition, most studies indicated that a short duration of symptoms before treatment resulted in a favorable outcome. The impact of the duration of inpatient treatment is unclear because of ambiguous findings across the outcome studies and no definite conclusions could be drawn as to whether lower weight at presentation had long-term effects on outcome.

Furthermore, it is quite clear that vomiting, bulimia, and purgative abuse imply an unfavorable prognosis whereas hyperactivity and dieting as weight-reduction measures did not have any prognostic significance. A small number of studies also showed that premorbid developmental and clinical abnormalities, including eating disorders during childhood, carry the risk for a poor outcome of anorexia nervosa. On the other hand, a good parent–child relationship may protect the patient from a poor outcome.

In addition, the data clearly show that chronicity leads to poor outcome, a finding that implies that there are cases of anorexia nervosa in which treatment is refractory. Some studies provided evidence that the features of histrionic personality disorder indicate a favorable outcome. Furthermore, the features of coexisting

Table 5
Frequency of studies with identified prognostic factors of anorexia nervosa

	Favorable Prognosis (N)	Unfavorable Prognosis (N)	Not Significant (N)
Early age at onset of illness	13	2	14
Short duration of symptoms	14	0	7
Short duration of inpatient treatment	7	0	7
Heavy weight loss	0	8	8
Hyperactivity and dieting	1	9	7
Vomiting	0	—	2
Bulimia and purgative abuse	0	11	2
Pre-morbid developmental or clinical abnormalities	0	4	—
Good parent–child relationship	8	—	3
Chronicity	0	0	0
Hysterical personality	8	7	1
Obsessive-compulsive personality	0	6	1
			8
High socioeconomic status	6	0	8

obsessive-compulsive personality or compulsivity add to chronicity. In a recent 12-year course and outcome predictors analysis, based on a parsimonious empirically based model, 4 predictors of outcome explaining 45% of the variance were identified, that is, sexual problems, impulsivity, long duration of inpatient treatment, and long duration of an eating disorder.[6] Clearly, chronicity is the major background factor in these findings. Finally, no definite conclusions can be drawn from the outcome studies as to the relevance of socioeconomic status.

Adolescent Patients

The just reported findings from follow-up studies in anorexia nervosa have mostly included the full age range at onset of the disorder. When only the adolescent age range at onset was considered, it became clear that the course of the disorder in these young patients might be different from that of those with later onset of the disorder. The smaller series of young patients in the author's review of follow-up studies[5] showed a less serious outcome than that with a mixed group of studies containing patients with either adolescent or later onset of anorexia nervosa. However, adolescent onset was not unequivocally supported as a favorable prognostic factor in all studies.

Given these limited and partly contradictory findings, it seems worthwhile to have a closer look at the outcome of adolescent onset patients, based on more recent findings. The latter stem from the, so far, largest outcome study performed with patients who had an adolescent onset of anorexia nervosa. Within the International Collaborative Outcome Study of Eating Disorders in Adolescence (ICOSEDA), the author and his associates studied the clinical features, treatment, and outcome in consecutive cohorts of adolescent patients at 5 sites in former West Berlin and East Berlin, Germany, Zurich, Switzerland, Sofia, Bulgaria, and Bucharest, Romania.[7]

All samples consisted of series of consecutively admitted patients who were initially seen in the 80s and early 90s at the 5 sites. All 338 patients fulfilled the ICD-10 Classification of Mental and Behavioural Disorders criteria for the various forms of eating disorders. The samples were predominantly composed of anorectic patients, with only the Berlin sample and the Zurich sample having 10% each of patients suffering from either bulimia or atypical eating disorders. Almost all patients were female (between 90% and 100%). The mean age at admission for the entire sample was 14.7 ($\pm$ 1.9 SD) years, and the mean age at onset of the disorder was 13.9 ($\pm$ 1.7 SD) years.

The entire cohort of patients was invited for follow-up assessment. The dropout rate at follow-up was acceptable in the West Berlin (10%) and Sofia (1.3%) samples and was non-existent in the Bucharest sample. In contrast, the dropout rate was sizeable in both the East Berlin (43.2%) and the Zurich (43.8%) samples. Thus, extensive analyses, based on comparison of participants and nonparticipants in the East Berlin sample and the Zurich sample, were mandatory to see whether refusal resulted in a serious bias of these follow-up samples. As a result of comparisons across 92 individual items, it was concluded that dropout was not due to any serious selection bias. The follow-up sample comprised a total of 241 patients, which was reassessed with semi-structured personal interviews at a mean age of 21.8 ($\pm$ 3.2 SD) years, after a mean follow-up period of 6.4 ($\pm$ 3.0 SD) years.

As one would expect from a collaborative study with such diverse cultural sites and health systems, the provided treatment varied considerably both in terms of types of intervention and quantity of treatment. On average, the entire sample had spent 6% of the total follow-up period as inpatients and 23% as outpatients. Taken together, the total time spent in any form of treatment amounted to 30% of the entire follow-up period. Half of the sample required a second hospitalization, a quarter a third, 10% a fourth, and 5% a fifth hospitalization. Significant predictors of readmission were a combination of family psychopathology, history, and treatment variables, including paternal alcoholism, history of AN in the family, eating disorder in infancy, periodic overactivity, lower weight increase at first admission, and lower body mass index (BMI) at first discharge. Clearly, readmissions carried the risk for later poor psychosocial and psychiatric outcomes.[8]

In this young sample, the average crude mortality rate was only 2.9% and thus lower than that calculated for the previously reported analysis of the literature, which was 5%.[5] The outcome of the eating disorder itself was also more favorable. Around 80% of the sample had a normalization of the core symptoms of weight, eating behavior, and menstruation at follow-up. On the diagnostic level, a total of 70% was free from any eating disorder whereas 10% still suffered from anorexia nervosa and another 20% had either bulimia nervosa or an atypical eating disorder.

In the ICOSEDA the author also looked at the psychosocial status and other psychiatric disorders than the eating disorder at follow-up. Findings based on a comparison of different outcome criteria are shown in **Table 6**. West Berlin data are missing in this table because no other psychiatric disorder than the eating disorder was assessed in this patient group. Starting from the previously described mean frequency of no eating disorder in 70% of the total sample, one can see from the table that a good or fair psychosocial outcome was observed in a similar mean proportion of 71%, with only a statistical trend for any differences across sites. Three quarters of the entire sample did not have another psychiatric disorder at follow-up. The rate was significantly lower for the Zurich sample. The other psychiatric disorders in the sample were affective disorders (N = 25), OCD (N = 8), anxiety disorder (N = 8), somatoform disorders (N = 9), substance abuse (N = 3), schizophrenia (N = 2), and other disorders (N = 21). Among those who had an eating disorder at follow-up, 40% also had an associated other psychiatric disorder.

The outcome is worse if one combines the criteria, as one can also see from **Table 6**. Only slightly more than half of the patients are free from both an eating

Table 6
Comparison of different outcome—criteria in 4 samples of adolescent onset eating disorder (N = 191)

	East Berlin, Germany (N = 67) %	Zurich, Switzerland (N = 36) %	Sofia, Bulgaria (N = 47) %	Bucharest, Romania (N = 41) %	Total (N = 191) %
No eating disorder	79	64	81	54	70
Good or fair psychosocial outcome	82	67	64	64	71
No other psychiatric disorder	86	56	81	73	76
No eating disorder or other psychiatric disorder	67	44	68	42	55
No eating disorder, no other psychiatric disorder, and good or fair psychosocial outcome	62	42	57	34	51

disorder and any other psychiatric disorder, with the Zurich and the Bucharest patients having even significantly lower rates than the other 2 groups. When considering the most complex outcome measure, that is, the combination of being free from an eating disorder and any other psychiatric disorder and enjoying a good or fair psychosocial outcome, then only half of the sample fulfills this optimal criterion of mental health. This most complex outcome criterion is significantly worse in the Zurich and in the Bucharest sample than in the other 2 samples.

Finally, prognostic factors were also analyzed in the ICOSEDA. In contrast to previous studies, an exhaustive list of potential predictors of the outcome were tested and various outcome criteria were considered. In addition, multiple regression analyses were performed to control for an overlap of prognostic factors and to identify the essential associations. In these extended analyses, only a few out of 17 predictors were significant. The BMI at follow-up was predicted by the BMI at initial assessment and treatment adherence (in terms of a negative association with rejection of premature termination of treatment). A more complex criterion, namely, an eating disorder score composed of 5 core symptoms (ie, dieting, vomiting, bulimic episodes, laxative abuse, and irregular menstruation), was more abnormal, with longer duration of outpatient treatment and rejections or premature termination of treatments. The same 2 variables and another psychiatric disorder than the eating disorder at follow-up jointly also predicted the total outcome score, which was composed of the eating disorder symptoms and 5 additional psychosocial items reflecting sexuality and the quality of social relationships.

Thus, the consideration of a large list of prognostic factors in rather parsimonious analytic models resulted in few significant predictors of the outcome in this young sample of patients. Irrespective of the outcome criterion, the most consistent finding was the unfavorable role that rejection or premature termination of treatment played for the long-term course of the eating disorders. Second, the findings point to a treatment-refractory subgroup, because the outcome deteriorated with increasing duration of outpatient treatment. Both findings are indicative of the pivotal function that treatment variables have for the outcome of adolescent eating disorders.

Other more recent outcome studies on adolescent patients support the general finding that the course of anorexia nervosa is more favorable in this young age group than in older patients. This has been shown for various European patient series. In a controlled study from Germany with a prospective 10-year follow-up, 69% were fully recovered and none of the patients died. However, half of the patients had an axis I disorder, whereas almost a quarter met the full criteria for a personality disorder, and depressive, anxious, and obsessive-compulsive features were more common in the long-term recovered patients than in the controls.[9,10] Similarly, a 9-year follow-up study in Norway found a high recovery rate of 82% and no mortality but frequent axis I diagnoses at follow-up and substantially more internalizing problems in former patients than in their siblings.[11,12] A favorable outcome of adolescent onset anorexia nervosa in terms of recovery was also reported by 2 studies from Sweden. However, these findings were associated with poor psychosocial outcomes, frequent depression, and other psychiatric problems in a sizeable proportion of the subjects.[13–15] Finally, the findings of 2 North American studies also concurs with the conclusion that younger age is associated with better prognosis.[16,17]

Conclusions

The analysis of a large body of follow-up studies across various age groups and several studies addressing more specifically the age range of adolescence lead to various conclusions as to the long-term course of anorexia nervosa. As a first general conclusion, one has to state that anorexia nervosa is a mental illness with a serious course and outcome in many afflicted individuals. This conclusion is based on the high crude mortality rate that increases with the length of follow-up and is corroborated by an analysis of an almost 18-fold increase in mortality in patients with anorexia nervosa, including a high suicide rate[18] and other register-based findings of an increased rate of premature death due to anorexia nervosa.[19,20] This conclusion is also supported by the high rate of chronic courses, which may be expected in approximately 20% of the cases across all ages at onset of the disorder. The seriousness of the course of anorexia nervosa is further documented by the fact that at follow-up more than half of the patients showed either a complete or a partial eating disorder in combination with another psychiatric disorder or another psychiatric disorder without an eating disorder. A 40% probability of a comorbid mental disorder can be expected in the younger patients with an eating disorder at follow-up.

The second conclusion has to address the mitigating factors of the outcome of anorexia nervosa. Age at onset of the disorder and duration of follow-up are definitely important. Onset of the disorder during adolescence is associated with lower crude mortality rates and a better outcome of the eating disorder per se. However, there is a relatively high rate of other psychiatric disorders in former adolescent patients at follow-up. It is less certain whether other psychiatric disorders, including comorbid disorder at follow-up, occur at a lower rate than that in patients who are older at onset of the disorder. The data based on comparable methods are simply lacking for this type of comparison. Furthermore, it must also be kept in mind that onset of anorexia nervosa before puberty has a poor outcome as shown in clinical reports based on old studies.[21,22] The other mitigating factor, namely, duration of follow-up, shows a clear trend of an improved global outcome of anorexia nervosa with increasing course so that there is also substantial hope, even for some rather complicated cases.

Third, there is limited knowledge of how intervention actually affects the course of anorexia nervosa. It may be that an early intervention, short duration of inpatient treatment, and adherence to the treatment program are prognostically favorable. However, all these variables may only reflect latent clinical factors in terms of severity of the disorder and patient characteristics. Clearly, the scarcity of controlled intervention studies with a sufficient duration of follow-up represents a major obstacle in the field of outcome research in anorexia nervosa. A notable exception is the London family therapy study with its documentation that treatment effects were kept at a 5-year follow-up.[23]

Finally, our understanding of the prognosis of anorexia nervosa has serious limitations. Quite obviously, vomiting, bulimia and purgative abuse, chronicity, and obsessive-compulsive features represent unfavorable prognostic factors, whereas hysterical personality features represent the only favorable prognostic factor that has been documented with very little conflicting evidence in the literature. However, the lack of replication of the factors in the data of the ICOSEDA data set with adolescent onset patients and a rigorous control of overlapping effects of various prognostic factors ask for a more conservative interpretation. In the same way, the variability in the findings on various other prognostic factors precludes any delineation of clear and simple rules as to the individual prognosis in a patient suffering from anorexia nervosa.

Despite the fact that more recent prospective outcome studies[16,17,24] have analyzed time trends of certain features of anorexia nervosa and, thus, focused more on the process rather than on the outcome, much has still to be learned about the continuity and discontinuity of anorexia nervosa and the factors influencing this process.

BULIMIA NERVOSA

Due to its characteristic peak of onset in early adulthood, there is only a small body of literature on bulimia nervosa in adolescence. So far, there have been no separate follow-up studies on this group of young patients. Furthermore, the available outcome studies do not allow the separation of findings that are relevant for adolescent patients only. Thus, the following description reports findings on the course and prognosis of bulimia nervosa without considering separate age groups.

Natural Course

Only a small series of longitudinal studies have used either screening measures of a 2-stage approach with a sequence of screening and interview that provide information on the natural history of bulimia nervosa. Several screening studies indicate that, in general, there is remarkable stability of symptoms and diagnoses across time.[25–30]

Studies using the 2-stage approach consolidate the impression of stability in the natural course of bulimia nervosa. Based on a consecutive series of adults who attended general practice, King[31] found a high stability of diagnostic status at follow-up 12 to 18 months later. At the second follow-up 2 to 3 years after the first assessment,[32] 3 of 5 of the original patients were still diagnosed as being bulimic, and there was little change in patients with the full syndrome of bulimia nervosa or in those with partial syndromes between the first and second follow-up. Lewinsohn and colleagues[33] observed an increase in lifetime prevalence rates for bulimia nervosa of 0.8% in adolescence to 2.8% in young adulthood.

In a large sample of female adolescents, Patton and colleagues[28] diagnosed bulimia nervosa or partial syndromes and calculated a mean point prevalence rate for these 2 categories of 2.1% across teens and of 1.9% in young adulthood. Finally, Keller and colleagues[34] also reported high rates of chronicity, relapse recurrence, and psychosocial morbidity in 30 women with bulimia nervosa. Their findings show that almost one-third of the subjects remained in the index episode after entry into the study.

Outcomes

Several reviews of the course and outcome of bulimia nervosa have been published in the recent past. Whereas the reviews by Keel and Mitchell[3] and Steinhausen[35] covered the outcome literature until 1997, the most recent and exhaustive review by Quadflieg and Fichter[36] also included 8 recent studies that had been published between 1997 and 2002.

The author's review covered 24 outcome studies with a total of 1,383 patients who were followed up at a mean of 31 months in 15 studies containing this information (Steinhausen, 1999).[35] The onset of the disorder had been between 14 and 22 years and the patients had been predominantly treated on an outpatient basis including some sort of psychotherapy with additional drug treatment in 6 studies and psychopharmacotherapy alone in 2 studies. In these 24 studies, crude mortality rates amounted to 0.7 % (range, 0%–6%) and were only slightly higher than those reported by Keel and Mitchell,[3] that is, 0.3% (range, 1%–3%). These figures predominantly indicate the frequencies of individuals with bulimia nervosa who were dead at follow-up. There is less information on mortality that is directly attributable to bulimia nervosa. Quadflieg and Fichter[36] in their review obtained crude death rates of 0% to 3.1% after varying follow-up periods of 2.0 to 11.5 years. So far, there are no studies reporting standardized mortality rates.

The major outcome parameters of bulimia nervosa based on the review of 24 outcome studies by Steinhausen[35] were 47.5% (range, 22%–66%) for recovery, 26% (range, 0%–67%) for improvement, and 26% (range, 0%–43%) for chronification. According to the review by Keel and Mitchell,[3] controlled treatment studies as compared with ordinary follow-up studies resulted in higher short-term recovery rates after 6 or 12 months (53% or 48% in contrast to 31%). However, this superiority was markedly lower after a follow-up interval of 5 years (54% versus 48%). Strong evidence for continuation of early adolescent bulimia nervosa was revealed in 1 more recent study showing that there was a 9-fold increase in risk for late adolescent bulimia nervosa and a 20-fold increase in risk for adult bulimia nervosa.[37]

According to some recent studies, the average recovery rate in adulthood is around 48% (eg, the study by Fairburn and colleagues[38]) whereas other studies greatly exceed this figure. A good outcome was seen in 58% in a 4-year follow-up on bulimia nervosa including subthreshold cases.[4] Even higher recovery rates were obtained by Ben-Tovim and colleagues,[39] who included less impaired outpatients from secondary and tertiary services only and found a recovery rate of 77%, and in the follow-up study by Fichter and Quadflieg[40] with a recovery rate of 55% after 2 years and 71% after 6 years, after intensive inpatient treatment in a primary service hospital. The high recovery rate was kept even after 12 years, with 70% showing no major eating disorder and few transitions to anorexia nervosa or binge-eating disorders.[41] However, a large international collaborative study observed higher rates of crossover in the eating disorders, that is, in 32 of the 88 patients, anorexia was followed by bulimia, and the reverse order was seen in 93 of 350 of eating disordered patients, with crossover occurring for most of the affected individuals by the fifth year of the illness.[42] High instability across the eating disorders was also observed within a 30-month follow-up of adult patients, with just a third of the patients retaining their original diagnosis.[43,44]

In contrast to anorexia nervosa, there is no strong association between recovery and duration of follow-up in bulimia nervosa. Quadflieg and Fichter[36] found a moderate correlation coefficient of $r = 0.26$ and concluded that, presumably, no stable recovery rate can be expected for the first 5 to 6 years after intake into a study on the long-term course of bulimia nervosa. After about 10 years, a proportion of two-thirds to three-quarters of former patients with bulimia nervosa can be expected to show at least partial recovery.

At present, the data on the chronicity and relapse rate are still far from being conclusive. The estimated relapse rate of 30% for bulimia nervosa in a time period of

6 months to 6 years by Keel and Mitchell[3] and the average progression to a chronic disease state of 26% by Steinhausen[35] do not allow the differentiation between chronic cases, with no remission at any point of the follow-up period and cases showing a relapse at the time of the follow-up assessment. In addition, the large variability in the findings precludes any definite conclusion as to the association of duration of follow-up and poor outcome.

A few studies analyzed the crossover from bulimia nervosa to anorexia nervosa. However, a lack of diagnostic accuracy and that of diagnostic hierarchy rules before the fourth edition of the Diagnostic and Statistical Manual of Mental Disorders (DSM-IV) may have led to an overestimation of figures. Recent studies indicate rather low frequencies of crossover to anorexia nervosa between 0.6% and 14.1% and varying length of follow-up.[36] In contrast, the crossover to eating disorders not otherwise specified (EDNOS) is much higher and amounts to figures between 1.6% and 26% in various studies and also depends on the duration of follow-up.[36] These high rates may well reflect chronic cases of eating disorders.

Only a few studies have assessed other psychiatric disorders than bulimia nervosa, so the figures calculated by Steinhausen[35] may only be tentative. According to this review, 25% (range, 9%–37%) of the patients hadan affective disorder, 5% (range, 2%–18%) a neurotic/anxiety disorder, 0.7% (range, 3%–5%) a personality disorder, and 10% (range, 2%–26%), a substance use disorder.

The psychosocial outcome in bulimia nervosa has also received only limited interest in follow-up studies. Better social outcome tends to match recovered and improved eating disorders outcome, and the patient groups tend to function less well than community control samples at follow-up. Furthermore, patients with bulimia nervosa tend to function better in terms of their social adjustment rather than their personal and sexual relationships.[36]

Prognostic Factors

The 2 recent reviews by Steinhausen[35] and Quadflieg and Fichter[36] allow a summary of the current knowledge on the significance of various prognostic factors. Findings based on relatively few studies are summarized in **Table 7**. The overall picture of the prognosis in bulimia nervosa is even less clear than in anorexia nervosa. Those studies that indicate a favorable function of some prognostic factors like younger age at onset, short duration of illness before treatment, severity of the disorder, or a positive history of alcohol abuse are clearly outbalanced by a similar or even higher number of studies with no significant findings. Borderline personality symptoms clearly stand out among the unfavorable factors because of a replicated status in various studies. Comorbid psychiatric disorders, such as depression, anxiety disorder, or alcohol abuse, also have a negative effect on outcome. The same is true also for low self-esteem whereas findings on impulsiveness are equivocal. However, all these findings on the prognostic function of comorbid disorders and personality features need further replication.

Summary and Conclusions

After the first description of bulimia nervosa by Russell,[1] the outcome of bulimia nervosa has only been studied since 1983. Thus, the number of outcome studies and their sample size is considerably smaller than in anorexia nervosa. Nevertheless, some major conclusions can be drawn from these analyses and some comparisons can be made between the outcomes of the two disorders.

Quite obviously, treatment of bulimia nervosa is efficient in the short term, whereas the longer-term outcome shows a similar, though only slightly, better, result than that

Table 7
Frequencies of studies with identified prognostic factors in bulimia nervosa

Prognostic Factors	Favorable	Unfavorable	Not Significant
Younger age at onset	2	—	6
Short duration of illness before treatment	6	—	6
Severity of the disorder	4	—	3
Premorbid anorexia nervosa	—	—	6
Premorbid substance abuse	—	—	3
Premorbid obesity	—	—	1
Family history of alcohol abuse	1	1	1
Family history of depression	—	1	2
Coexistent borderline personalizing symptoms	—	6	1
Coexistent depression	—	2	—
Coexistent anxiety disorder	—	1	—
Coexistent alcohol abuse	—	1	—
Low self-esteem	—	2	—
Impulsiveness	—	1	1

in anorexia nervosa. Unfortunately, the rates of relapse and chronicity of bulimia nervosa are still considerable. However, the rate of mortality is low, and anorexia nervosa is certainly the more dangerous and deadly eating disorder. Diagnostic crossover from bulimia nervosa to anorexia nervosa or the more recently introduced binge-eating disorder is a rather rare phenomenon, whereas the high rates of EDNOS may explain a large proportion of chronic courses. Social adjustment and the quality of personal relationships normalize in most of the affected patients. However, there is a substantial number of women who suffer not only from persistent bulimic symptoms but also from social and, most notably, from sexual impairment.

At present, the study of prognostic factors in bulimia nervosa does not allow any definite conclusions because the picture is diverse and partly also contradictory. Sampling bias (eg, the inclusion of a high rate of chronic cases) and lack of control for overlapping risk factors by use of adequate analytic models may have contributed to this limitation and have to be overcome in future research. Similar to anorexia nervosa, it would be most hazardous to delineate any conclusions from research to the prognosis of an individual patient.

Because most studies on the course of bulimia nervosa are of recent origin, they have profited more strongly from prospective rather than retrospective samples that have been used in many follow-up studies of anorexia nervosa. However, there are also limitations as precisely addressed in the review by Quadflieg and Fichter.[36] These limitations include the heterogeneity of the diagnostic definition reflecting the changes in psychiatric nosology in the recent past and the variations in the definition of outcome measures, as is true also for outcome studies of anorexia nervosa. Similarly, further limitations pertain to outcome studies of both eating disorders, namely, the lack of studies on the natural course without treatment and an insufficient focus on the process rather than the outcome of the disorder. As a consequence, it is not clear how long a given person suffered from the disorder nor is there differentiation between relapse or chronic state of the disorder at follow-up. Finally, so far the outcome of bulimia nervosa has not yet been studied in males.

Future studies have to address these limitations. It may be expected that with more systematic diagnostic categories, standardized assessment procedures, control of interventions, longer follow-up periods, and a stronger focus on the process of change in the individual patients, a more refined picture of the outcome of bulimia nervosa will emerge. It is hoped that these future studies will also concentrate on young patients with onset of the disorder during adolescence.

REFERENCES

1. Russell G. Bulimia nervosa: an ominous variant of anorexia nervosa. Psychol Med 1979;9:429–48.
2. Rathner G. Aspects of the natural history of normal and disordered eating and some methodological considerations. In: Herzog W, Deter H-C, Vandereycken W, editors. The course of eating disorders: long-term follow-up studies of anorexia and bulimia nervosa. Berlin: Springer-Verlag; 1992. p. 273–303.
3. Keel P, Mitchell JE. Outcome in bulimia nervosa. Am J Psychiatry 1997;154: 313–21.
4. Bogh EH, Rokkedal K, Valbak K. A 4-year follow-up on bulimia nervosa. Eur Eat Disord Rev 2005;13:48–53.
5. Steinhausen H-C. The outcome of anorexia nervosa in the 20th century. Am J Psychiatry 2002;159:1284–93.
6. Fichter MM, Quadflieg N, Hedlund S. Twelve-year course and outcome predictors of anorexia nervosa. Int J Eat Disord 2006;39(2):87–100.
7. Steinhausen H-C, Boyadjieva S, Griogoroiu-Serbanescu M, et al. The outcome of adolescent eating disorders. Findings from an international collaborative study. Eur Child Adolesc Psychiatry 2003;12(Suppl 1):S91–8.
8. Steinhausen HC, Grigoroiu-Serbanescu MG, Boyadjieva S, et al. Course and predictors of rehospitalization in adolescent anorexia nervosa in a multisite study. Int J Eat Disord 2008;41(1):29–36.
9. Holtkamp K, Muller B, Heussen N, et al. Depression, anxiety, and obsessionality in long-term recovered patients with adolescent-onset anorexia nervosa. Eur Child Adolesc Psychiatry 2005;14(2):106–10.
10. Herpertz-Dahlmann B, Müller B, Herpertz S, et al. Prospective 10-year follow-up in adolescent anorexia nervosa–course, outcome, psychiatric comorbidity, and psychosocial adaptation. J Child Psychol Psychiatry 2001;42(5):603–12.
11. Halvorsen I, Andersen A, Heyerdahl S. Good outcome of adolescent onset anorexia nervosa after systematic treatment. Intermediate to long-term follow-up of a representative county-sample. Eur Child Adolesc Psychiatry 2004; 13(5):295–306.
12. Halvorsen I, Andersen A, Heyerdahl S. Girls with anorexia nervosa as young adults self-reported and parent-reported emotional and behavioural problems compared with siblings. Eur Child Adolesc Psychiatry 2005;14(7):397–406.
13. Nilsson KB, Hagglof B. Long-term follow-up of adolescent onset anorexia nervosa in northern Sweden. Eur Eat Disord Rev 2005;13:89–100.
14. Wentz E, Gillberg C, Gillberg C, et al. Ten-year follow-up of adolescent-onset anorexia nervosa: psychiatric disorders and overall functioning scales. J Child Psychol Psychiatry 2001;42(5):613–22.
15. Ivarsson T, Råstam M, Wentz E, et al. Depressive disorders in teenage-onset anorexia nervosa: a controlled longitudinal, partly community-based study. Compr Psychiatry 2000;41(5):398–403.

16. Strober M, Freeman R, Morrell W. The long-term course of severe anorexia nervosa in adolescents: survival analysis of recovery, relapse, and outcome predictors over 10–15 years in a prospective study. Int J Eat Disord 1997;22: 339–60.

17. Herzog DB, Dorer DJ, Keel PK, et al. Recovery and relapse in anorexia and bulimia nervosa: a 7.5-year follow-up study. J Am Acad Child Adolesc Psychiatry 1999;38(7):829–37.

18. Nielsen S, MØller-Madsen S, Isager T, et al. Standardized mortality in eating disorders—a quantitative summary of previously published and new evidence. J Psychosom Res 1998;44:413–34.

19. Millar HR, Wardall F, Vyvyan JP, et al. Anorexia nervosa mortality in Northeast Scotland, 1965–1999. Am J Psychiatry 2005;162(4):753–7.

20. Birmingham CL, Su J, Hlynsky JA, et al. The mortality rate from anorexia nervosa. Int J Eat Disord 2005;38(2):143–6.

21. Russell G. Anorexia nervosa of early onset and its impact on puberty. In: Cooper PJ, Stein A, editors. Feeding problems and eating disorders in children and adolescents. Chur (Switzerland): Harwood Academic Publishers; 1992. p. 85–112.

22. Russell JD, Kopec-Schrader E, Rey JM, et al. The Parental Bonding Instrument in adolescent patients with anorexia nervosa. Acta Psychiatr Scand 1992;86(3): 236–9.

23. Eisler I, Dare C, Russell GF, et al. Family and individual therapy in anorexia nervosa. A 5-year follow-up. Arch Gen Psychiatry 1997;54(11):1025–30.

24. Steinhausen H-C, Seidel R, Winkler Metzke C. Evaluation of treatment and intermediate and long-term outcome of adolescent eating disorder. Psychosom Med 2000;30:1089–98.

25. Yager J, Landsverk J, Edelstein CK. A 20-month follow-up study of 628 women with eating disorders. I. Course and severity. Am J Psychiatry 1987;144:86–94.

26. Drewnowski A, Yee DK, Krahn DD. Bulimia in college women—incidence and recovery rates. Am J Psychiatry 1988;145:733–5.

27. Johnson C, Tobin DL, Lipkin J. Epidemiologic changes in bulimic behavior among female adolescents over a five-year period. Int J Eat Disord 1989;8: 647–55.

28. Patton GC, Coffey C, Sawyer SM. The outcome of adolescent eating disorders: findings from the Victorian adolescent health cohort study. Eur Child Adolesc Psychiatry 2003;12(Suppl 1):S25–9.

29. Striegel-Moore RH, Silberstein LR, Frensch P, et al. A prospective study of disordered eating among college students. Int J Eat Disord 1989;8:499–509.

30. Steinhausen H-C, Gavez S, Winkler Metzke C. Psychosocial correlates, outcome, and stability of abnormal adolescent eating behavior in community samples of young people. Int J Eat Disord 2005;37:1–8.

31. King MB. Eating disorders in a general practice population. Prevalence, characteristics and follow-up at 18 months. Psychol Med Monogr Suppl 1989;14(Suppl): 1–34.

32. King MB. The natural history of eating pathology in attenders to primary medical care. Int J Eat Disord 1991;10:379–88.

33. Lewinsohn PM, Striegel-Moore RH, Seeley JR. Epidemiology and natural course of eating disorders in young women from adolescence to young adulthood. J Am Acad Child Adolesc Psychiatry 2000;39:1284–92.

34. Keller MB, Herzog DB, Lavori PW, et al. The naturalistic history of bulimia nervosa: extraordinarily high rates of chronicity, elapse, recurrence, and psychosocial morbidity. Int J Eat Disord 1992;12:1–9.

35. Steinhausen H-C. Eating disorders. In: Steinhausen H-C, Verhulst F, editors. Risks and outcomes in developmental psychopathology. Oxford (UK): Oxford University Press; 1999. p. 210–30.
36. Quadflieg N, Fichter MM. The course and outcome of bulimia nervosa. Eur Child Adolesc Psychiatry 2003;12(Suppl 1):99–109.
37. Kotler LA, Cohen P, Davies M, et al. Longitudinal relationships between childhood, adolescent, and adult eating disorders. J Am Acad Child Adolesc Psychiatry 2001;40(12):1434–40.
38. Fairburn CG, Cooper Z, Doll HA, et al. The natural course of bulimia nervosa and binge eating disorder in young women. Arch Gen Psychiatry 2000;57:659–65.
39. Ben-Tovim DI, Walker K, Gilchrist P, et al. Outcome in patients with eating disorders: a 5-year study. Lancet 2001;357:1254–7.
40. Fichter MM, Quadflieg N. Six-year course of bulimia nervosa. Int J Eat Disord 1997;22(4):361–84.
41. Fichter MM, Quadflieg N. Twelve-year course and outcome of bulimia nervosa. Psychol Med 2004;34(8):1395–406.
42. Tozzi F, Thornton LM, Klump KL, et al. Symptom fluctuation in eating disorders: correlates of diagnostic crossover. Am J Psychiatry 2005;162(4):732–40.
43. Milos G, Spindler A, Schnyder U, et al. Instability of eating disorder diagnoses: prospective study. Br J Psychiatry 2005;187:573–8.
44. Eddy KT, Dorer DJ, Franko DL, et al. Diagnostic crossover in anorexia nervosa and bulimia nervosa: implications for DSM-V. Am J Psychiatry 2008;165:245–50.

Index

Note: Page numbers of article titles are in **boldface** type.

A

Abuse, substance, adolescent eating disorders and, 41
ADHD. See *Attention-deficit hyperactivity disorder (ADHD)*.
Adolescent(s)
    eating disorder not otherwise specified in, cognitive-behavioral therapy for, 154
    eating disorders in. See Binge eating disorder; Bulimia nervosa; *specific eating disorders, e.g.,* Anorexia nervosa.
Adolescent anorexia nervosa. See *Anorexia nervosa.*
Adolescent eating disorders. See *Eating disorders.*
Affective disorders, adolescent eating disorders and, 39
Amenorrhea
    reproductive function related to, 119–120
    secondary, defined, 119
Anorexia nervosa, 25–26, 32–33
    body weight and, 11–13
    classification of, 34–35
    comorbidity of, 26
    diagnostic criteria for, 32
    dopamine and, 104
    epidemiology of, 26, 36
    family interventions in, **159–173**
        history of, 159–160
        multiple-family day treatment, 166–169
        randomized controlled trials of, 162–164
        stages of treatment, 165–166
        theoretic model of, 164–165
        uncontrolled open studies of, 161
    food taste and, 102
    leptin levels in, 118–119
    leptin-mediated neuroendocrine alterations in, **117–129**
        amenorrhea and reproductive function effects of, 119–120
        bone formation effects of, 120–121
        HPA axis in, 119
        hyperactivity, 121–122
        neuronal function effects of, 122
    natural course of, studies of, 225–226
    neuroimaging in, 100–101
    neurotransmission/receptor functioning in, 104–105
    outcome of, 232–235
    prognostic factors for, 229–232
    psychological and behavioral characteristics associated with, 25–26
    serotonin and, 104–105

Child Adolesc Psychiatric Clin N Am 18 (2008) 243–255
doi:10.1016/S1056-4993(08)00092-8

childpsych.theclinics.com

Anorexia nervosa (*continued*)
    stimulus provocation in, 102
    treatment of
        body image therapy in, 138
        coercive pressure in, 132–133
        cognitive behavioral approaches in, **147–158.** See also *Cognitive-behavioral therapy, in adolescent anorexia and bulimia nervosa.*
        day care management in, 134–135
        family-based interventions in, 139–141
        further research on, 141
        group psychotherapy in, 138–139
        individual psychotherapy in, 137–138
        inpatient, 131–132
            full-time, vs. outpatient treatment, 133–134
        involuntary, 132–133
        multimodal approach in, 135–141
        nutritional counseling in, 136–137
        nutritional rehabilitation in, 136
        outpatient, vs. full-time inpatient treatment, 133–134
        overview of, **131–145**
        pharmacotherapy in, 175–178
        settings in, 131–135
    visual presentation of food/drinks and, 102
Anxiety disorders, adolescent eating disorders and, 40
Anxiety management, in eating disorders prevention, 75–76
Arkansas Child and Adolescent Obesity Initiative, 213
ASDs. See *Autistic spectrum disorders (ASDs).*
Attentional biases, weight- and shape-related, reducing of, in eating disorders prevention, 76
Attention-deficit hyperactivity disorder (ADHD), adolescent eating disorders and, 41–42
Autistic spectrum disorders (ASDs), feeding problems in, 19–20

B

Behavior(s)
    eating, biology of, 96–97
    eating-disordered
        in overweight youth, seqeulae of, 59
        psychiatric aspects of, 60–61
    feeding, problematic, eating disorders related to, 70
    sedentary, changes in, for obesity in children and adolescents, 194–195
    suicidal, obesity and, 53–54
    weight control, inappropriate, 57–58
Behavioral modification techniques, for obesity in children and adolescents, 192–194. See also *Obesity, behavioral modification techniques for.*
Behavioral therapy, evidence-based, for obesity in children and adolescents, **189–198.** See also *Obesity, evidence-based behavioral treatment of.*
Bias(es), attentional, weight- and shape-related, reducing of, in eating disorders prevention, 76
Binge eating disorder
    body weight and, 10–11

comorbidity of, 26
described, 26
epidemiology of, 26
neuroimaging in, 108
psychiatric comorbidity with, 58–59
Body composition, 3–9
    developmental aspects related to, 9–10
Body fat distribution, 3–9
Body image, bulimia nervosa and, 103
Body image therapy, in adolescent anorexia nervosa management, 138
Body weight
    anorexia nervosa and, 11–13
    binge eating disorder and, 10–11
    bulimia nervosa and, 10
    developmental aspects related to, 9–10
    eating disorders and, 10–13
    parental overemphasis on, eating disorders related to, 70–71
Bone formation, leptin-mediated neuroendocrine alterations in anorexia nervosa effects
    on, 120–121
Breakfast eating, in eating disorders prevention, 75
Bulimia nervosa, 26, 33–34, 236–240
    body image and, 103
    body weight and, 10
    classification of, 34–35
    comorbidity of, 26
    described, 26
    diagnostic criteria for, 33
    disgust and, 103
    dopamine and, 105
    epidemiology of, 26, 36
    natural course of, 236
    neuroimaging in, 101
    neurotransmission/receptor functioning in, 105–106
    opioids and, 105–106
    outcomes of, 236–238
    prognostic factors for, 238
    reward and, 103–104
    serotonin and, 105
    stimulus provocation in, 102–104
    treatment of
        cognitive behavioral approaches in, **147–158.** See also *Cognitive-behavioral
            therapy, in adolescent anorexia and bulimia nervosa.*
        pharmacotherapy in, 178–179

C

Centers for Disease Control and Prevention (CDC), on obesity, 179–180
Childhood
    eating disorders of, **17–30.** See also *Eating disorders, of infancy and childhood.*
    feeding disorders of, 18–20
Children, PICA in, 20–21

Coercive pressure, in adolescent anorexia nervosa management, 132–133
Cognitive development, cognitive-behavioral therapy and, 148–149
Cognitive-behavioral therapy
    cognitive development and, 147–149
    described, 148
    in adolescent anorexia and bulimia nervosa
        case formulation in, 151
        developmental considerations, 148–150
        discussion of, 154–155
        engagement in, 150–151
        evidence base for, 152–154
        general principles of, 150
        guided self-care, 153
        internet-based, 153–154
        motivation in, 150–151
        parental involvement in, 152
        planning in, 151
        treatment motivation, 150
        working toward change in, 151
        writing in, 151
    social development and, 149
Community-based programs, in prevention of obesity in children and adolescents,
    216–218
Contracting, for obesity in children and adolescents, 193
Counseling, nutritional, in adolescent anorexia nervosa management,
    136–137
Criticism(s), weight- and shape-related, eating disorders related
    to, 73–74

D

Day care treatment, in adolescent anorexia nervosa management, 134–135
Decisional balance, for obesity in children and adolescents, 192–193
Depression
    obesity and, 54–55
    weight gain associated with, 54–55
Dietary change, for obesity in children and adolescents, 194
Diffusion-weighted imaging, in obesity, 108
Disability(ies), learning, feeding problems in context of, 19–20
Disgust, bulimia nervosa and, 103
Distress tolerance
    eating disorders related to, 71–73
    in eating disorders prevention, 75–76
Dopamine
    anorexia nervosa and, 104
    bulimia nervosa and, 105
Drink(s), visual presentation of, anorexia nervosa and, 102
Drug(s)
    in eating disorders management, **175–187**
    in obesity management, **175–187**
Dysphagia, functional, in infants and children, 24

E

Eating
    breakfast, in eating disorders prevention, 75
    selective, in infants and children, 22–23
Eating behavior, biology of, 96–97
Eating disorder(s), **31–47.** See also Binge eating disorder; Bulimia nervosa; *specific types, e.g.,* Anorexia nervosa.
    acute phase of, structural brain findings in, 97–98
    ADHD and, 41–42
    affective disorders and, 39
    anxiety disorders and, 40
    assessment of, 42–43
    body weight and, 10–13
    causes of, gene-environment relationships influencing, 69–73
    characteristics of, 199
    classification of, 31–32
    cognitive-behavioral therapy in, 147–148. See also *Cognitive-behavioral therapy, in adolescent anorexia and bulimia nervosa.*
    comorbidity of, 20, 37–38
    defined, 1–3, 31–32
    described, 31
    diagnostic issues in, **1–16**
    eating disorder not otherwise specified, 34
    environmental factors in, **75–78**
        buffering effects for high-risk groups
            distress tolerance/anxiety management, 75–76
            reducing weight- and shape-related attentional biases, 76
        buffering factors for high-risk groups, 75–76
        clinical implications of, 76–78
    epidemiology of, 36–37
    family interventions in, history of, 159–160
    genetic factors in, **67–75**
        clinical implications of, 76–78
        described, 67–69
        integrating risk factor research with, 69–73
        scenario of, 69
    management of, pharmacotherapy in, **175–187**
    medical alterations in, 38
    neuroimaging in, **95–115**
        food as stimulus in, 102
        functional imaging, 100
        in resting state, 100–101
        MRS, 99
        nuclear imaging techniques, 102
        PET, 100–101
        SPECT in, 100–101
        stimulus provocation in, 101–104
        structural brain findings in, 97–98
    neurotransmission/receptor functioning in, 104–106
    OCD and, 40–41

Eating (*continued*)
  of infancy and childhood, **17–30**
    anorexia nervosa, 25–26
    binge eating, 26
    bulimia nervosa, 26
    FAED, 23
    feeding disorders, 18–20
    food phobias, 23–24
    food refusal, 24–25
    functional dysphagia, 24
    PICA, 20–21
    rumination disorder, 21–22
    selective eating, 22–23
  osteopenia and, 37–38
  osteoporosis and, 37–38
  outcomes of, **225–242.** See also Bulimia nervosa; *specific disorders,*
    e.g., Anorexia nervosa.
  personality traits and, 42
  prevention of, **199–207**
    programs for
      meta-analysis of, 200
      successful
        defining of, 200
        features of, 200–201
        Girl Talk, 203
        healthy weight intervention, 202–203
        promising programs, 204
        Sorority Body Image Program, 202
        Student Bodies, 203
        The Body Project, 202
        Weigh to Eat, 203
  psychiatric comorbidity and, 38–42
  psychiatric comorbidity with, 56–58
  substance abuse and, 41
  symptoms of, 35–36
  types of, 1
Eating disorder not otherwise specified, 34
  cognitive-behavioral therapy for, 154
  epidemiology of, 37
Eating pathology, characteristics of, 199
Eating-disordered behavior
  in overweight youth, seqeulae of, 59
  of parents, child eating disorders related to, 70
  psychiatric aspects of, 60–61
Energy intake, increased, obesity due to, 88–89
Engagement, in cognitive-behavioral therapy for adolescent anorexia and bulimia
    nervosa, 150–151
Enteral feeding, for feeding disorders of infancy and childhood, 20
Environment
  in eating disorders, **75–78.** See also *Eating disorders, environmental factors in.*
  obesity related to, **87–89**

Environmental/stimulus control, for obesity in children and adolescents, 193–194
Evidence-based behavioral treatment, for obesity in children and adolescents,
    189–198. See also *Obesity, evidence-based behavioral treatment of.*

F

FAED. See *Food avoidance emotional disorder (FAED).*
Family(ies), role in adolescent anorexia nervosa, **159–173.** See also *Anorexia nervosa,*
    family interventions in.
Family meals, in eating disorders prevention, 75
Family-based interventions, in adolescent anorexia nervosa management, 139–141
FDA. See *Food and Drug Administration (FDA).*
Feeding behaviors, problematic
    eating disorders related to, 70
    in ASDs, 19–20
Feeding disorders
    comorbidity of, 20
    feeding problems in context of neurodevelopmental disorders or learning disability,
        19–20
    of infancy and childhood, 18–20
        epidemiology of, 20
        subclassification and measurement of, 18–19
Fluoxetine Bulimia Nervosa Collaborative Study Group, 179
fMRI. See *Functional MRI.*
Food, visual presentation of, anorexia nervosa and, 102
Food and Drug Administration (FDA), on obesity management, 180–182
Food avoidance emotional disorder (FAED), in infants and children, 23
Food phobias, in infants and children, 23–24
Food refusal, in infants and children, 24–25
Food taste, anorexia nervosa and, 103
Functional dysphagia, in infants and children, 24
Functional imaging, in eating disorders, 100
Functional MRI (fMRI), in obesity, 107

G

Gene-environmental relationships, eating disorders related to, 69–73
    active correlations, 74–75
    buffering effects for high-risk groups
        breakfast eating, 75
        family meals, 75
    evocative correlations, 73–75
    life events and distress tolerance, 71–73
    media, 74
    parental overemphasis on child weight and shape, 70–71
    parental role model of eating disordered behavior, 70
    peer group selection, 75
    problematic feeding behaviors, 70
    teasing, 73–74
    temperamental style, 73
    weight- and shape-related criticism, 73–74

Genetics
   in eating disorders, **67–75.** See also *Eating disorders, genetic factors in.*
   obesity related to, **83–87.** See also *Obesity, genetic factors in.*
Girl Talk, 203
Goal setting, by client, for obesity in children and adolescents, 193
Group psychotherapy, in adolescent anorexia nervosa management, 138–139

H

Health Promotion Board, 213
Healthy weight intervention, in eating disorders prevention, 202–203
HPA axis. See *Hypothalamic-pituitary adrenal (HPA) axis.*
Hyperactivity, leptin-mediated neuroendocrine alterations in anorexia nervosa and,
   121–122
Hypothalamic-pituitary adrenal (HPA) axis, in leptin-mediated neuroendocrine alterations
   in anorexia nervosa, 119
Hypothalamus, abnormality of, obesity and, 107

I

Individual psychotherapy, in adolescent anorexia nervosa management, 137–138
Infancy, eating disorders of, **17–30.** See also specific disorder and *Eating disorders,
   of infancy and childhood.*
International Obesity Taskforce, 214

L

Learning disabilities, feeding problems in context of, 19–20
Leptin
   described, 117–118
   levels of, in anorexia nervosa, 118–119
   obesity and, 107
Leptin-mediated neuroendocrine alterations, in anorexia nervosa, **117–129.** See also
   Anorexia nervosa, leptin-mediated neuroendocrine alterations in.
Life events tolerance, eating disorders related to, 71–73
Lifestyle, self-monitoring of, for obesity in children and adolescents, 193

M

Magnetic resonance imaging (MRI), functional, in obesity, 107
Magnetic resonance spectroscopy (MRS)
   in eating disorders, 99
   in obesity, 99–100
Marketing, social, in prevention of obesity in children and adolescents, 217–218
Media, eating disorders related to, 74
Medication(s), obesity due to, 89
Monogenic obesity, 85–86
Motivation, in cognitive-behavioral therapy for adolescent anorexia and bulimia nervosa,
   150–151
MRS. See *Magnetic resonance spectroscopy (MRS).*
Multiple-family day treatment, for anorexia nervosa in adolescents, 166–169

N

National Healthy Lifestyle program, 213
Neurodevelopmental disorders, feeding problems in context of, 19–20
Neuroendocrine system, alterations in, leptin-mediated, in anorexia nervosa, **117–129.** See
    also *Anorexia nervosa, leptin-mediated neuroendocrine alterations in.*
Neuroimaging
    in anorexia nervosa, 100–101
    in binge eating disorder, 108
    in bulimia nervosa, 101
    in eating disorders, **95–115.** See also *Eating disorders, neuroimaging in.*
    in obesity, **95–115.** See also *Obesity, neuroimaging in.*
Neuronal function, leptin-mediated neuroendocrine alterations in anorexia nervosa effects
    on, 122
Neurotransmission/receptor functioning, in eating disorders, 104–106
Nuclear functional imaging, in obesity, 106
Nuclear imaging techniques, in eating disorders, 102
Nutritional counseling, in adolescent anorexia nervosa management, 136–137
Nutritional rehabilitation, in adolescent anorexia nervosa management, 136

O

Obesity
    behavioral modification techniques for, 192–194
        clinical outcomes of, 195
        contracting in, 193
        decisional balance, 192–193
        dietary change, 194
        dropout/noncompliance with, 195
        environmental/stimulus control, 193–194
        goal setting by client in, 193
        physical activity changes, 194–195
        problem-solving barriers, 193
        psychosocial outcomes, 195
        relapse prevention, 194
        rewards for reaching goals in, 193
        sedentary behavior changes, 194–195
        self-monitoring of lifestyle, 193
        weight status as outcome, 195
    causes of, 180
    definitions associated with, 179–180
    depression and, 54–55
    described, 1–3, 189–190
    diagnosis of, 179–180
    diagnostic issues in, **1–16**
    diffusion-weighted imaging in, 108
    eating-disordered hehaviors associated with, seqeulae of, 59
    environmental factors in, **87–89**
        decreased physical activity, 88
        described, 87–88
        increased energy intake, 88–89

Obesity (*continued*)
    medications, 89
  epidemic of, 209
  evidence–based behavioral treatment of, **189–198.** See also *Obesity, behavioral modification techniques for.*
    health professionals role in, 190–191
    parents' role in, 191–192
  fMRI in, 107
  food and reward and, 107
  functional neuroimaging in, 106–108
  genetic factors in, **83–87**
    formal aspects, 84–85
    molecular findings, 85–87
    monogenic obesity, 85–86
    polygenic obesity, 86–87
    syndromal obesity, 85
  hypothalamus abnormality and, 107
  inequalities in, addressing of, 218–219
  leptin and brain activation and, 107
  management of, pharmacotherapy in
    FDA-recommended, 180–182
    investigational targets for, 183
    non–FDA-approved, 182–183
    orlistat in, 182
    sibutramine in, 181–182
    weight change related to, 183
  monogenic, 85–86
  neuroimaging in, **95–115**
    MRS in, 99–100
    structural imaging, 99–100
  novel therapies for, 196
  parental perception of, 51–52
  perception of, 50–52
  polygenic, 86–87
  prevention of, **209–223**
    community capacity–building approach to, 216
    community-based programs in, 216–218
    food and beverage marketing to children in, 214
    food service policies in, 214–215
    interventions in
      cost-effectiveness of, 218
      effectiveness of, 218
    paradigms for, 210–212
      clinical approach, 210
      "free" market approach, 211–212
      human rights approach, 212
      public health approach, 210–211
      risks/benefits approach, 212
    political leadership in, 213
    population-based strategies in, 212–213
    "safety" of community programs in, 216–217

        scaling up community action in, 217
        school programs in, 216–218
        social marketing in, 217–218
        supportive policies in, 213–216
        transport policies in, 215–216
        urban planning in, 215–216
    primary health care providers perception of, 52
    psychiatric aspects of, **49–65**
    psychiatric comorbidity with, 55–59
    psychological aspects of, **49–65**
    quality of life of children and adolescents with, 52–53
    radical therapies for, 196
    receptor/NT and, 107–108
    resting state and, 106
    self-esteem and, 53
    self-perception of, 51
    serotonergic mechanisms and, 108
    suicidal behavior associated with, 53–54
    suicide associated with, 53–54
    symptom provocation and, 106
    syndromal, 85
Obsessive-compulsive disorder (OCD), adolescent eating disorders
        and, 40–41
OCD. See *Obsessive-compulsive disorder (OCD)*.
Opioid(s), bulimia nervosa and, 105–106
Orlistat, in obesity management, 182
Osteopenia, adolescent eating disorders and, 37–38
Osteoporosis, adolescent eating disorders and, 37–38
Overweight, described, 3

P

Parent(s), eating disordered behavior of, child eating disorders related to, 70
Parental involvement, in cognitive-behavioral therapy for adolescent anorexia
        and bulimia nervosa, 152
Peer group selection, eating disorders related to, 75
PET. See *Positron emission tomography (PET)*.
Phobia(s), food, in infants and children, 23–24
Physical activity
        changes in, for obesity in children and adolescents, 194–195
        decreased, obesity due to, 88
PICA, in infants and children, 20–21
Polygenic obesity, 86–87
Positron emission tomography (PET), in anorexia nervosa, 100–101
Prader-Willi syndrome (PWS), 85
Problem-solving barriers, for obesity in children and adolescents, 193
Psychiatric disorders, adolescent eating disorders and, 38–42
Psychotherapy
        group, in adolescent anorexia nervosa management, 138–139
        individual, in adolescent anorexia nervosa management, 137–138

Q

Quality of life, of obese children and adolescents, 52–53
Quitlines, 212

R

Radical treatments, for obesity in children and adolescents, 196
Receptor/NT, obesity and, 107–108
Rehabilitation, nutritional, in adolescent anorexia nervosa management, 136
Relapse prevention, for obesity in children and adolescents, 194
Reproduction, amenorrhea effects on, 119–120
Reward(s)
    bulimia nervosa and, 103–104
    food, obesity and, 107
    for reaching goals, in obesity management in children and adolescents, 193
Rumination disorder, in infants and children, 21–22

S

School programs, in prevention of obesity in children and adolescents, 216–218
Sedentary behavior, changes in, for obesity in children and adolescents, 194–195
Selective eating, in infants and children, 22–23
Self-esteem, of obese children and adolescents, 53
Self-perception, of obesity, 51
Serotonin
    anorexia nervosa and, 104–105
    bulimia nervosa and, 105
Shape-related attentional biases, reducing of, in eating disorders prevention, 76
Shape-related criticism, eating disorders related to, 73–74
Sibutramine, in obesity management, 181–182
Single-photon emission computed tomography (SPECT), in eating disorders, 100–101
Social development, cognitive-behavioral therapy and, 149
Social marketing, in prevention of obesity in children and adolescents, 217–218
Sorority Body Image Program, 202
SPECT. See *Single-photon emission computed tomography (SPECT)*.
Structural brain findings, in acute phase of eating disorders, 97–98
Structural imaging, in obesity, 99–100
Student Bodies, 203
Substance abuse, adolescent eating disorders and, 41
Suicidal behavior, obesity and, 53–54
Suicide, obesity and, 53–54
Sydney Principles, in prevention of obesity in children and adolescents, 214–215
Syndromal obesity, 85

T

TAF program, 213
Taste, food, anorexia nervosa and, 103
Teasing, eating disorders related to, 73–74
Temperamental style, eating disorders related to, 73

The Body Project, 202
Trim and Fit (TAF) program, 213

W

Weigh to Eat, 203
Weight, body. See *Body weight.*
Weight change, as factor in pharmacotherapy management of obesity, 183
Weight classes, 3–9
Weight control behavior, inappropriate, 57–58
Weight gain, depression and, 54–55
Weight-related attentional biases, reducing of, in eating disorders prevention, 76
Weight-related criticism, eating disorders related to, 73–74
Writing, in cognitive-behavioral therapy for adolescent anorexia and bulimia nervosa, 151

Moving?

Make sure your subscription moves with you!

To notify us of your new address, find your **Clinics Account Number** (located on your mailing label above your name), and contact customer service at:

E-mail: elspcs@elsevier.com

800-654-2452 (subscribers in the U.S. & Canada)
314-453-7041 (subscribers outside of the U.S. & Canada)

Fax number: 314-523-5170

Elsevier Periodicals Customer Service
11830 Westline Industrial Drive
St. Louis, MO 63146

*To ensure uninterrupted delivery of your subscription, please notify us at least 4 weeks in advance of move.